Magnetic resonance (MR) imaging and spectroscopy are powerful tools in demonstrating and monitoring pathological processes of the brain and spinal cord. This is a rapidly advancing field with development of new techniques which provide greater pathological specificity and functional information than was previously thought possible. Multiple sclerosis (MS), a common and as yet incurable disease of the central nervous system, is being studied intensively using these techniques. They perform a major role in facilitating the diagnosis, understanding the mechanisms of symptoms and monitoring the effect of new treatments. Compiled by experts in the field, this extensively illustrated text provides a comprehensive review of the benefits and limitations of MR in the study of MS. Coverage ranges through the overall contributions of MR, the variety of techniques available, diagnosis and differential diagnosis, MR as a predictor of clinical course, MR views of pathophysiology and finally monitoring the efficacy of new treatments. This book will prove an invaluable aid to all neurologists, neuroradiologists and neuroscientists with an interest in MS.

MAGNETIC RESONANCE IN MULTIPLE SCLEROSIS

Magnetic Resonance in Multiple Sclerosis

David H Miller *Institute of Neurology, London*

Jürg Kesselring *Rehabilitation Centre, Valens, Switzerland*

W Ian McDonald *Institute of Neurology, London*

Donald W Paty *University of British Columbia*

Alan J Thompson *Institute of Neurology, London*

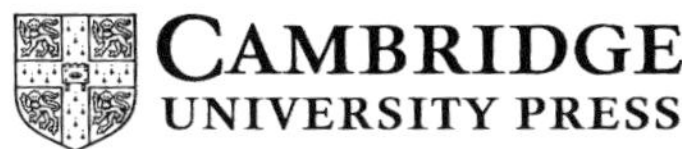

CAMBRIDGE
UNIVERSITY PRESS

PUBLISHED BY THE PRESS SYNDICATE OF THE UNIVERSITY OF CAMBRIDGE
The Pitt Building, Trumpington Street, Cambridge CB2 1RP, United Kingdom

CAMBRIDGE UNIVERSITY PRESS
The Edinburgh Building, Cambridge CB2 1RU, United Kingdom
40 West 20th Street, New York, NY 10011-4211, USA
10 Stamford Road, Oakleigh, Melbourne 3166, Australia

First published 1997

Printed in the United Kingdom at the University Press, Cambridge

Typeset in Adobe Minion 10/13pt

A catalogue record for this book is available from the British Library

Library of Congress Cataloguing in Publication data

Magnetic resonance in multiple sclerosis/David H. Miller . . . [*et al.*].
        p.   cm.
    Includes bibliographical references and index.
    ISBN 0 521 47325 x (hardback)
    1. Multiple sclerosis – Magnetic resonance imaging. 1. Miller, David H. (David Hugh)
    [DNLM: 1. Multiple Sclerosis – diagnosis. 2. Nuclear Magnetic Resonance – diagnostic use.
WL 360 M1963 1997]
    RC377.M24 1997
    616.8′3407548–dc20   96-21044 CIP
    DNLM/DLC
    for Library of Congress
ISBN 0 521 47325 x hardback

Contents

1 **The impact of magnetic resonance in multiple sclerosis**

W Ian McDonald

1.1 Introduction

A profound change in the attitude of neurologists to multiple sclerosis has taken place over the past decade following the introduction of magnetic resonance (MR) techniques to clinical research and practice about 15 years ago. The prevailing sense that the physician's role was essentially supportive has changed to one that is more positive. Though the capacity to control the disease, to alter favourably the long-term prognosis, remains uncertain, there is a sense that real progress is now possible. This notion derives partly from the apparent success of recent therapeutic endeavours such as the use of interferon-β-1b in relapsing-remitting multiple sclerosis, and partly from the evident power of MR techniques to help illuminate our understanding of the disease mechanisms and to monitor the effects of treatment on at least some elements of the pathological process. This chapter will look at two questions: in what ways has our knowledge increased, and how justified are we in our present enthusiasm?

1.2 The contribution of MRI

It was at once clear from the first small study of MR images of the brain in multiple sclerosis [Young *et al.* 1981] that the technique had a much greater sensitivity in demonstrating abnormalities than any other existing method, and that the distribution of lesions closely resembled that seen at post-mortem. That the changes in MR signal corresponded with plaques was soon shown by MRI–pathological correlations in formalin-fixed brain [Stewart *et al* 1986; Ormerod *et al,* 1987].

1.2.1   Diagnosis

The diagnostic potential of MRI was immediately appreciated. Possible problems soon became apparent when it was discovered that apparently healthy individuals have areas of abnormal signal in the deep white matter of the cerebral hemispheres with an increasing frequency from the age of 50 onwards. Several sets of criteria have been developed which considerably increase diagnostic reliability [Fazekas *et al.* 1988; Paty *et al.* 1988], but it is unfortunately true that in non-neurological settings multiple sclerosis is still all-too-often diagnosed incorrectly through failure to apply either or both the now standard clinical [Poser *et al.* 1983] and MRI diagnostic criteria (see Chapter 3); the latter cannot, of course, be sufficient to make a diagnosis of multiple sclerosis without the former. One of our aims in writing this book will have been achieved if as a result of reading it, these errors, which have caused much unnecessary distress to patients, become less frequent.

Where MRI has proved to be particularly valuable is in the ready recognition of congenital and neoplastic structural abnormalities which may simulate the progressive forms of multiple sclerosis and which can often be readily treated. Good examples are the Arnold Chiari malformation and neurofibroma compressing the spinal cord.

1.2.2   Prognosis

The temptation to make a diagnosis of multiple sclerosis in a patient with an isolated neurological syndrome of the kind seen in multiple sclerosis (e.g. optic neuritis) when additional asymptomatic lesions are seen in the brain in a distribution characteristic of those seen in multiple sclerosis, is understandable. But without the clinical criteria of dissemination in time being fulfilled it is not possible to do so. Nevertheless, long-term follow-up – now reaching ten years – has shown that the risk of early development of multiple sclerosis in those with such additional lesions is substantially higher than in those without. The latter are however not spared. There has been a significant increase in the number of those with truly isolated lesions who have developed multiple sclerosis in the second quinquennium of follow-up [O'Riordan *et al.* 1996a]. Nevertheless, in selecting patients for trials of treatment aimed at delaying or preventing the development of the disseminated disease, the different risks of those with and those without asymptomatic lesions at presentation would be useful in selecting high-risk patients.

Thus the first major way in which MRI has changed our view of multiple sclerosis is in the improvement it has led to in early and secure diagnosis and in assigning prognosis. These matters are taken up in detail in later chapters.

1.2.3   Pathogenesis

The second major way in which magnetic resonance techniques have increased our understanding of demyelinating disease is through their contribution to the study of pathogenesis in man. The earliest rational conjecture about the primary event in the development of the new lesion in multiple sclerosis was that of Rindfleisch [1863], who postulated on the basis of post-mortem studies that it was inflammation. Charcot [1868] rejected the notion, but it gained increasing favour in modern times as the mechanism of lesion formation was elucidated in chronic relapsing experimental allergic encephalomyelitis (EAE) (which bears histological similarities to multiple sclerosis [Lassmann 1983] and is a T-cell mediated inflammatory demyelinating disease). Occasional biopsies of lesions in patients with multiple sclerosis presenting in unusual ways (e.g. with raised intracranial pressure) lent general support to this idea [Youl *et al.* 1991a]. Convincing evidence for it in the human disease has come from the use of serial gadolinium-diethylenetriamine pentacetic acid (Gd-DTPA) enhanced MRI. Studies of EAE have shown that Gd-DTPA, which does not normally cross the blood–brain barrier in cerebral white matter, does so contemporaneously with the appearance of histological evidence of inflammation [Hawkins *et al.* 1990a, 1991].

The study of a patient with multiple sclerosis who died unexpectedly ten days after a Gd-DTPA enhanced MRI led to the demonstration that enhancing lesions were associated with inflammation, whereas non-enhancing lesions were not [Katz *et al.* 1993]. Though this observation was on a single case, it provides strong supporting evidence for the view derived from comparative studies of EAE and human post-mortem material that gadolinium-DTPA enhancement in multiple sclerosis reflects a breakdown in the blood–brain barrier in association with inflammation.

1.2.3.1 *The acute lesion*

Using a variety of quantitative MRI methods and magnetic resonance spectroscopy (MRS), the details of which are given elsewhere in this book, it has been possible to define the broad sequence of pathological events in the development of the new lesion [McDonald *et al.* 1992; McDonald 1993, 1994]. In relapsing-remitting and secondary progressive multiple sclerosis, the earliest detectable event is a focal breakdown of the blood–brain barrier which, for the reasons just given, is interpreted as signifying the presence of inflammation. Oedema develops and reaches a peak at about 4–6 weeks. The breakdown in the blood–brain barrier is repaired at about this time and the oedema is subsequently absorbed to leave a smaller residual area of abnormality. MR spectroscopy shows that demyelination commences in the inflammatory phase of the lesion, and there is electrophysiological evidence in optic neuritis that it occurs very early in it [S. Jones, R. Kapoor, WI McDonald, unpublished observations].

1.2.3.1.1 *Changes in conduction* What of the functional evolution of the lesion? This has been elucidated, as the pathological evolution of the lesion was, by comparing the results of animal experiments with observations using related techniques in man.

It is appropriate here to remind the reader of some basic facts about the properties of experimentally demyelinated nerve fibres, since an understanding of them is crucial to an understanding of the poor correlation between the presence of areas of abnormal

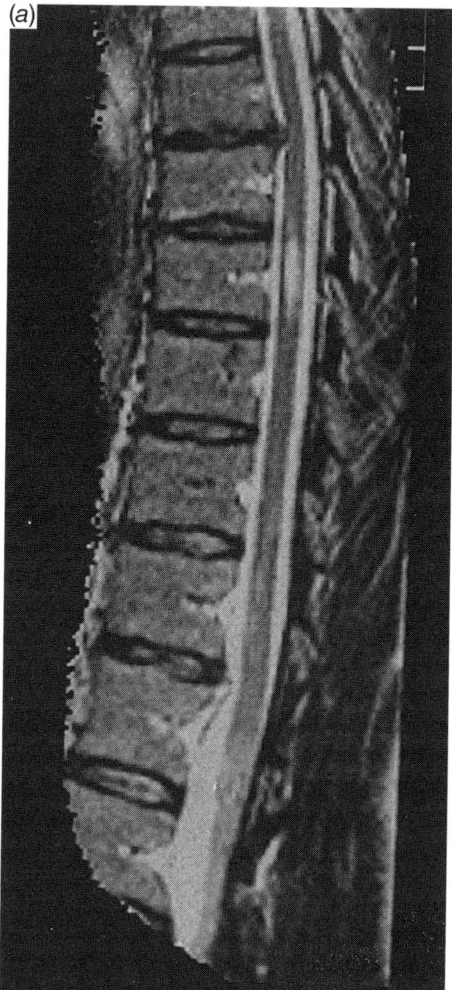
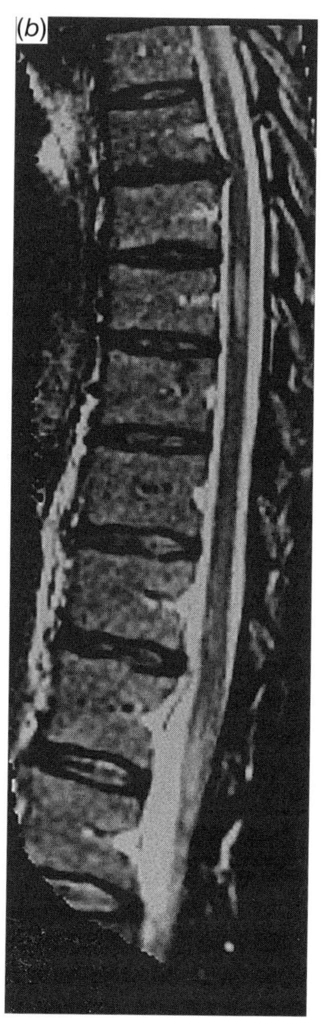

Figure 1.1 *T2-weighted images of the thoracic spinal cord in a patient with multiple sclerosis. Figure 1a was obtained early in an acute relapse when the patient was paraplegic and incontinent. Figure 1b, which is indistinguishable apart from background contrast, was taken a month later when the only residual neurological impairment was an extensor plantar response.*

MRI signal and functional deficit, even in clinically eloquent areas such as the spinal cord and the optic nerve (Figure 1.1).

It has long been known that demyelination by any method produces complete conduction block when it is extensive enough. However, some days after the induction of certain non-inflammatory acute demyelinating lesions conduction is restored [Bostock & Sears 1978; Smith *et al.* 1982]. There is good evidence that in the peripheral nervous system this results from the insertion of new sodium channels (on which propagation of the nerve impulse depends) into the demyelinated portions of the axon [England *et al.* 1990]. Recently, evidence has been obtained that the same process occurs in experimentally demyelinated central nerve fibres [Black *et al.* 1991]. It is thus of exceptional interest that a marked increase in sodium channel density has been demonstrated at post-mortem in plaques containing many surviving axons, using a method depending on the binding of the sodium channel marker saxitoxin [Moll *et al.* 1991]. It thus seems likely that an increased density of sodium channels in the demyelinated axons makes an important contribution to the recovery which is so characteristic of the early relapses of multiple sclerosis.

Optic neuritis provides an ideal opportunity to explore the relationship between function, electrophysiological changes and MRI appearances in human disease. Youl *et al.* [1991b] showed that the well-known reduction in amplitude of the visual evoked potential (largely due to conduction block) occurred during the inflammatory phase of the lesion, as shown by Gd-DTPA enhancement. That demyelination was present was shown by the delay in the residual cortical response. After enhancement ceased (presumably signifying a decline in the intensity of inflammation) the amplitude of the evoked potential increased, indicating reversal of conduction block. But in keeping with established knowledge, the responses remained delayed and by an amount corresponding with that seen in conduction in persistently demyelinated axons in experimental studies [Bostock & McDonald 1982]. Visual acuity recovered to normal or close to it at the same time.

Two further conclusions can be drawn from these observations. First, clinical recovery occurred without remyelination, as shown by the persistence of a delay in the visual evoked potential. A variable amount of remyelination does occur in multiple sclerosis [Prineas *et al.* 1993a, b] and would undoubtedly contribute to recovery [Smith *et al.* 1981] but the usual persistence of delayed evoked potentials in the face of virtually full clinical recovery (on which the diagnostic use of evoked potentials depends) shows that remyelination is not essential for at least the initial phase of recovery.

Secondly, inflammation *per se* probably contributes to conduction block: delay, indicating demyelination, was present early and late, but the substantial reduction in amplitude indicating conduction block occurred only during the early phase at the time of the enhancement. How the inflammatory process affects conduction remains to be determined. One possibility is that soluble products such as cytokines might block existing or new sodium channels [Brosnan *et al.* 1989; Brinkmeier *et al.* 1992]. Another is that such substances might inhibit the formation or insertion of new channels.

1.2.3.2   *The chronic lesion*

Less is understood about the chronic lesion and its effect on function. The central unsolved question is why the initial excellent recovery processes become less effective as time goes by. It has repeatedly been affirmed since the time of Charcot [1868] that axonal degeneration is a prominent feature of some lesions at post-mortem [Bielschowsky 1903; Dawson 1916; Greenfield & King 1936; Adams & Kubic 1952; Lassmann *et al.* 1994]. Given the limited recovery which is possible following extensive Wallerian degeneration in individual pathways, it seems likely that this process contributes to the irrecoverable deficit characteristic of the later stages of multiple sclerosis. There is increasing evidence that this is so. Two lines are particularly persuasive. First, MR spectroscopy provides evidence for a relationship between ataxia and axonal loss in the cerebellum [Davie *et al.* 1995]. Secondly, Losseff *et al.* [1996a] have reported a graded relationship between disability as measured on the Kurtzke extended disability status scale and atrophy of the spinal cord at C2. It is likely that axonal loss makes an important contribution to the atrophy.

In summary, the exploitation of MR techniques has given valuable insights into the dynamics of the pathological and physiological evolution of the new lesion in multiple sclerosis, and promises to do so in the chronic lesion.

1.2.4   Monitoring treatment

The third contribution that magnetic resonance techniques have made to our understanding of the problems of multiple sclerosis is through their use to monitor treatment. Intuitively it seemed from the time of the earliest reports that MRI would be useful in this context because areas of altered signal corresponded with lesions. The intuition was strengthened when it was shown that Gd-DTPA enhancement provided an index of disease activity. But a closer look soon revealed difficulties. Marked variations in the area of individual lesions were seen to occur over a matter of weeks [Willoughby *et al.* 1989]. This problem was overcome by making long-term serial measurements: a net increase in the area of abnormal signal over a year or two clearly indicated a net increase in the total area of pathological tissue. But as the North American β-interferon 1b study showed most strikingly, this corresponded only weakly with an increase in disability [Paty *et al.* 1993]. The limited correlation between the extent of abnormal signal and disability was already well known and was indeed to be expected, first on the basis of past post-mortem evidence of multiple sclerosis in individuals who were not known to be symptomatic during life [Phadke & Best 1983], secondly on the basis of a few moments' reflection on the pathophysiology of demyelinated nerve fibres, and thirdly on the mechanism of magnetic resonance changes in multiple sclerosis and their distribution. A prominent site of predilection for lesions is the periventricular region, which is not clinically eloquent, at least as far as physical disability is concerned (though careful specific testing has revealed a correlation with impairment of cognitive function [Rao *et al.* 1989; Ron & Feinstein 1992]). It is, moreover, not surprising that there is a poor correlation between the presence of chronic lesions on conventional T2-weighted or proton density-weighted images in vulnerable areas such as the optic nerve and the spinal cord, and a corresponding clinical effect (often there is no residual deficit). The MRI changes on such images depend on changes in the relative amount, physico-chemical state and distribution of water (see Chapter 2), and give no indication about the integrity of myelin or axons, or about the electrical properties of axons on which function depends. There is, on the other hand, a good correlation between acute deficits and the presence of Gd-DTPA enhancement and conduction block in clinically eloquent regions such as the optic nerve, the pyramidal tract and the brain stem.

These comments have several implications. First, given that standard MRI techniques have poor specificity in discriminating the different elements of the pathological process in multiple sclerosis (inflammation, demyelination, axonal degeneration, gliosis), and none at all in assessing the electrical properties of nerve fibres, they are bound to have limited value in predicting the effect of putative treatments on disability. Where standard methods (including change in area of abnormality on proton density/T2-weighted images and especially Gd-DTPA enhancement) come into their own is in deciding whether a putative treatment has an effect on the acute elements of the pathological process. This has clearly been shown for interferon-β-1b [Paty *et al.* 1993; Stone *et al.* 1995a]; the failure to demonstrate an effect on disability raises the possibility that the chronic elements of the process which lead to disability are left relatively unmodified.

1.3   Is our enthusiasm justified?

It is now time to see whether our enthusiasm about progress in understanding multiple sclerosis and our optimism about the future are justified. The answer is clearly in the affirmative as far as diagnosis and differential diagnosis are concerned, as later chapters in this book show. True, difficulties remain in some cases, but numerically they represent a small proportion compared with that of 20 years ago.

What of our understanding of pathogenesis? Here the progress has been striking, but many questions remain. What is the initiating event in the development of the disease? What is the mechanism of relapse: does the crucial event take place in the brain or systemically, or both? What terminates the inflammatory process? What, besides axonal degeneration, contributes to irrecoverable disability: is there secondary failure of compensatory mechanisms leading to re-establishment of conduction block in persistently demyelinated fibres (as occurs in the peripheral nervous system)? Might remyelination, which is manifestly not necessary for recovery from the acute deficit associated with a new lesion, be crucial to preventing such secondary failure? What is it that triggers axonal loss: does recurrent inflammation involving the same fibres at the same or different levels increase the likelihood of degeneration? If so, what is it about the inflammatory process that leads to failure of the mechanisms maintaining axonal integrity?

Many of these questions will require other approaches (e.g. pathological, immunological and physiological) for their elucidation, but some are likely to yield to MR techniques currently being exploited. A central aim in this work is to improve the specificity of magnetic resonance in identifying different elements of the pathological process. Magnetisation transfer imaging and diffusion imaging, for example, both have the potential to allow differentiation of demyelination and axonal degeneration.

Finally, are we right to be so optimistic about the value of MR techniques in monitoring treatment? I have described the difficulties. What are the prospects that they can be overcome and that MR techniques can be used to predict disability in the future? A better understanding of the mechanism of irrecoverable deficit – currently the focus of basic research in the NMR Unit at the Institute of Neurology, London – will help in the selection of the optimum methods for monitoring the effects of treatment. It seems likely that a number of complementary techniques will be needed. At present measurement of spinal cord area, and, in the brain, magnetisation transfer imaging, diffusion imaging and quantifying areas of low signal on T1-weighted images [van Walderveen *et al.* 1995], are promising. Some of these techniques are time consuming and at present this general approach is limited by the time required to obtain data from large areas of the brain and spinal cord at each imaging session. Fortunately this difficulty is likely to be diminished by the exploitation of echo-planar imaging. MR spectroscopy also offers promise as a means of monitoring the effects of treatment on neuronal loss, but remains time consuming and is not widely available. It promises, however, to be invaluable in the investigation of mechanisms of action of putative treatments.

To sum up, I believe that our enthusiasm about recent progress is justified and that our optimism about the future will be also, provided the powerful tools we now have are used rationally and the results viewed critically, taking care to correlate them with clinical measures, and with pathology and disordered physiology in experimental and human disease.

2 Magnetic resonance techniques relevant to the study of multiple sclerosis

David H Miller

2.1 General remarks

The first demonstrations of nuclear magnetic resonance (NMR) in condensed matter were published 50 years ago by Bloch [1946] and Purcell [1946]. For this discovery both were awarded the 1952 Nobel prize in physics. Applications of NMR were initially confined to physics and chemistry. The first NMR images of an object were published almost 30 years later by Lauterbur [1973]; these were formed by projection reconstruction in a manner similar to CT.

The production of satisfactory images from humans required the development of large-bore magnets with very homogeneous magnetic fields, together with an efficient method of spatial localisation of the acquired NMR signals. These requirements were met in the early 1980s when the first whole-body imagers were built and two-dimensional Fourier transformation was used to constitute the images [Edelstein *et al.* 1980].

MRI scanners are in essence large magnets; their use is therefore contraindicated in patients with cardiac pacemakers and berry aneurysm clips. The field strength of MR imagers in clinical use varies from 0.02 to 4.0 tesla (T). Signal-to-noise ratio is proportional to the square root of field strength, so that at low fields sensitivity to small lesions, as often occur in multiple sclerosis, is reduced.

To produce an NMR signal an atomic nucleus must be mobile and contain an odd number of protons or neutrons. MR images are constituted from the NMR signals derived from such nuclei after the application of a radio-frequency excitation pulse. Conventional MR images are obtained from the ^{1}H nuclei in *water* and *fat*, because of their great abundance in the living organism. In routine clinical work, the usual resolution of such images is about 1 mm $\times$ 1 mm in plane with a 5 mm slice thickness. Much lower resolution images can be obtained from certain other metabolites containing mobile protons, e.g. *N*-acetyl aspartate (spectroscopic imaging, see Section 2.5), or from other NMR visible nuclei, e.g. ^{31}P and ^{23}Na.

2.2   Brain MRI

2.2.1   Unenhanced proton density (PD) and T2-weighted sequences

On conventional ^{1}H MR images, different tissues, normal or pathological, are discriminated by differences in the density and macromolecular environment of their mobile protons – in the brain these are almost all water protons since the lipid protons in myelin are relatively immobile and therefore produce negligible NMR signal.

The intensity of tissue signals is influenced by three main parameters: proton density (PD) and T1 and T2 relaxation times. T1 and T2 define the rate at which the NMR signals decay after the radio-frequency excitation pulse ceases (T1=longitudinal relaxation, i.e. parallel to the magnetic field; T2=transverse relaxation, i.e. perpendicular to the magnetic field). Although all three contribute to some extent in any MR image, strategies are employed to allow one or other to have a major influence on the image. Thus sequences are often described as PD-, T1- or T2-weighted (Figure 2.1). Tissues display greater variations in their T1 and T2 relaxation than their proton density, and most sequences in clinical use (including the so-called PD-weighted sequence) have an important degree of T1 or T2 weighting.

The first clinical MR images in multiple sclerosis used a T1-weighted inversion recovery sequence, which showed normal white matter as high intensity and lesions as low intensity [Young *et al.* 1981]. However, it was soon realised that PD- and T2-weighted spin echo (SE) sequences were more sensitive in detecting multiple sclerosis lesions (seen as high signal regions surrounded by lower signal normal white matter) [Lukes *et al.* 1983; Runge *et al.* 1984; Ormerod *et al.* 1987]. The PD- and T2-weighted SE sequences use a long repetition time (TR, usually 2–3s) between each radio-frequency excitation pulse. At shorter echo times (TE) of 15–40 ms, T2 weighting is partly offset by T1 weighting such that the signal from the cerebrospinal fluid (CSF) is low, and proton density makes a significant contribution to the overall image so that the sequence is conventionally described as PD-weighted. With longer TEs (80–120 ms), T2 weighting is dominant and CSF signal is high (this is sometimes referred to as a heavily T2-weighted sequence; for clarity we simply call it the T2-weighted sequence). Sequences with a shorter TE (PD-weighted) detect more lesions, especially in the periventricular region, because of the improved contrast between high signal lesions and low signal CSF [Ormerod *et al.* 1987](Figure 2.1).

Since the early 1980s, PD- and T2-weighted SE sequences have been the most widely used for routine diagnostic studies in multiple sclerosis (they are usually acquired simultaneously as a double echo sequence), although recently a modification called fast (or turbo) spin echo (FSE) has become popular, because it requires a fraction of the time to obtain a very similar looking image (Figure 2.2). FSE is based on the Rapid Acquisition with Relaxation Enhancement (RARE) sequence first described by Hennig [1986]. In essence, the technique acquires a multi-echo train (typically 4, 8, 16 or more echoes) following each radio-frequency excitation. A different phase encoding pulse is applied in conjunction with each echo, which allows multiple 'lines' of image data to be collected after

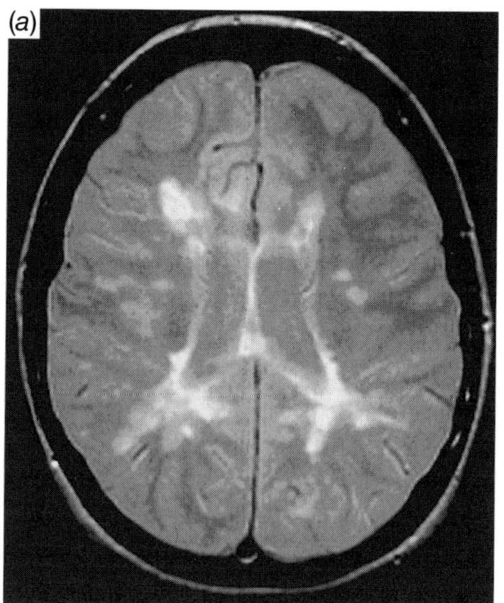

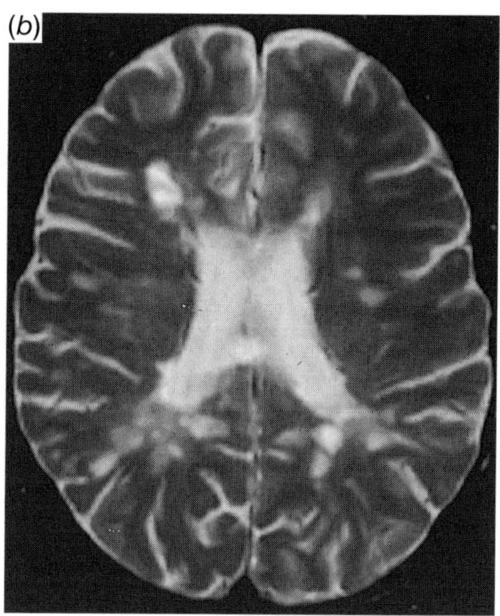

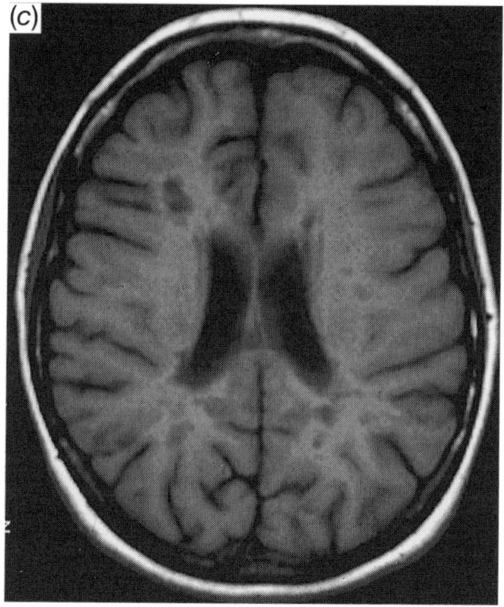

Figure 2.1 *Spin echo images in a 38-year-old female patient with multiple sclerosis. (a) PD-weighted (b) T2-weighted and (c) T1-weighted. Compared to normal white matter, lesions are hyperintense on PD and T2-weighted images and iso- or hypointense on T1-weighted images, while CSF is iso- or hypointense on PD-, hyperintense on T2- and hypointense on T1-weighted images.*

each excitation. Thus the total time required is radically reduced compared with an SE sequence; if all other parameters are kept constant, imaging time is reduced approximately 16-fold if a 16 echo train is used, or eight-fold if an eight echo train is employed. (Because of the way in which multi-slice images are acquired, the actual time saving is often not quite as great as this.) The ordering of the phase-encoding steps determines the effective echo time (TE_{ef}). The resulting T2 contrast is very similar, but not identical, to that obtained with conventional SE [Melki *et al.* 1991, 1992], and FSE has been shown to have a similar

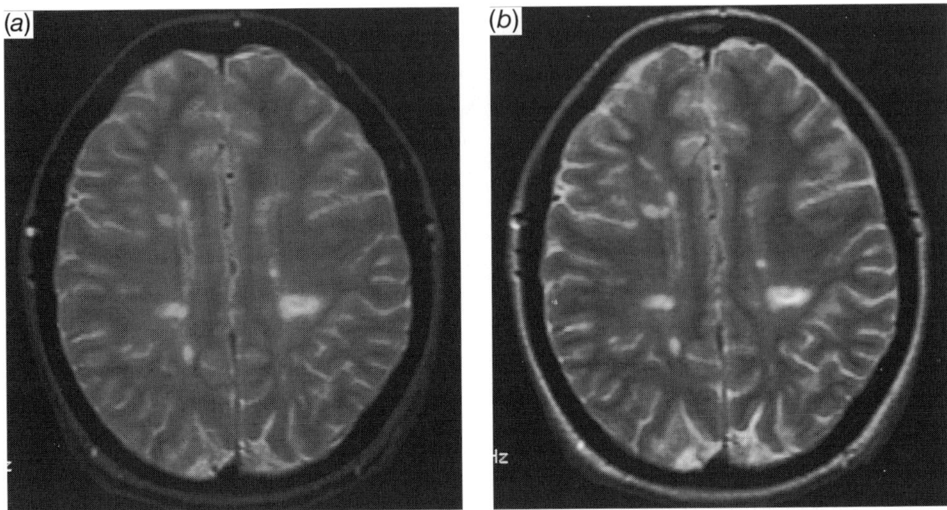

Figure 2.2 *T2-weighted (a) spin echo and (b) fast spin echo brain images in a 26 year-old female with multiple sclerosis. High signal lesions are depicted with an equal sensitivity.*

sensitivity to SE in detecting a variety of brain [Jones *et al.* 1992; Ahn *et al.* 1992] and spinal cord [Sze *et al.* 1992] pathologies, including multiple sclerosis [Thorpe *et al.* 1994a] (Figure 2.2). As with conventional SE, FSE sequences with a short TE (PD-weighted) detect more multiple sclerosis lesions than those with a long TE [Thorpe *et al.* 1994a].

2.2.1.1   *FLAIR and fast FLAIR*

The fluid attenuated inversion recovery sequence (FLAIR) makes use of an inversion pulse followed by a long inversion time (usually 2–2.5 s) which nulls the signal from CSF; a long echo time (e.g. 140–160 ms) is then employed to achieve a high degree of T2-weighting. Some early reports suggested that the conventional or fast FLAIR sequence detects many more multiple sclerosis lesions than standard PD/T2-weighted sequences [Hajnal *et al.* 1992; Thomas *et al.* 1993; Rydberg *et al.* 1994], though other reports were less encouraging [Thorpe *et al.* 1994b; Baratti *et al.* 1994].

A disadvantage of conventional FLAIR is the long acquisition time (a TR of 6 s or longer is usual). This is overcome by using a fast FLAIR sequence, although this still takes 2–3 times longer to acquire than an equivalent FSE sequence. Both FLAIR and fast FLAIR have other disadvantages: (i) a lower signal-to-noise ratio due to the use of long echo times; (ii) partial saturation of tissues due to a long inversion time (TI) following the inversion pulse; (iii) a degree of hyperintensity of periventricular white matter is a normal finding, and this sometimes compromises detection of MS lesions; (iv) CSF flow artefacts are sometimes troublesome.

Thorpe [1994b] performed a quantitative comparison of fast FLAIR versus FSE in the brain using a TE optimised for lesion/white matter contrast on the fast FLAIR sequence

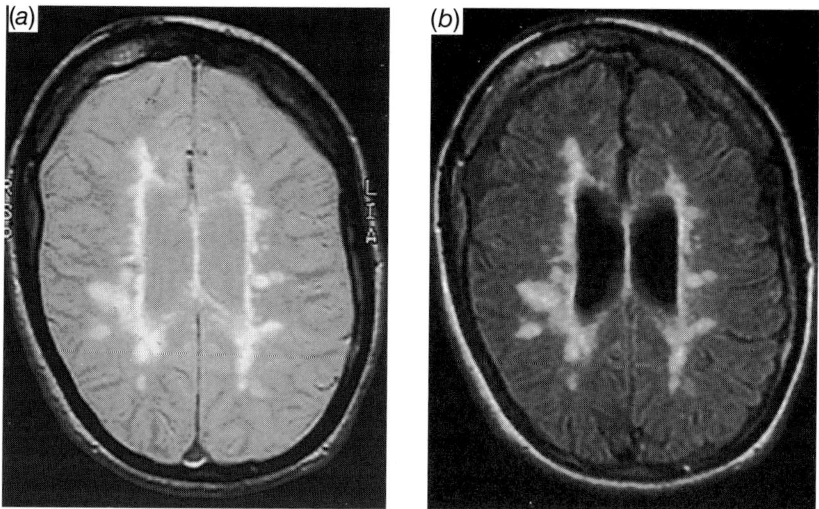

Figure 2.3 *(a) PD-weighted fast spin echo (b) fast FLAIR images in a 31 year-old female with multiple sclerosis. Note the greater suppression of CSF signal and generally increased lesion–white matter contrast seen using fast FLAIR.*

and a short TE_{ef} for the FSE sequence. He found similar numbers of lesions using either sequence; of a total of 479 lesions, 144 were missed on fast FLAIR and 140 on FSE. Lesion/white matter and lesion/grey matter contrast-to-noise ratios (CNR) were measured from 119 lesions. Lesion/white matter CNR was virtually identical (9.4 ± 3.3 and 9.3 ± 3.4 for FSE and fast FLAIR respectively); lesion/grey matter CNR was superior for fast FLAIR (7.2 ± 2.8 cf. 3.9 ± 2.7). This suggested that fast FLAIR would be better at picking up lesions that occur in the cortex or basal ganglia (Figure 3.5).

Rydberg and colleagues [1994] studied 41 patients with a variety of brain pathologies, including 9 with multiple sclerosis, using fast FLAIR and conventional SE. Considerably more white matter lesions were seen on the fast FLAIR sequence in virtually all the multiple sclerosis patients (Figure 2.3). The NMR parameters used by Rydberg were quite different from those of Thorpe (e.g. TR was 11 s versus 6 s). These two preliminary studies suggested that the findings on fast FLAIR are much dependent on the NMR parameters used, but that with optimisation [Rydberg *et al.* 1995], it may be an important new method for improving the detection of multiple sclerosis lesions.

Two recent studies have further clarified the sensitivity of fast FLAIR in detecting multiple sclerosis brain lesions. Filippi *et al.* [1996a] studied 7 multiple sclerosis patients with a fast FLAIR and conventional SE sequence. They found that fast FLAIR detected 28% more lesions than conventional SE, with most of the additional lesions located in the cortical-subcortical area. There was a trend for fast FLAIR to detect fewer lesions in the posterior fossa.

Gawne-Cain *et al.* [1997] studied 32 multiple sclerosis patients with 5 mm axial contiguous slices using conventional SE and a fast FLAIR sequence optimised for the detection of MS lesions according to the work of Rydberg *et al.* [1995]. Gawne-Cain and colleagues found that, overall, the two sequences detected similar number of lesions, but fast FLAIR detected fewer lesions in the posterior fossa (66 versus 138, $p = 0.001$), fewer small discrete cerebral white matter lesions (671 versus 829, $p = 0.002$), more subcortical lesions (542 versus 306, $p < 0.001$) and more large discrete lesions (419 versus 385, $p = 0.0006$). The increased detection of subcortical lesions on fast FLAIR can be expected because of improved lesion/grey matter contrast. Its poorer detection of small discrete lesions might be due to point spread function associated with the RARE technique. Paired lesion T2 estimations found significantly lower T2 values for posterior fossa lesions, and this, along with flow artefact effects, probably contributes to the poorer performance of fast FLAIR in the posterior fossa.

In summary, conventional PD/T2-weighted SE and fast FLAIR appear to have complementary value in the detection of multiple sclerosis brain lesions, the former being more sensitive in the posterior fossa and the latter more sensitive in the supratentorial regions, especially cortical/subcortical areas.

2.2.1.2 *Pathological specificity of PD/T2-weighted and FLAIR/fast FLAIR sequences*
An important limitation of PD/T2-weighted and FLAIR/fast FLAIR sequences is their low pathological specificity. Multiple sclerosis plaques are readily seen because they have a higher density and mobility of water protons than normal white matter. However, this is equally the case for other white matter pathologies such as infarcts and granulomas. Furthermore, any of the main pathological features of plaques may result in an increase in water content and mobility. It occurs in new lesions as a direct consequence of blood–brain barrier breakdown, with the associated inflammatory oedema, or in chronic lesions as result of an increased extracellular space secondary to demyelination and axonal loss, or to gliosis, which increases intracellular water content.

The contribution of each pathological feature to functional impairment in multiple sclerosis is not established, although demyelination and axonal loss are probably important. Demyelination can produce conduction block [McDonald & Sears 1970] which, however, may be reversible [Bostock & Sears 1978; Moll *et al.* 1991]. It is likely that axonal loss, which can be marked in chronic lesions [Adams 1989; Lassman *et al.* 1994], makes an important contribution to irreversible disability. To further elucidate the pathophysiological basis of clinical deficits, it is important to develop MR techniques which can identify specific pathological features in multiple sclerosis lesions, especially demyelination and axonal loss. Sections 2.2.2 to 2.2.6 review a number of techniques that may increase pathological specificity.

2.2.2 Gadolinium enhancement

Gadolinium-containing intravenous MRI contrast agents, such as gadolinium-diethylenetriaminepentacetic acid (Gd-DTPA), produce enhancement by reducing proton mobility in areas in which they accumulate (e.g. regions with an abnormal blood–brain barrier). The paramagnetic effect of such agents produces marked shortening of the T1 relaxation time of nearby water protons, and this appears as an area of high signal on T1-weighted sequences (enhancement is also seen, but less well, on PD/T2-weighted sequences [Barkhof *et al.* 1992a]). In multiple sclerosis, gadolinium enhancement is a regular finding in new lesions [Miller *et al.* 1988a](see Figures 3.7–3.9 and 6.2). It has also been correlated with the acute inflammatory phase of lesion development in chronic experimental allergic encephalomyelitis [Hawkins *et al.* 1990a], an experimental model of multiple sclerosis, and in multiple sclerosis itself [Nesbit *et al.* 1991; Katz *et al.* 1993; Rodriguez *et al.* 1993].

The free gadolinium ion is highly toxic and therefore it must be chelated. The chelates used in contrast agents bind gadolinium with an extremely high affinity. Side effects are infrequent; nausea, headache and local injection site pain occur in a small percentage, and anaphylaxis is exceedingly rare, occurring in only about one per 100,000 cases [Niendorf 1991]. Serial administration at standard dose (0.1 mmol/kg) seems safe, and some multiple sclerosis patients have undergone monthly contrast enhanced scans for up to five years without adverse effects (JA Frank, NIH, personal communication). Higher doses (e.g. 0.3 mmol/kg) or the application of a magnetisation transfer pulse (see Section 2.2.4) to the T1-weighted sequence have both been shown to increase the number and intensity of enhancing lesions in a number of brain pathologies including multiple sclerosis [Finelli *et al.* 1994a; Mathews *et al.* 1994; Filippi *et al.* 1995a; Metha *et al.* 1995, Filippi *et al.* 1996b].

2.2.3   Relaxation time measurement

As mentioned in Section 2.2.1, contrast is achieved in routine MRI by utilising the major differences which occur in the T1 and T2 relaxation times of different tissues. It is possible to go a step further and measure the actual relaxation time in milliseconds [Larsson *et al.* 1988]. Measurement of T1 or T2 requires a minimum of two sequences with different repetition (TR) or echo times, respectively. A multi-echo sequence, with 16 or more echo times, can be used to accurately plot T2 relaxation. Mathematical analysis of the T2 relaxation curve provides additional information about water compartments; mono-exponential relaxation suggests that water is predominantly in a single compartment with a uniform relaxation time, while bi-exponential relaxation suggests that there are two substantial compartments with different relaxation times. Analysis of T2 relaxation curves, using a multi-echo sequence with a short inter-echo interval, has revealed a very fast-relaxing compartment in normal white matter (T2<10 ms) which is not present in plaques; this has been tentatively ascribed to water protons bound to normal myelin [MacKay *et al.* 1994]. Experimental studies have revealed characteristic changes in T1 and T2 with gliosis (moderately elevated T1 and mono-exponential T2 relaxation) and oedema (markedly elevated T1 and bi-exponential T2 relaxation)[Barnes *et al.* 1986, 1987, 1988]. In multiple sclerosis plaques, oedema has been reported in two types of lesion: (i) new lesions in which there is breakdown of the blood–brain barrier with vasogenic oedema [Adams 1989]; (ii) chronic lesions in which there is a markedly expanded extracellular space in association with extensive axonal loss [Barnes *et al.* 1991]. Thus, quantitative relaxation time measurement has the potential to characterise specific pathological features in MS, namely oedema, gliosis, demyelination, and, in chronic lesions, axonal loss (the last inferred by the presence of oedema).

2.2.4   Magnetisation transfer imaging

Proton density (PD) and T1 and T2 relaxation times are the main determinants of tissue contrast in conventional MR images. Only relatively mobile or *free* water protons (about 80% of the total in normal brain, with a T2 of about 50 ms) are MR visible on conventional PD-, T1- and T2-weighted images. Immobile water protons, which are tightly bound to macromolecular structures such as proteins and lipid membranes, have extremely short T2 relaxation times ($<$1 ms) and are therefore not visible [Edzes & Samulski 1977].

Exchange of magnetisation between free water and bound water after selectively saturating the bound water pool reduces T1 and the equilibrium magnetisation. The magnitude of this effect is an indicator of the amount and complexity of macromolecular structure present and is called the magnetisation transfer (MT) ratio [Wolff & Balaban 1989; Eng *et al.* 1991; Balaban & Ceckler 1992]. Myelin is the most complex macromolecular structure in normal white matter and it has therefore been proposed that the extent of demyelination in multiple sclerosis might be quantified by measuring MT ratios. Although direct pathological confirmation that this is so is lacking, experimental studies have shown that major reductions in the MT ratio are observed where there is loss of myelin and/or Wallerian degeneration (in the latter situation an early rise in MT ratio is followed by a fall)[Dousset *et al.* 1994, 1995; Lexa *et al.* 1993].

MT images are derived from sequences (either SE or gradient echo) which are acquired with and without the application of a prepulse to selectively saturate the broad resonance of immobile macromolecular protons. MT images of the brain can be obtained in 10–20 minutes and with good resolution (e.g. 1 mm $\times$ 2 mm in plane and 5 mm thick slices [Gass *et al.* 1994]). The MT ratio measurements obtained are quantitative and highly reproducible (to $\pm$ 1%). MT imaging thus looks to be a promising method for monitoring destructive (and functionally disabling) pathological features in multiple sclerosis lesions.

2.2.5   Unenhanced T1-weighted spin echo imaging

The commonly used T1-weighted SE sequence (which uses a short TR of about 500–700 ms and a short TE of about 15–20 ms) depicts most MS lesions as isointense with normal brain. This arises because the signal loss due to a moderately prolonged T1 relaxation time is offset by increased signal due to increased proton density (water content) and T2 within the lesion. Lesions with a markedly prolonged T1 relaxation time appear as hypointense regions (Figure 2.1), since the T1 effect is dominant. Very long T1 relaxation times arise when there is loss of tissue structure and a markedly expanded extracellular space. Hypointense multiple sclerosis lesions on T1-weighted images have lower magnetisation transfer ratios than isointense lesions [Hiehle *et al.* 1995; Loevner *et al.* 1995]. Thus, it is likely that hypointensity on T1-weighted SE images is a marker of tissue destruction.

2.2.6 Diffusion imaging

The diffusion coefficient of water depends critically on its environment; it is highest in free water, and is reduced when water is confined to small spaces. Measurement of the apparent diffusion coefficient (ADC) using MR techniques has the potential to probe the size, shape and orientation of water spaces within the brain, and thus provide pathological insights distinct from those obtained from other NMR parameters [Doran & Bydder 1990].

The most common method for obtaining diffusion-weighted MR images uses a pair of magnetic field gradient pulses in an SE sequence [Tanner & Stejskal 1968]. The first pulse encodes the spatial position of each mobile proton as a phase angle. The second pulse reverses the encoding completely if the proton does not change position. However, if the proton moves due to diffusion, some phase dispersion of the spin echo occurs. The amount of phase dispersion provides a measure of the ADC.

Diffusion-weighted imaging sequences require the use of large and rapidly changing field gradients, and are performed optimally at high magnetic fields. Unfortunately, the images are very susceptible to artefacts caused by even small amounts of patient motion. Such motion artefacts can be avoided by obtaining ultra-fast images (in a few seconds) using echo planar techniques [Turner *et al.* 1990]; however, the equipment for echo planar imaging is not yet widely available.

A localised, non-imaging method has been developed that is less susceptible to motion artefacts, and provides a rapid measurement of ADC, since no phase information is required to construct an image [Horsfield *et al.* 1994]. The ADC can be measured in several directions, by altering the direction of the diffusion gradient; this gives information on the orientation and anisotropy of the diffusion spaces. Normal white matter tracts reveal *anisotropic* diffusion, i.e. diffusion along the fibre tracts is greater than that perpendicular to the fibres [Doran & Bydder 1990]. Anisotropy is most marked in the corpus callosum, where the ADC parallel to the fibres is 3–4 times greater than that perpendicular [Horsfield *et al.* 1994]. The ADC can also be measured for a variety of diffusion times; this gives information on the size of the diffusion spaces.

In multiple sclerosis, MR studies of diffusion appear promising as a means of assessing the structural integrity of white matter tracts – it is possible that an alteration in ADC and the degree of anisotropy will occur in the presence of demyelination and/or axonal loss. Axonal loss may be necessary for loss of anisotropy to occur, since it has been shown experimentally that an unmyelinated bundle of nerve fibres (the garfish olfactory nerve) displays anisotropy [Beaulieu & Allen 1994]. One study of multiple sclerosis lesions showed an increase in ADC, in some instances approaching that of pure water, but did not evaluate anisotropy [Larsson *et al.* 1992]. The results of further studies are awaited with interest.

2.3   Spinal cord MRI

2.3.1   Importance of spinal MRI in multiple sclerosis

MRI has revolutionised the investigation of patients with clinical disorders of the spinal cord, including multiple sclerosis. It has largely superseded myelography, being in comparison less invasive and offering much greater discrimination of soft tissue detail. Detection of spinal cord lesions in multiple sclerosis is of particular relevance since they are often the major cause of disability (paraplegia and sphincter disturbance); using current MRI techniques it is possible to detect multiple cord lesions in the majority of patients [Kidd *et al.* 1993]. Current strategies for spinal cord MRI are now reviewed.

2.3.2   Motion artefact suppression

Artefacts from CSF pulsation or cardiac motion can be troublesome. Several approaches have been developed to minimise these artefacts. One is cardiac gating, in which each repetition of the radio-frequency excitation is time-locked to the cardiac cycle. Another strategy is to use a bipolar rephasing gradient, which with appropriate timing can effectively nullify some motion artefacts. A third approach is to eliminate artefact from intrathoracic or intra-abdominal motion by applying a pulse to saturate protons anterior to the spine. Many of the artefacts arise from CSF motion and a fourth strategy is to apply a sequence in which signal from CSF is suppressed. The fast FLAIR sequence looks promising in this regard, although artefacts from CSF flow can still occur, and this sequence appears insensitive in detecting MS lesions in the cord (Stevenson *et al.* 1997).

2.3.3   Receiver coils

Because of the greater signal-to-noise ratio, surface coils applied over the spine are more effective than the conventional body coil for demonstrating spinal pathology.

2.3.3.1   *Conventional spinal surface coils*

The cervical cord is usually studied using a saddle-shaped coil, and the thoracolumbar cord using a flat coil. The coils are relatively large but cover at most a field of view (FOV) of 30 cm. Thus, examination of the whole spinal cord is time consuming, as it is necessary to perform a two-stage procedure. In addition, signal-to-noise ratio decreases with increasing size of the surface coil, and the relatively large conventional spinal coils provide suboptimal signal-to-noise from the the cord. These limitations have been partly overcome by the introduction of multi-array spinal coils.

2.3.3.2   *Multi-array coils*

Multi-array coils consist of a series of smaller surface coils, each with its own data acquisition hardware, linked together electronically to provide a composite image which combines the high signal-to-noise of a small surface coil with the greater coverage of a much larger coil [Roemer *et al.* 1990]. In London, we have been using a General Electric prototype spinal multi-array of six partly overlapping coils. The two most rostral coils are saddle-shaped and cover the upper cervical cord. The remaining four coils are flat and rectangular (14 $\times$ 11 cm) and extend from the mid-cervical to the sacral region. Data can be collected simultaneously from any four adjacent coils and integrated to form a single sagittal or coronal image. The four most rostral coils cover an FOV of 48 cm, which encompasses the entire spinal cord in all but a few very tall individuals. The whole spinal cord can be imaged with high signal-to-noise in a single acquisition (Figure 2.4).

2.3.3.3   *Image uniformity correction*

The sagittal images produced using the spinal multi-array coils do not have uniform sensitivity along their length. Near the centre of the individual coils (in this example (Figure 2.4) note especially the posterior fossa and mid-thoracic regions) signal is slightly higher than at the edges of the coils. This gives the images a 'stripy' appearance and can on occasions impede the detection of focal intrinsic cord lesions. A uniformity correction algorithm can be applied [Tofts *et al.* 1995] in which a uniform phantom is imaged using the same pulse sequences and the signal intensities of the spinal images are then divided by the intensities of the phantom. The resulting image has a much more uniform appearance along its length (Figure 2.4).

2.3.4   Sequences

2.3.4.1   *PD- and T2-weighted conventional spin echo*

Even if the spinal multi-array is used, conventional PD- and T2-weighted SE images which cover the entire spinal cord in the sagittal plane still take an appreciable time to generate: approximately 11 minutes for a typical dual echo SE sequence, TR=2500 ms, TE=30 ms and 80 ms, one excitation, a 512 $\times$ 256 matrix (which is required to obtain adequate resolution over a large rectangular FOV, 48 cm in the supero-inferior (S/I) direction and 24 cm in the antero-posterior (A/P) direction). Furthermore, the resulting images of the spinal cord have been affected by motion artefacts when phase encoding is performed in the A/P direction. These artefacts, derived from pulsatile motion of the heart, blood vessels and CSF, are distributed in the phase-encoding direction; some are therefore superimposed on the spinal cord. They need to be eliminated if one is reliably to detect small intrinsic cord lesions, as occur in multiple sclerosis. The use of bipolar rephasing ('flow compensated') gradients, ECG gating and anterior saturation bands reduce, but do not abolish, these artefacts. Phase encoding in the S/I direction does appreciably reduce artefacts within the cord, because they are distributed in an S/I direction from their source (and therefore are not superimposed on the cord). However, using

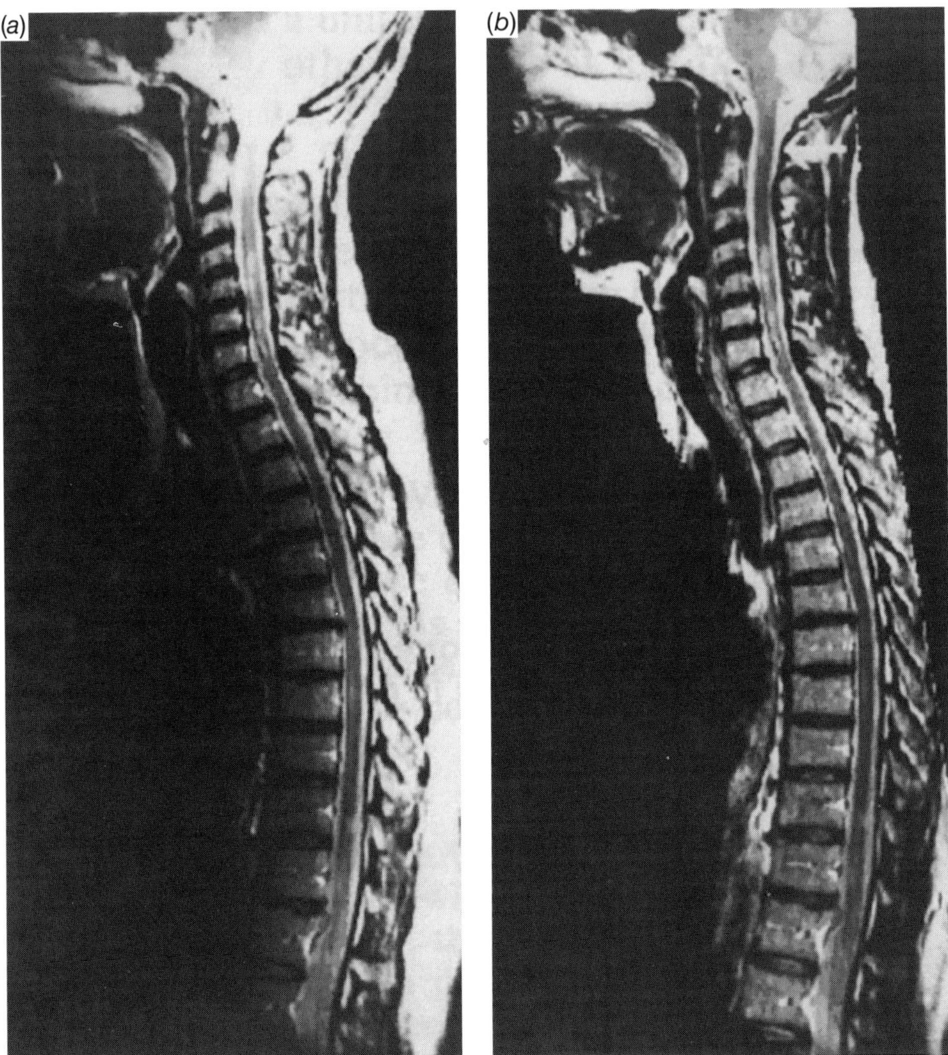

Figure 2.4 *Sagittal T2-weighted fast spin echo image of whole spinal cord (a) before and (b) after correction for image nonuniformity. These images were obtained using a multi-array receiver coil provided by General Electric Medical Systems, Milwaukee, USA. (From Tofts et al. 1995.)*

S/I phase encoding doubles the imaging time to 22 minutes because a square 48 cm $\times$ 48 cm FOV is required.

2.3.4.2   *T2-weighted fast spin echo*

The difficulty in detecting intrinsic cord lesions in a reasonable period of time has largely been resolved by the use of FSE. Provided S/I phase encoding is used (there is a good deal of motion artefact on FSE images with A/P phase encoding), high resolution (512 $\times$ 512

matrix with 48 cm FOV), artefact-free, T2-weighted sagittal FSE images of the entire
spinal cord can be obtained in about five minutes (Figure 2.4). The sagittal spinal FSE
images with S/I phase encoding are less prone than conventional SE to artefacts resulting from CSF pulsation, despite the lack of linear flow compensation in the FSE
sequence. This may be because the rapid dephasing and rephasing of spins by the multi-
echo train makes FSE less sensitive to motion. Thus, for the detection of small intrinsic
cord lesions with an increased T2 (e.g. an area of inflammatory demyelination), FSE
appears to be the sequence of choice.

2.3.4.3   *T2-weighted gradient echo*

An alternative approach is to use a gradient echo (GE) sequence with proton density and
T2 weighting. GE images are obtained more rapidly than SE because of the shorter
repetition times (typical parameters for a GE sequence with T2 weighting: TR = 400 ms,
TE = 30 ms, flip angle = 12°). However, GE images have lower signal-to-noise ratios than
SE because of the low flip angle, and they are prone to artefacts from magnetic field inho-
mogeneity and local susceptibility variations (e.g. at bone–soft tissue interfaces). Sagittal
GE sequences are appreciably less sensitive than SE or FSE in detecting intrinsic cord
lesions [Enzmann & Rubin 1988]. Lesions are shown with better contrast when a
magnetisation transfer pulse is applied to the GE sequence [Finelli *et al.* 1994b]. The GE
sequence has also proved useful for defining the boundary between the cord and subarachnoid CSF on axial images, and for measuring spinal cord cross-sectional area
[Thorpe *et al.* 1993]. An inversion-prepared, volume-acquired T1-weighted GE sequence,
which suppresses CSF signal, allows the construction of thin axial slices from which
highly reproducible measurements of cord area can be obtained [Losseff *et al.* 1996a].

2.3.4.4   *Short inversion time inversion recovery (STIR)*

Theoretically, the combination of T1- and T2-weighting of STIR might be expected to
increase the detection of multiple sclerosis lesions compared to a conventional T2-
weighted sequence. In practice, the gains, in either the brain or spinal cord, are minimal
[Dorwat *et al.* 1986; Thorpe *et al.* 1994c], and are more than offset by the lower signal-to-
noise and greater propensity to motion artefact from high signal CSF using the STIR
sequence.

2.3.4.5   *Fluid attenuated inversion recovery (FLAIR)*

One report indicated a major increase in the number of spinal multiple sclerosis lesions
detected using FLAIR when compared to conventional T2-weighted SE [Thomas *et al.*
1993]. However, compared with other series [Wiebe *et al.* 1992; Kidd *et al.* 1993], the
sensitivity of the T2-weighted sequence in this study was unusually low: only six lesions
were seen in 16 patients. This suggests that the T2-weighted images were suboptimal. A
study comparing fast FLAIR and FSE in the cervical spinal cord has been recently performed in 10 multiple sclerosis patients, and in fact revealed that fast FLAIR is much less
sensitive in this region (Stevenson *et al.* 1997). Whereas a total of 33 lesions were seen on
FSE, only two were seen with fast FLAIR.

2.3.5   Future developments

While the combination of spinal multi-array coils and FSE provides rapid and good quality sagittal T2-weighted images of the whole spinal cord and is proving useful in the investigation of patients with spinal cord disease, resolution within the cord is still limited. It is not yet possible to detect individual white matter tracts, the distinction of white and grey matter is often poor, and axial FSE sequences are of poor quality due to motion artefact. There are also theoretical reasons why small objects, especially those with a short T2, may be lost on FSE sequences [Constable & Gore 1992], although most multiple sclerosis lesions have a relatively long T2 and visibility on FSE should be as good as on SE.

Better resolution within the cord is desirable since it may improve diagnosis of intrinsic cord diseases, increase our understanding of their pathophysiology, and perhaps even allow the effects of treatment to be monitored. Various developments of MRI technology may allow these aims to be achieved. These include the implementation of 3D FSE sequences, the use of higher field scanners (4 T), increasing the number of component coils in the multi-array coil and increasing the maximum imaging matrix to 1024 (currently it is 512, which gives a pixel size of just under 1 mm^2 with a 48 cm field of view). Reduction of motion artefacts will also be important. The application of effective flow compensation techniques to FSE may allow sagittal images to be obtained with A/P phase encoding (and consequently in half the time) and may also improve axial image quality.

2.4   Optic nerve MRI

2.4.1   Importance of optic nerve MRI in multiple sclerosis

Optic neuritis is a frequent manifestation of multiple sclerosis. It is the presenting symptom in about 25% of cases, and over 50% of young adults presenting with optic neuritis subsequently develop clinically definite MS [Francis *et al.* 1987]. The typical clinical picture is of a young adult developing unilateral visual loss and pain on eye movement over several days, followed by gradual recovery towards normal vision over the next few weeks; in about 15% there is little or no recovery. This characteristic syndrome is due to an acute inflammatory/demyelinating lesion in the optic nerve. Neuro-ophthalmological examination allows precise assessment of the evolving clinical deficit. Visual evoked potentials (VEPs) provide a measure of nerve conduction through the symptomatic lesion, and are abnormal, with prolonged latency and/or reduced amplitude responses in over 90% of cases [Halliday 1982]. The significance of detecting such lesions on MRI is that it offers a unique opportunity to explore pathophysiological mechanisms of relapse, recovery and failure to recover in multiple sclerosis; this might be achieved by correlating serial clinical, VEP and MRI data during an episode of acute optic neuritis [Youl *et al.* 1991b].

2.4.2 Sequences

2.4.2.1 *Conventional T2-weighted spin echo*

Using conventional T1- and T2-weighted sequences, there has been little success in detecting the small intrinsic lesions of optic neuritis; this is due to the dominant high signal from surrounding orbital fat, and the presence of chemical shift artefact at the nerve–fat interface. Two main sequences have been used to suppress orbital fat signal: STIR and fat suppressed SE or FSE

2.4.2.2 *STIR (short inversion time inversion recovery)*

The TI is set at about 150 to 175 ms, which is the null point for the longitudinal T1 relaxation of fat (the T1 of fat is much shorter than water)[Johnson *et al.* 1987]. A conventional SE sequence follows the inversion pulse and the final image is obtained with both T1- and T2-weighting. A limitation of STIR is the rather low signal-to-noise ratio and resolution. It takes about 11 minutes to complete a scan with a 256 $\times$ 256 matrix, 20 cm field of view, and enough contiguous, coronal slices to examine the optic nerves from the globe to the chiasm. The resolution (approximately 1 mm $\times$ 1mm in plane and 5 mm thick slices) gives a poor delineation between the CSF-containing sheath which surrounds the optic nerve and the nerve itself. Nevertheless high signal in the nerve is seen in over 80% of patients with acute optic neuritis [Miller *et al.* 1988b] (Figure 3.14).

2.4.2.3 *Fat suppressed SE and FSE*

Chemical shift selective pulses are used to saturate the fat signals [DH Lee *et al.* 1991; Miller *et al.* 1993a; Gass *et al.* 1995]. These can be applied to conventional T2-weighted SE or FSE sequences. Effective fat suppression is achieved, and such approaches also demonstrate intrinsic lesions in the optic nerve in optic neuritis patients with a sensitivity similar to or slightly exceeding that of STIR when a similar matrix and field of view is used. An advantage of FSE is that a higher resolution (512 $\times$ 512, 16 cm field of view and 3 mm thick slices) can be obtained with complete coverage of the anterior visual pathway on coronal images in clinically acceptable times (10–11 minutes). This higher resolution (in plane 0.4 $\times$ 0.4 mm) clearly delineates the nerve from its surrounding CSF-containing sheath (Figure 2.5), and using such an approach, there is a clear depiction of demyelinating lesions (Figure 3.15), including features such as swelling or partial cross-sectional involvement of the optic nerve [Gass *et al.* 1995]. Enlargement and elongation of the CSF space around the nerve, as occurs in benign intracranial hypertension, is readily demonstrated [Gass *et al.* 1995] (Figure 2.6).

Fat suppression can also be applied to T1-weighted SE sequences, and is useful for detecting gadolinium enhancement of orbital or optic nerve lesions [Hendrix *et al.* 1990; Tien *et al.* 1991; Simon 1993], although the degree of fat suppression is less complete than with T2-weighted sequences. Nevertheless, this approach is preferable to STIR for the demonstration of enhancement, since T1 shortening due to gadolinium uptake on the latter results in an area of signal loss.

With the approaches described above, there is still a limitation. Ocular motion will inevitably occur over a 10-minute period, even in well-motivated subjects. In future, the use of echo planar techniques providing images in a matter of seconds may well overcome motion artefacts. Resolution will be further improved using 3D FSE sequences. Another strategy is a double inversion recovery sequence – this uses a short TI to suppress orbital fat and a long TI (e.g. 2000 ms) to suppress CSF [Redpath *et al.* 1993]. Thus an image of the nerve in isolation from surrounding CSF and fat is obtained. This sequence is yet to be evaluated in optic nerve diseases.

2.4.3   Coils

With such a small structure as the optic nerve, signal-to-noise ratio (SNR) is an important consideration. Conventional surface coils for orbital imaging maybe monocular (circular) or binocular. These provide better SNR for the superficial few centimetres of the optic nerve within the orbits, but poorer SNR at the greater depth of the chiasm, when compared with a conventional head coil. A two piece multi-array coil consisting of

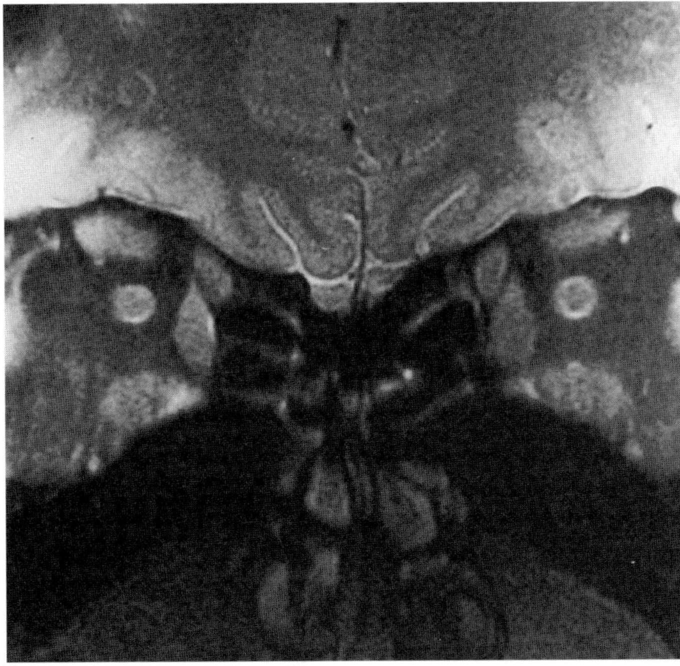

Figure 2.5 *Coronal high resolution T2-weighted image (slice thickness 3 mm, in-plane resolution 0.4 × 0.4 mm) in a healthy volunteer through the orbits and optic nerves using a fast spin echo sequence and a multi-array receiver coil provided by General Electric Medical Systems, Milwaukee, USA. Note the normal appearance of a thin layer of CSF contained within the optic nerve sheath around the nerve.*

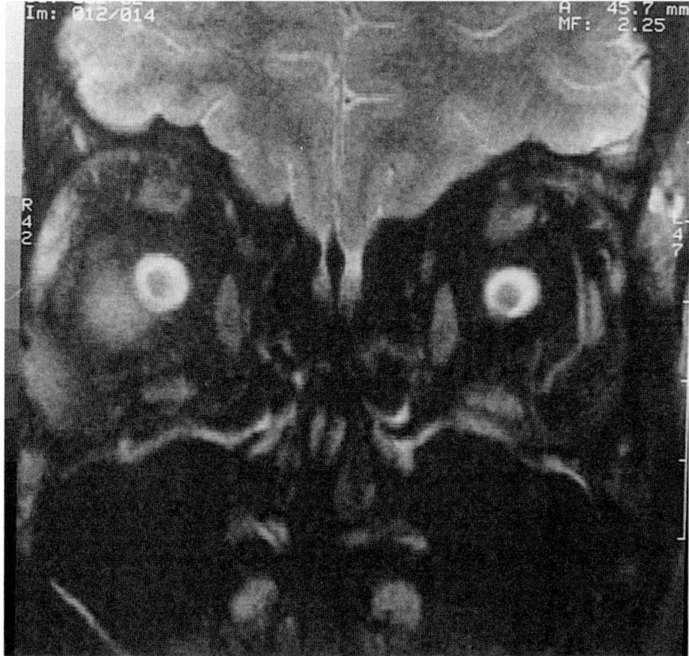

Figure 2.6 *Coronal T2-weighted fast spin echo image through the orbits in a patient with benign intracranial hypertension. Note the expanded CSF-containing optic nerve sheaths. (From Gass et al. 1995.)*

a pair of 3-inch circular coils has been developed specifically for imaging the temporo-mandibular joints. We have found that applying these coils (provided by GE Medical Systems, Milwaukee, USA) over the temples at the level of the orbits provides a composite image of the optic nerves with high SNR from the globe to the chiasm. In the future, more complex multi-array coils (e.g. four coils forming a semicircle around the front of the head at the level of the orbits) will increase SNR and image quality further.

2.4.4   Slice orientation

Axial and sagittal slices section the nerve longitudinally, whereas coronal slices image it more cross-sectionally. However, the nerve often runs a tortuous course and coronal slices are not truly perpendicular as the nerve travels medially towards the chiasm (about 15° from the anteroposterior axis). We nevertheless prefer coronal imaging to either sagittal or axial orientations, as it is less prone to partial volume contamination from surrounding tissues when visualising the nerve. It is possible to obtain oblique slices more perpendicular to the nerve. In the future, 3D FSE sequences will improve resolution (1 mm thick slices will be possible) and allow truly perpendicular sections through the nerve.

2.5   MR spectroscopy

2.5.1   Importance of spectroscopy in multiple sclerosis

MR spectroscopy (MRS) is a technique which allows the study and quantitation in vivo of metabolites containing NMR-visible nuclei. The two nuclei studied most often are proton (^{1}H) and phosphorus (^{31}P)

2.5.2   Proton MR spectroscopy

Proton spectroscopy studies mobile proton-containing metabolites apart from water. These are present at millimolar concentration in the nervous system, compared to water which has a concentration of approximately 80 moles/litre. Thus, to visualise the NMR signals from such metabolites it is necessary to effectively suppress the water signal, which otherwise dominates the spectrum making it impossible to discriminate the smaller metabolite peaks nearby. It is also necessary to study relatively large volumes of interest in order to obtain sufficient SNR. For proton spectroscopy this is usually between 1–8 ml. Thus in multiple sclerosis, only large lesions can be studied without the influence of partial volume effects.

At long echo times (135 or 270 ms), metabolites with long T2s are detected; in normal brain the three major peaks are attributable to *N*-acetyl-containing compounds, particularly *N*-acetyl aspartate (NAA), choline-containing compounds (Cho) and creatine/phosphocreatine (Cr) (Figure 2.7). A peak due to lactate (Lac) is not visible under resting conditions, when its concentration is less than 1 mmol/litre, but it may appear with brain activation (e.g. in the striate cortex in response to flashing light) or in a variety of pathological processes. NAA is the second most abundant amino acid in the central nervous system. Its function is uncertain, but it is contained almost entirely within neurones in the adult brain [Birken & Oldendorf 1989]. It is therefore of particular interest in multiple sclerosis as being a putative marker of axonal integrity [Arnold *et al.* 1990; Miller *et al.* 1991a]; loss of axons occurs in chronic multiple sclerosis lesions and may be an important cause of irreversible disability.

Proton spectroscopy at short echo times (e.g. 10–30 ms) detects additional metabolites with short T2s. These include mobile lipids, proteins, inositol, glucose and a number of neurotransmitters such as glutamate, glutamine and gamma aminobutyric acid (Figure 2.7). Little, if any, NMR signal is obtained from the proteins and lipids of intact myelin because of their relative immobility. The ability to detect mobile lipid resonances within multiple sclerosis lesions on proton MRS provides a non-invasive tool with which to monitor myelin breakdown directly [Wolinsky *et al.* 1990; Larsson *et al.* 1991; Grossman *et al.* 1992; Koopmans *et al.* 1993a; Davie *et al.* 1994a].

Quantitation of metabolites has often been based on ratio measurements using the Cr peak as an internal standard. It is clear however that the concentration of Cr may alter in a number of pathological states including multiple sclerosis [Davies *et al.* 1995].

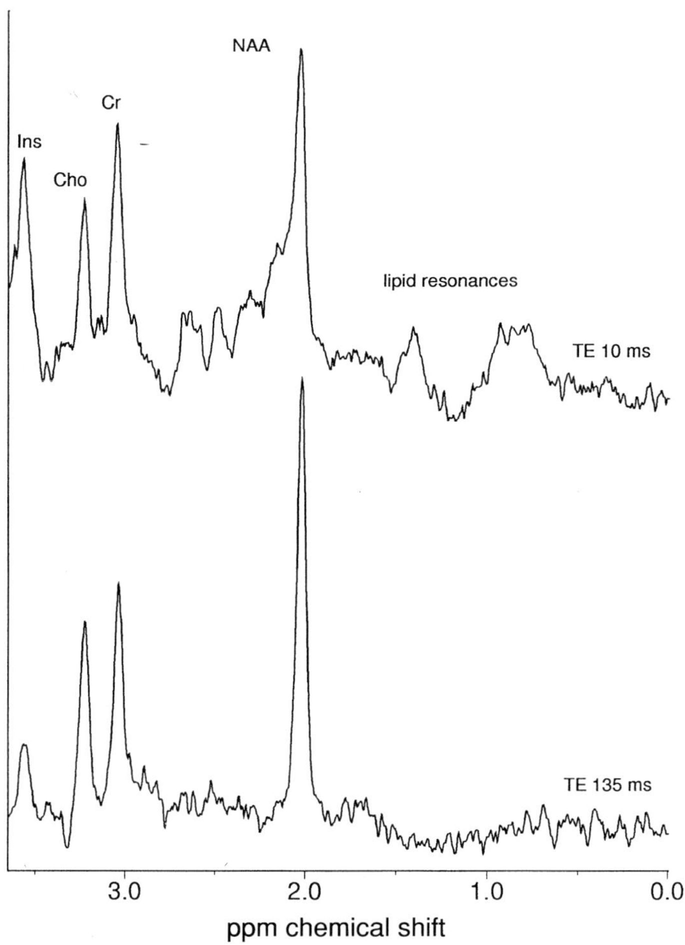

Figure 2.7 *Proton MR spectrum obtained from normal white matter of an adult volunteer using short (TE 10 ms, top) and long (TE 135 ms, bottom) echo times.*

Techniques are now increasingly being used which provide an absolute measurement of metabolite concentrations. Such methods usually employ the water peak as a standard of known concentration.

In vivo spectroscopic examinations normally involve a single small (1–8 ml) region of interest (voxel). Given that multiple sclerosis is a multifocal disease, there is a need for techniques which survey the disease in a more global manner. One approach is to acquire a single, large voxel which includes much of the cerebral white matter. This approach shows promise – serial changes in NAA have been identified in the absence of corresponding alterations on conventional images [Arnold *et al.* 1994]. An alternative strategy is spectroscopic imaging. Single slice spectroscopic images with a voxel size of about 1 cc can be obtained in a 30-minute examination [Arnold *et al.* 1992]. Multi-slice spectroscopic images are also feasible and have been successfully applied in a study of adrenoleucodystrophy by an experienced group of workers [Kruse *et al.* 1994].

2.5.3 Phosphorus MR spectroscopy

The major metabolite peaks visible on ^{31}P MRS are those due to alpha, beta and gamma ATP, inorganic phosphorus (Pi), phosphocreatine (PCr), phosphomono- (PME) and phosphodiesters (PDE). Because the ^{31}P nucleus has an intrinsically lower NMR sensitivity than the ^{1}H nucleus, and because of the low concentration of ^{31}P-containing metabolites, large voxels need to be studied – typically $3 \times 3 \times 3$ cm (27 cc). This severely restricts the utility of this technique for the evaluation of multiple sclerosis lesions. Nevertheless a number of abnormalities have been reported both in lesions and normal appearing white matter. These have included an increase in PCr in lesions [Minderhoud *et al.* 1992], an elevated pH and PDE level in a large, acute MS lesion [Cadoux-Hudson *et al.* 1991], and a reduction in the phospholipid broad component in lesions and normal appearing white matter [Husted *et al.* 1994a]. It has been suggested that the last finding might be due to reduced concentrations of myelin phospholipids. Because of its low resolution, further applications of ^{31}P spectroscopy in multiple sclerosis will probably be limited.

2.6 Image analysis

Image analysis-assisted techniques to analyse MRI data have a number of potential applications in multiple sclerosis. These include: (i) quantification of lesion load in studying the natural history of the disease and its modification by treatment; (ii) co-registration of multiple types of MR images in order to correlate different MR parameters.

2.6.1 Quantification of lesion load

The electronic image data (on tape or disc) can be displayed on an appropriate computer, e.g. a Sun workstation. Lesion load can then be measured in a relatively simple though time consuming fashion by manual outlining of lesions. A highly trained individual can measure multiple sclerosis lesion load on conventional PD-weighted images with a reproducibility of about 94%, and such an approach has been used successfully in the North American trial of interferon β-1b in relapsing-remitting multiple sclerosis [Paty *et al.* 1993]. In order to provide quicker analysis, and to improve reproducibility and objectivity, much effort has gone into developing more fully automated methods for lesion segmentation. A semi-automated threshold technique, applied after correction

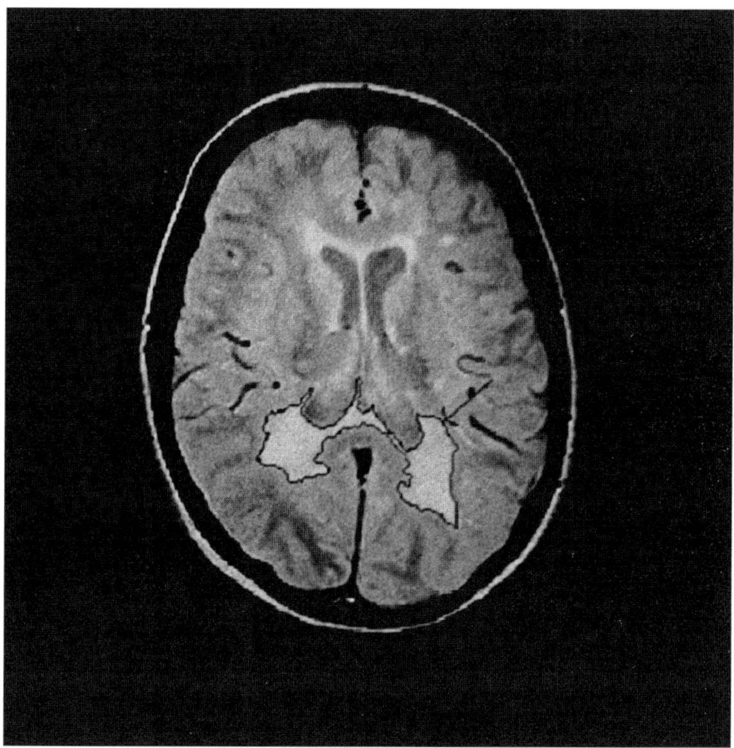

Figure 2.8 *PD-weighted image of a patient with multiple sclerosis showing two posterior parietal periventricular lesions outlined using the semi-automated 'contour' technique.*

for image nonuniformity to PD-weighted images, has been shown to improve reproducibility [Wicks *et al.* 1992; Filippi *et al.* 1995b], although the technique is very threshold dependent and considerable editing is needed to deal with areas of normal brain which were segmented (false positives) and low signal lesions which were not segmented (false negatives).

Semi-automated local threshold or edge detection techniques can be applied to each lesion (e.g. seed growing or Contour). These are time consuming but are more objective than manual outlining, since it is the program that defines the edge of each lesion. Using one such technique called Contour (provided by D Plummer, University College Department of Medical Physics) at The National Hospital, three relatively inexperienced observers have demonstrated intra-rater reproducibilities of 96–98% and an inter-rater reproducibility of 95%, these values being considerably higher than those obtained by manual outlining [Grimaud *et al.* 1996] (Figure 2.8).

Efforts to achieve more fully automated lesion segmentation have employed a variety of approaches including the use of multiparametric data (e.g. PD-, T2– and T1-weighted data) to improve the separation of pathological from normal tissue [Cline *et al.* 1990;

Jackson *et al.* 1993; Simmonds *et al.* 1993; Mitchell *et al.* 1994; Guttman *et al.* 1994; Cohen *et al.* 1995; Johnston *et al.* 1996]. While such techniques offer promise for the future, at present there is no totally reliable, fully automated technique. It is prudent that whatever method is used, the final step in analysis should be an expert review of the segmented images, with careful editing as and where needed.

The accuracy of lesion load measurement is improved by obtaining thinner slices (e.g. from 5 to 3 mm) due to reduction in partial volume errors [Kapouleas *et al.* 1993; Filippi *et al.* 1995c]. In the future, three-dimensional FSE should allow even more accurate lesion quantitation with slices as thin as 1 mm being possible; in addition, it will avoid 'apparent' changes in lesion size which can occur with poor repositioning – such spurious changes can be quite marked, especially if lesions are small [Goodkin *et al.* 1992].

2.6.2   Co-registration of MR images

It is often useful to compare several different types of MR data (e.g to evaluate the relationship between magnetisation transfer ratio, apparent diffusion coefficient and T_2 decay), or to compare the same data sets collected serially (e.g. total lesion loads on conventional images during a treatment trial). In order to optimise such comparisons, precise anatomical co-registration of the data is required. When the data is collected during different scanning visits, or even during a single long session, image planes from one data set to the other are often not the same. These problems may in the future be largely resolved by using 3D sequences (such as 3D FSE for lesion load), or by ultra-fast imaging with echo planar methods. Another approach is to use algorithms which transform multiple sets of data on to a standardised stereotaxic space or atlas of the brain. Complex but increasingly accurate and automated algorithms are being developed for this purpose [Collins *et al.* 1994]. The application of such methods in MS should improve the quality of studies in which multiple sets of image data are being compared.

3 Spectrum of abnormalities in multiple sclerosis

David H Miller

3.1 Use of MRI in diagnosis

3.1.1 Introduction

Magnetic resonance imaging (MRI) has, in the last decade, become the single most valuable investigation in confirming the diagnosis of multiple sclerosis. The next two chapters concentrate on its use in the diagnosis and differential diagnosis of multiple sclerosis.

A crucial point is that multiple sclerosis is diagnosed primarily on clinical grounds. It should not be diagnosed from the results of MRI or any other laboratory investigation alone. The interpretation of MRI abnormalities should always be considered in the clinical context. A confident diagnosis of multiple sclerosis requires the demonstration of clinically disseminated central nervous system (CNS) white matter lesions both in time and space. MRI aids diagnosis by providing paraclinical evidence for dissemination in space; evoked potentials have a similar function, but MRI is far more sensitive. A characteristic pattern of cerebral white matter lesions in young adults greatly consolidates the clinical diagnosis, although it should be remembered that even 'classical' MRI patterns are not totally specific for multiple sclerosis.

3.1.2 MRI as a diagnostic tool using the Poser criteria (see also Table 3.1)

The most widely used criteria for MS are those of the Poser committee [Poser 1983; Poser *et al.* 1983]. Using these, a diagnosis of clinically definite multiple sclerosis requires there to have been at least two episodes of CNS symptoms separated by a minimum of one month, and signs on examination of at least two lesions involving anatomically separate regions of the CNS white matter. It is also required that the subject is aged 10–59 years, and that there is no better explanation for the clinical findings. If multiple sclerosis is definite on clinical grounds, it is not always necessary to perform MRI.

If there are multiple symptomatic episodes, but signs of only a single CNS lesion, the diagnosis is clinically probable. If the patient is a young adult, and MRI reveals multiple white matter lesions characteristic of multiple sclerosis, the diagnosis can be upgraded to clinically definite.

Table 3.1 *MRI and the Poser criteria (From Miller DH & Donald WI,* Clinical Neuroscience, 2, 215–224, 1994 © Wiley-Liss Inc 1994.*)*

	MRI	Poser classification
Two attacks; clinical evidence of two lesions	+	CDMS
	−	CDMS
Two attacks; clinical evidence of one lesion	**+**	**CDMS**
	−	CPMS
One attack; clinical evidence of one lesion	**+ (with new lesions developing)**	**CPMS**
	−	Not diagnostic
One attack; clinical evidence of one lesion +CSF OCBs	**+ (with new lesions developing)**	**LSDMS**
	−	Not diagnostic

Notes:
Situations in which a positive MRI scan permits a more certain diagnosis are shown in bold

If the presentation is with a clinically isolated progressive myelopathy of more than six months duration, and a compressive lesion has been excluded by spinal MRI or myelography, the presence of typical cerebral white matter lesions in a young adult allows a diagnosis of clinically probable multiple sclerosis.

If there has been a single episode characteristic of multiple sclerosis (e.g. acute unilateral optic neuritis, internuclear ophthalmoplegia, or partial myelopathy), the diagnosis can only be 'suspected' or 'possible'. MRI reveals multifocal white matter lesions indistinguishable from multiple sclerosis in 50–70% of such patients [Ormerod *et al.* 1986a; Ormerod *et al.* 1986b; Jacobs *et al.* 1986; Miller *et al.* 1987a]. This evidence of dissemination in space does not allow an immediate diagnosis of multiple sclerosis, as the same appearances can be produced by the less common monophasic demyelinating disease, acute disseminated encephalomyelitis (ADEM) [Kesselring *et al.* 1990]. However, disseminated MRI lesions are associated with a high risk of progression to clinically definite multiple sclerosis in the next 1–5 years [Ford *et al.* 1992; Morrissey *et al.* 1993a; Beck *et al.* 1993] (for further details see Chapter 5: Prognosis). If follow-up MRI after an interval of more than one month reveals new lesions, a diagnosis of clinically probable multiple sclerosis can be made, even in the absence of new clinical events. However, it is unknown whether the risk of future clinical events is influenced by the results of an early follow-up scan, and therefore the wisdom of obtaining this may be doubted in an otherwise asymptomatic individual. We do not perform such a study in routine clinical practice.

Examination of the CSF for oligoclonal bands remains a very useful investigation, particularly if either the clinical or MRI features are considered atypical or non-specific. CSF examination is particularly valuable in patients more than 50 years old, since brain

MRI is least specific in this age group. A patient with clinically probable multiple sclerosis *and* CSF oligoclonal bands is classified as laboratory supported definite multiple sclerosis.

3.2   Brain MRI in clinically definite multiple sclerosis

3.2.1   Frequency of abnormalities

Brain MRI abnormalities were reported in early studies to occur in between 75% and 100% of patients with clinically definite multiple sclerosis [Young *et al.* 1981; Lukes *et al.* 1983; Runge *et al.* 1984; Jackson *et al.* 1985]. The variable frequency of abnormalities probably reflects the stringency with which clinical criteria are applied in making a definite diagnosis, as well as variable sensitivities of different scanners. With strict application of the Poser criteria for clinically definite disease, and using only clinical features to classify cases (the results of MRI, CSF and evoked potentials were not considered), we found one or more focal brain MRI abnormalities in 113/114 (99%) and 197/200 (98.5%) of patients studied in two consecutive series at The National Hospital, London [Ormerod *et al.* 1987; Miller 1988] (Tables 3.2 and 3.3). This suggests that about 1% of patients with clinically definite multiple sclerosis will have a completely normal brain MRI. In the second series [Miller 1988], two patients had a single lesion and six others had only two lesions: thus two or fewer brain lesions were seen in 11 (5.5%) of 200 patients. Looked at another way, three or more brain lesions were seen in 95% of patients. There follows a review of the MRI findings reported in clinically definite multiple sclerosis, taking into account both The National Hospital and other series (see also Tables 3.2 and 3.3).

3.2.2   Cerebral white matter

Concordant with pathological observations, the classical MRI pattern is one of multiple white matter lesions, with a periventricular predominance (Figure 3.1). In The National Hospital series, 308/314 (98%) of patients had one or more lesions in contiguity with the lateral ventricles. The occurrence of multiple discrete white matter lesions without periventricular involvement is distinctly unusual, although the occurrence of discrete lesions *in addition* to periventricular ones is the rule rather than the exception. All parts of the lateral ventricles are commonly involved; lesions of the body and trigones are more frequent than in other regions. Lesions are usually irregular in shape, but sometimes have a rounded or oval appearance, a feature said to be relatively specific for multiple sclerosis [Horowitz *et al.* 1989]. The size of lesions is highly variable – most are small (less than 5 mm diameter), but sometimes very large lesions occur, even to the point of simulating a cerebral tumour (see Section 3.2.7).

Table 3.2 *Frequency of cerebral hemisphere white matter MRI abnormalities in 200 patients with clinically definite multiple sclerosis*

	No. of lesions	No. of patients (%)
Periventricular	0	4 (2)
	1	9 (4.5)
	≥2	187 (93.5)
Discrete from ventricles	0	15 (7.5)
	1	10 (5)
	≥2	175 (87.5)
All white matter regions	0	3 (1.5)
	1	4 (2)
	≥2	193 (96.5)

Table 3.3 *Distribution of brain MRI abnormalities in 200 patients with clinically definite multiple sclerosis*

	No. of patients	%
Periventricular		
Lateral ventricle	196	98
Body	194	97
Trigone	171	86
Occipital horn	149	75
Temporal horn	132	66
Frontal horn	117	59
Third ventricle	31	16
Fourth ventricle	106	53
Discrete cerebral white matter	185	93
Cortico-medullary junction	130	65
Internal capsule	83	42
Cerebral cortex	25	13
Basal ganglia	15	8
Brain stem	132	66
Pons	103	52
Midbrain	72	36
Medulla	29	15
Cerebellum	113	57

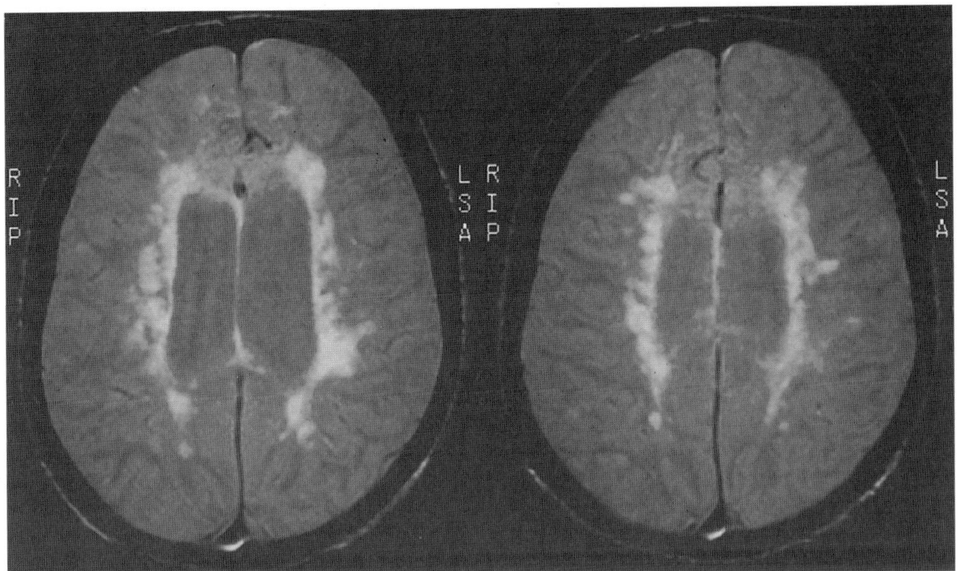

Figure 3.1 *Multiple sclerosis. PD-weighted image showing typical periventricular lesions. The lesions are multiple, asymmetrical, and mainly small, and of irregular, rounded or oval shape.*

Pathologically, the corpus callosum is frequently involved in multiple sclerosis [Brownell & Hughes 1962; Barnard & Trigg 1974; Allen 1991]. MRI abnormalities in this region are better seen on sagittal images [Wilms *et al.* 1991; Gean-Marton *et al.* 1991] (Figure 3.2). In one series, callosal lesions were seen in 93% and 55% of 42 MS patients on sagittal and axial images respectively [Gean-Marton *et al.* 1991]; in contrast, sagittal images of 127 control patients with periventricular white matter disorders of a different aetiology (usually vascular disease) revealed such lesions in only 2.4%, suggesting that this feature has a relatively high diagnostic value. Lesions were noted to have a particular predilection for the interface between the callosum and septum pellucidum. The high frequency of corpus callosum lesions in multiple sclerosis has been confirmed by other investigators [Simon *et al.* 1986].

Lesions at the corticomedullary junction are also relatively common in multiple sclerosis: in one post-mortem study, 17% of cerebral plaques were sited in this region [Brownell & Hughes 1962]. On MRI, lesions sometimes follow the curvature of a gyrus without involving the ribbon of cortical grey matter, giving the impression of relatively selective involvement of the subcortical U-fibres [Miller 1988] (Figure 3.3). Subcortical lesions may also occur in vascular disease, but usually as small punctate lesions or as larger areas of infarction which also extend into the cortex; in one form of vascular disease, Binswanger's subacute arteriosclerotic encephalopathy, sparing of the subcortical U-fibres is characteristic [Révèsz *et al.* 1989].

Lesions in the internal capsule were visible in 95/314 (30%) of patients in the National Hospital series. Vascular lesions also occur quite often in this region, so these lesions are of little diagnostic value.

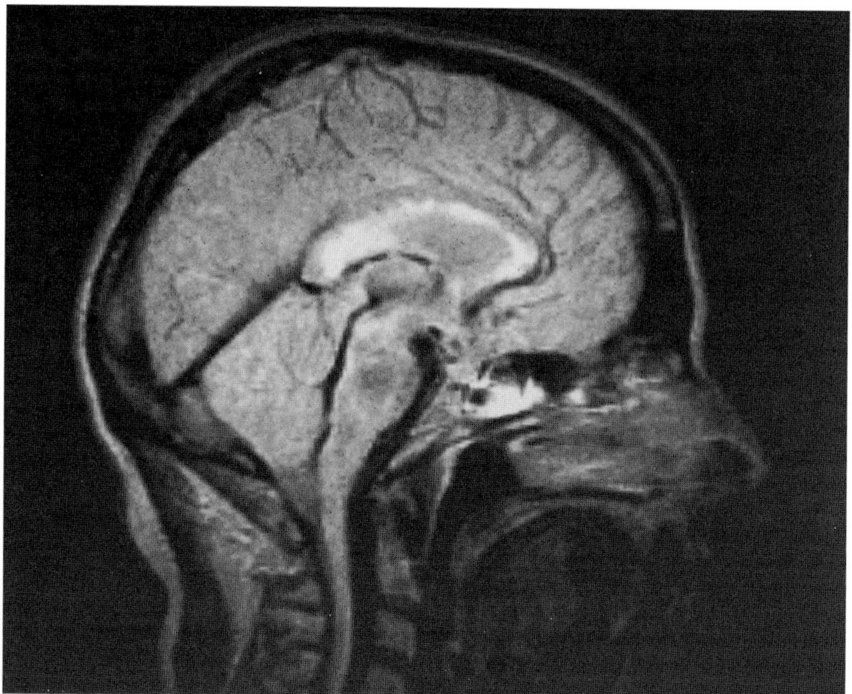

Figure 3.2 *Sagittal PD-weighted image showing corpus callosum lesions in a 43-year-old female with multiple sclerosis.*

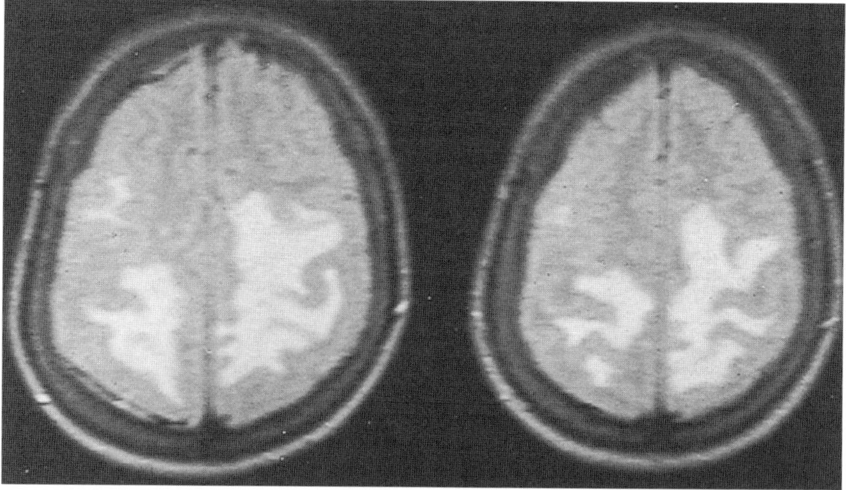

Figure 3.3 *PD-weighted image in a 37-year-old female with multiple sclerosis showing extensive subcortical white matter lesions extending to the corti-comedullary junction.*

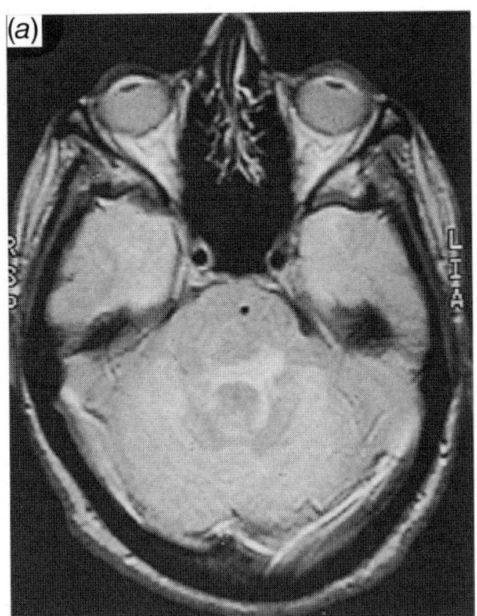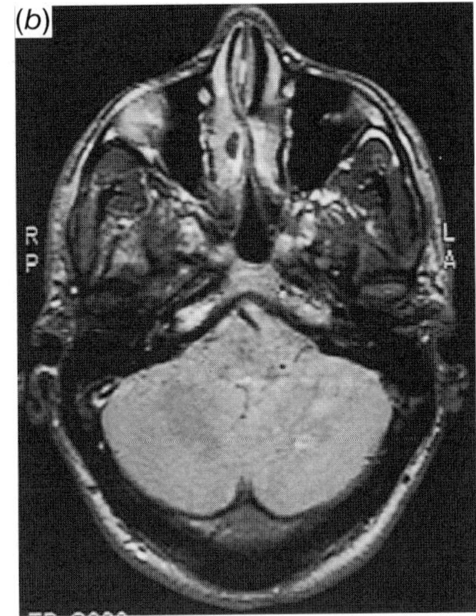

Figure 3.4 *PD-weighted images in multiple sclerosis patients showing (a) a lesion in the floor of the fourth ventricle and (b) cerebellar white matter lesions.*

3.2.3   Brain stem

Lesions in the brain stem were seen in 209/314 (67%) of patients in the National Hospital series. Any part of the brain stem may be affected, but the floor of the fourth ventricle is a particularly frequent and characteristic site of involvement (Figure 3.4a). Most lesions are small (typically a few millimetres in diameter), but much larger lesions can occur and there may be associated swelling in new lesions. Clinical brain stem syndromes are common in multiple sclerosis, and in most instances, an appropriately placed lesion is detectable on MRI [Bogousslavsky *et al.* 1986; Constantino *et al.* 1986; Barratt *et al.* 1988; Mochizuki *et al.* 1988; Curé *et al.* 1990; Bronstein *et al.* 1990a, b; Howard *et al.* 1992]. Some brain stem lesions in multiple sclerosis are superficial, abutting the subarachnoid space; in small vessel disease, abnormalities in the central pons are more characteristic.

3.2.4   Cerebellum

Lesions may occur in any part of the cerebellar white matter; 169/314 (54%) of National Hospital patients had one or more lesions. Most cerebellar lesions are small; their shape may be irregular, rounded or oval (Figure 3.4). Lesions are not often seen in the cerebellar cortex.

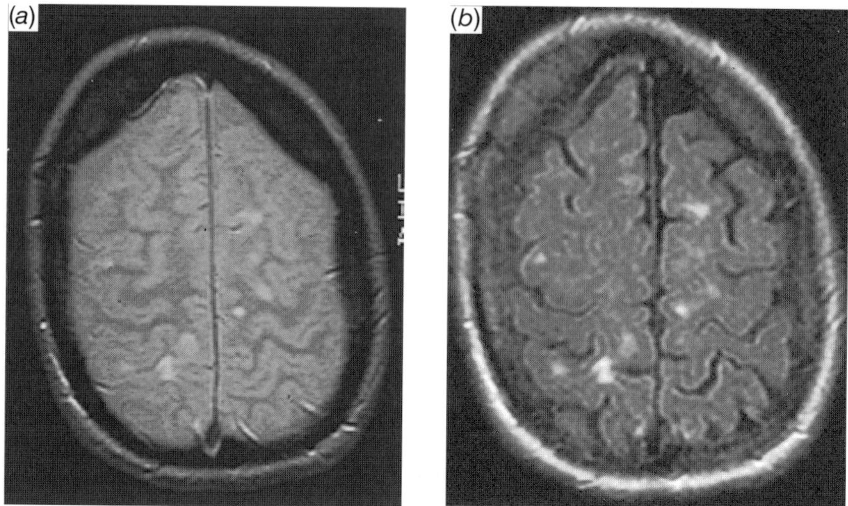

Figure 3.5 *Multiple sclerosis. (a) PD-weighted fast spin echo and (b) fast FLAIR images. Note the greater conspicuity of cortical/subcortical lesions using fast FLAIR.*

3.2.5   Cerebral cortex

In the post-mortem series of Brownell & Hughes [1962], 5% of plaques were restricted to the cerebral cortex. Unequivocal cortical lesions are rarely seen using conventional T2-weighted sequences, although because of partial volume effects, it is often difficult to determine whether or not subcortical white matter lesions have extended into the cortex. It is likely that PD- and T2-weighted scans miss small cortical lesions, because of the relatively high signal of normal cortex and because of partial volume contamination by medium or high signal CSF. Gadolinium enhancement has detected hitherto unsuspected cortical lesions [Miller *et al.* 1988a], but will only identify acute lesions with an abnormal blood–brain barrier (see Section 3.3). The FLAIR (or fast FLAIR) sequence, by suppressing signal from normal grey matter and CSF, does improve the detection of cortical plaques [Hajnal *et al.* 1992; Thorpe *et al.* 1994b; Boggild *et al.* 1995] (Figure 3.5).

3.2.6   Basal ganglia

Focal lesions in the basal ganglia were seen in only 44/314 (14%) of patients in the combined National Hospital series. Basal ganglia lesions are seen rather more frequently in cerebrovascular disease [Ormerod *et al.* 1987], a feature of some value in differential diagnosis.

One report indicated an abnormal degree of signal hypointensity on T2-weighted images in the putamen and thalamus of multiple sclerosis patients, when compared to healthy controls, and suggested that this was due to excessive iron deposition in these nuclei (iron induces local magnetic field inhomogeneities leading to accelerated T2 relaxation and thus low signal on T2-weighted images)[Drayer *et al.* 1987]. The same group also reported a correlation between the degree of basal ganglia hypointensity and white matter lesion load. It is clear that such an observation is non-specific, signal hypointensity being seen in a number of extrapyramidal diseases including multisystem atrophy [Pastakia *et al.* 1986], and indeed with normal aging [Milton *et al.* 1991]. It is known that brain iron concentrations are normally highest in basal ganglia nuclei, especially the pallidum, and that they increase with age [Hallgren & Sourander 1958; Hoeck *et al.* 1975].

In London we have recently compared 46 MS patients and 42 age matched controls and found no difference in the frequency or intensity of putaminal signal loss between the two groups; there was a slight reduction in thalamic signal in the patient group compared to controls, although there were no individuals in which this was marked [Grimaud *et al.* 1995]. There was no correlation between white matter lesion load and basal ganglia signal. In summary these findings, although much less impressive than those of Drayer, do not exclude the possibility of a slightly excessive accumulation of iron in the thalamus in multiple sclerosis.

It is not clear why iron normally accumulates in the basal ganglia. It is known that iron is resorbed by capillary endothelial cells in the thalamus and other basal ganglia after transferrin binds to a specific receptor on the cell surface [Hill & Switzer 1984; Dietrich & Bradley 1988]. It is then transported along axons to their sites of projection where the iron is subsequently released and stored in oligodendrocytes [Hill & Switzer 1984]. There can be marked loss of axons in multiple sclerosis [Adams 1989; Lassman *et al.* 1994], and this could conceivably lead to an increased accumulation of iron at the site of uptake in the basal ganglia. It is possible that axonal loss in the thalamus is greater than in other basal ganglia nuclei because it is a relay centre for sensory afferent pathways which are very frequently involved, clinically and pathologically, in MS.

3.2.7   Mass lesions

Occasionally, large lesions simulating tumours are seen [Youl *et al.* 1991a], the patient usually presenting with focal neurological deficits, seizures or raised intracranial pressure [Figure 3.6]. These have been biopsied on occasions and confirmed to be large regions of inflammatory demyelination, sometimes accompanied by considerable tissue destruction. A false positive diagnosis of cerebral tumour was more likely when only CT results were available, since MRI is more likely to reveal additional smaller lesions characteristic of multiple sclerosis, in addition to the presenting mass lesion.

Mass lesions can occur anywhere in the cerebral hemispheres. They frequently display ring enhancement, but sometimes the pattern of contrast uptake is homogeneous or irregular. Acute infratentorial lesions may also display mass effect; a lesion in the floor of the fourth ventricle may distort the shape of the adjacent ventricle. There is one case report of a large midbrain plaque causing obstructive hydrocephalus [Butler & Gilligan 1989].

3.3   Evolution of lesions

3.3.1   PD/T2-weighted MRI

Serial studies in patients with relapsing-remitting or secondary progressive MS have revealed new cerebral lesions appearing with a surprising frequency. Such lesions are usually asymptomatic – overall five to ten new lesions appear for every clinical relapse [Isaac *et al.* 1988; Willoughby *et al.* 1989; Koopmans *et al.* 1989a]. Scans have been performed as frequently as once a fortnight and a highly characteristic evolution has emerged. Lesions expand over a few days to weeks, generally reaching their maximum

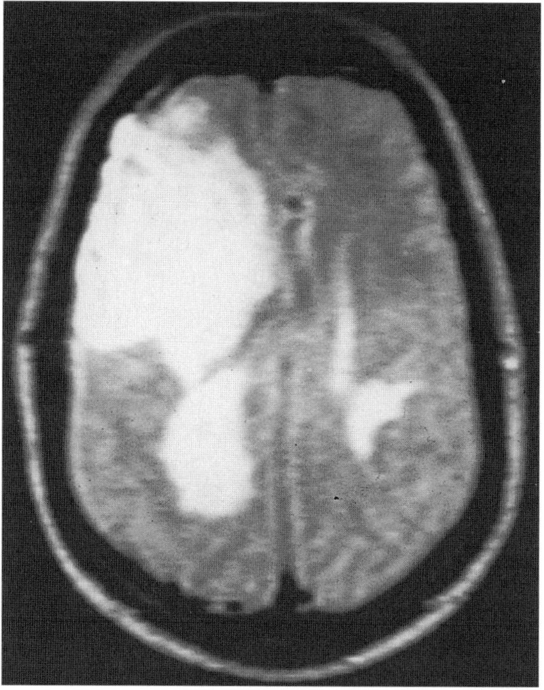

Figure 3.6 *PD-weighted image in a 56-year-old male with known multiple sclerosis who presented with obtundation and seizures. There is a large lesion causing mass effect in the right frontal lobe. Biopsy revealed a demyelinating lesion.*

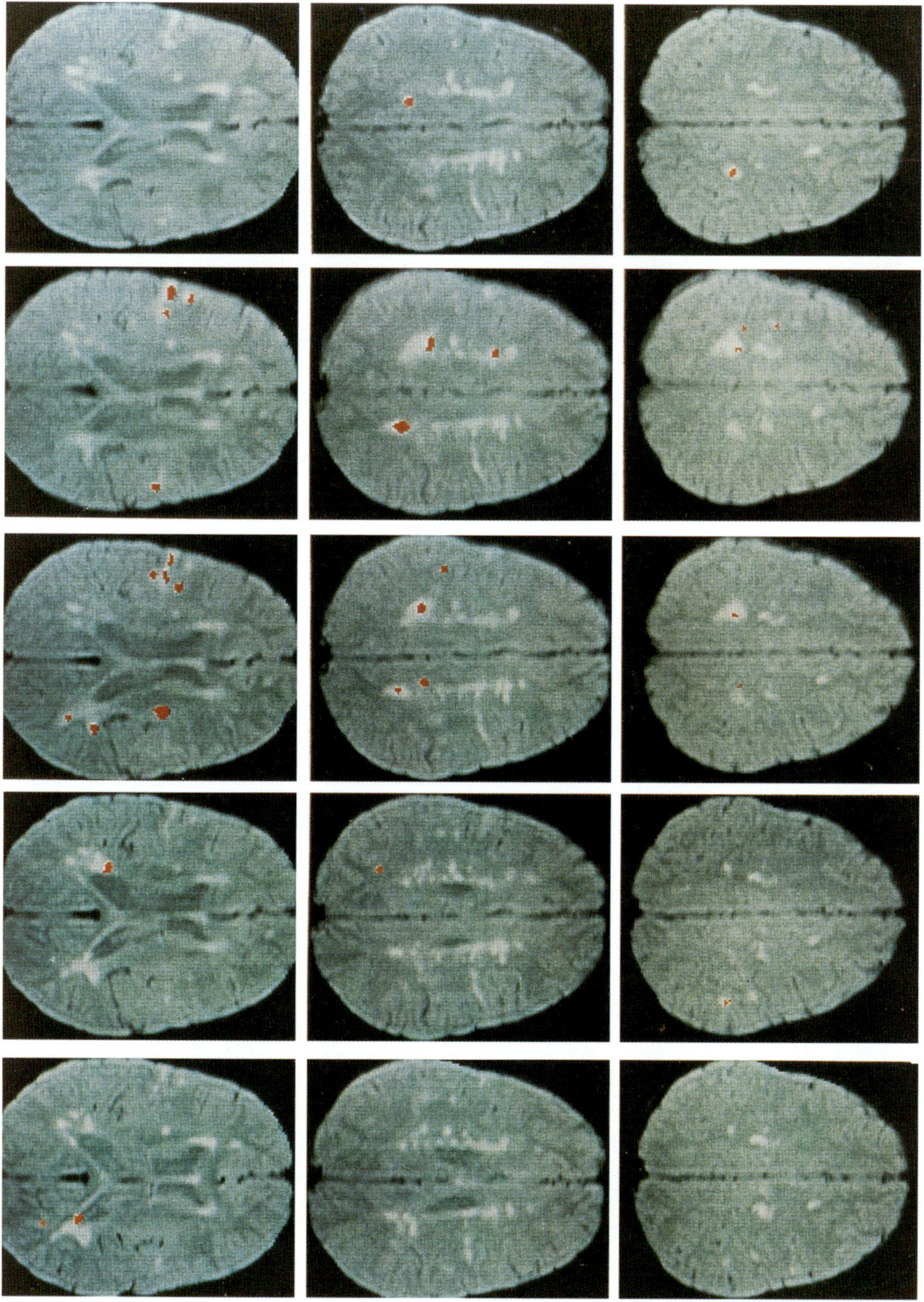

Figure 3.9 *Superimposed serial T2-weighted and gadolinium enhanced T1-weighted scans at monthly intervals in a 24-year-old patient with secondary progressive multiple sclerosis. New lesions on the T2-weighted scans are seen as high signal areas and areas of enhancement are superimposed in red.*

size within one month, at which time they start to get smaller. The phase of lesion waning again lasts a matter of weeks, the final stable size being attained in about two to three months. At low field, using 10 mm thick slices, 40% of such lesions disappeared altogether [Willoughby *et al.* 1989]; however, studies at higher fields and with thinner slices have shown that a residual, albeit small, abnormality almost invariably persists [Thompson *et al.* 1991].

It is also apparent that many new lesions are very small, and show little change in size after first appearing. Some larger new lesions have a 'halo' or 'target' appearance [Ormerod *et al.* 1987; Miller *et al.* 1988a], with a markedly hyperintense centre and a less hyperintense periphery. Occasionally, a thin ring of low signal intensity separates the two regions, and it has been suggested that this might be due to the effect of paramagnetic free radicals [Powell *et al.* 1992].

3.3.2   Gadolinium enhancement

In patients with relapsing-remitting or secondary progressive multiple sclerosis, most new lesions show gadolinium enhancement, indicating blood–brain barrier breakdown, which lasts about two to six weeks [Miller *et al.* 1988a; Bastianello *et al.* 1990; Harris *et al.* 1991; Thompson *et al.* 1991 & 1992; Barkhof *et al.* 1992b; Capra *et al.* 1992]. Enhancement occasionally precedes the appearance of an abnormality on the T2-weighted image [Kermode *et al.* 1990a] (Figure 3.7), but more often coincides with the emergence and expansion of the T2 lesion (Figure 3.8). Initially a small lesion enhances homogeneously, then if the lesion expands over the next few days to weeks, enhancement is seen as an expanding ring at or near the edge of the T2-weighted lesion [Kermode *et al.* 1990b; Guttmann *et al.* 1995]. Enhancement usually ceases after about one month, and subsequently the T2-weighted lesion becomes smaller. Persistent enhancement beyond one month is unusual (Figure 3.9). In the series reported from the National Institutes of Health in Washington [Harris *et al.* 1991], where a group of six relapsing-remitting patients was followed with monthly MRI for 8–11 months, there was a total of 94 new enhancing lesions. Of these, 69 (73%) enhanced on a single scan, 20 (21%) enhanced on two consecutive scans and only three and two lesions respectively enhanced on three and four consecutive scans. Our experience is fully in accord with this, although we have recently seen a case of clinically definite multiple sclerosis in whom many lesions showed persistence of enhancement for six months or longer (courtesy of Professor G Edan, Rennes, France) (Figure 3.10).

Gadolinium enhancement may also occur in old lesions seen on previous T2-weighted images (Figure 3.11). At any point in time, only a small minority of old lesions will enhance (or, as is often the case, none at all). As in new lesions, re-enhancement of old lesions generally lasts for only a few days or weeks; it may or may not be accompanied by enlargement of the original lesion on the T2-weighted image.

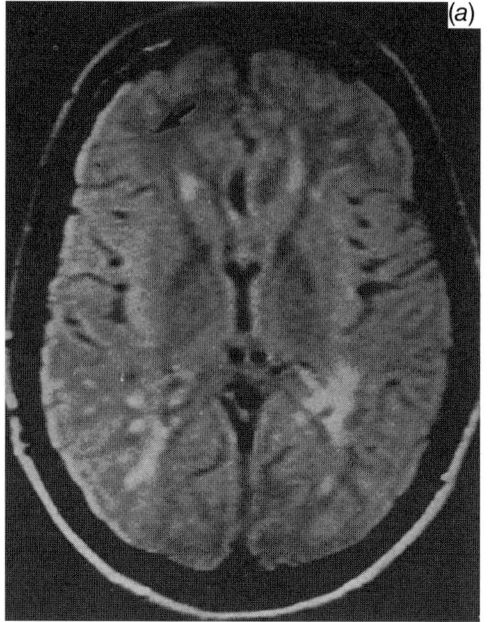
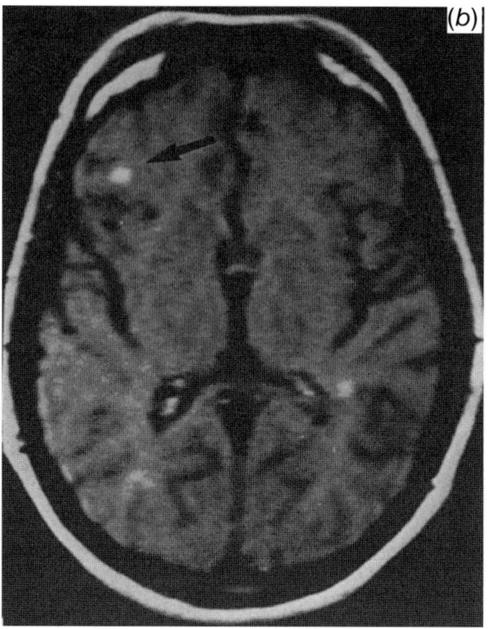
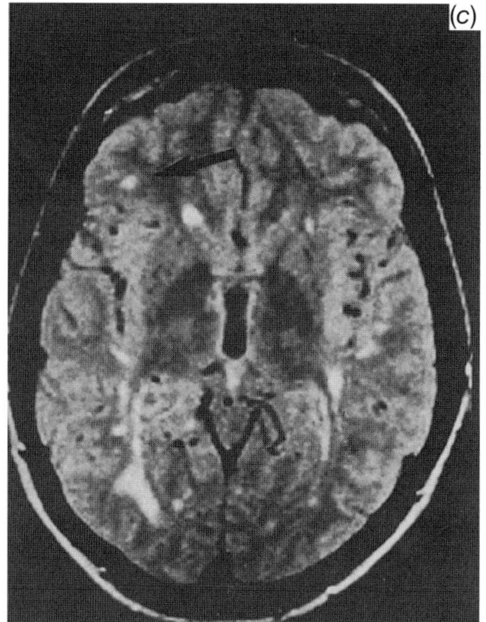

Figure 3.7 *A multiple sclerosis lesion displaying blood–brain barrier breakdown as the earliest visible abnormality. (a) PD-weighted image and (b) gadolinium enhanced T1-weighted image acquired at the same examination. There is an enhancing lesion in the right frontal lobe (arrowed, with no corresponding abnormality on the PD-weighted scan). (c) PD-weighted scan ten days later: a corresponding lesion has now appeared. (From Kermode et al. 1990a.)*

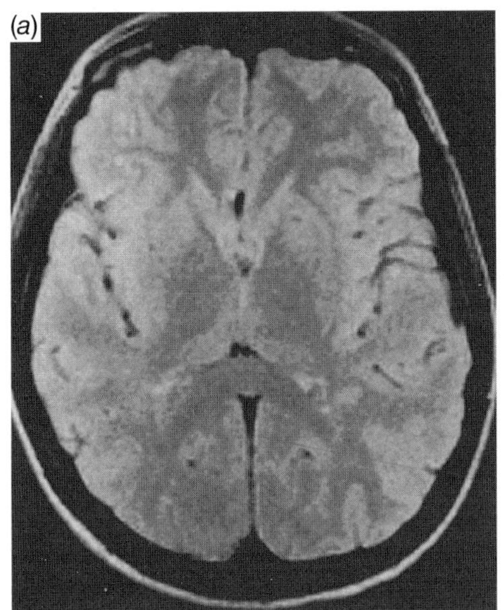

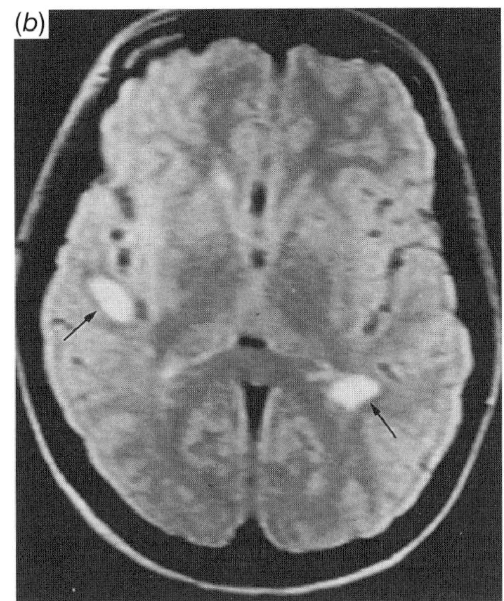

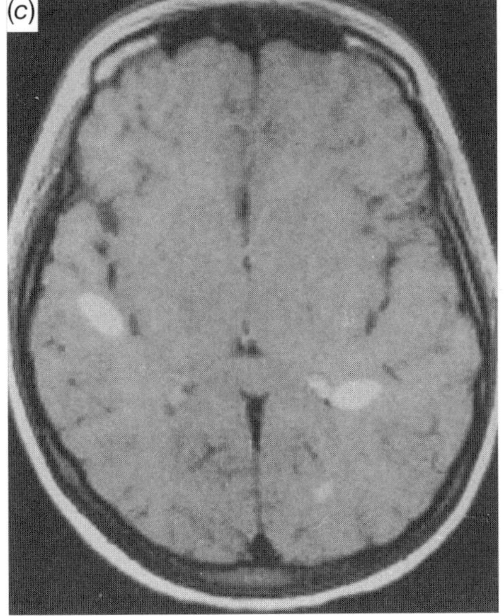

Figure 3.8 *New multiple sclerosis lesions displaying blood–brain barrier breakdown. PD-weighted scans (a) at first study and (b) three days later; note two large lesions have appeared adjacent to the left trigone and in the right temporal lobe (arrowed). (c) Gadolinium enhanced T1-weighted scan obtained at the same examination as the follow-up PD-weighted scan: both new lesions display homogeneous enhancement.*

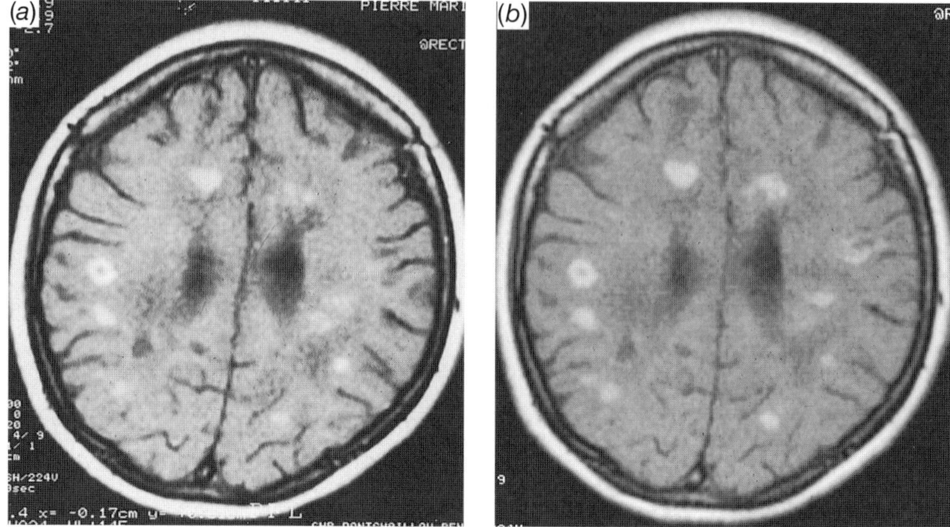

Figure 3.10 *Gadolinium enhanced T1-weighted scans demonstrating unusually longstanding enhancement of lesions in a 30-year-old female with clinically definite multiple sclerosis. Many enhancing lesions seen on the first study (a) are still enhancing six months later (b).*

3.3.3   Role of serial MRI or gadolinium enhancement in diagnosis

The pathophysiological basis and significance of the dynamic changes described in Sections 3.3.1 and 3.3.2 are discussed in Chapter 6. This section deals solely with implications for diagnosis.

Serial MRI can assist diagnosis in those patients in whom the criterion of dissemination in time has not been fulfilled; thus, if there has been a single episode suggestive of multiple sclerosis (e.g. optic neuritis), MRI at presentation reveals multiple cerebral lesions, and follow-up MRI after more than one month reveals new lesions, a diagnosis of clinically probable multiple sclerosis is possible using the Poser criteria. The added finding of oligoclonal bands in the CSF upgrades the diagnosis to laboratory supported definite multiple sclerosis.

If the first MRI is obtained several months after a single clinical episode, gadolinium enhancement may be helpful; if some lesions enhance, it is likely that they are new or at least that they are displaying new pathological activity, again suggesting that the process is disseminated in time. The duration of gadolinium enhancement may also assist diagnosis. It is exceptional for multiple sclerosis lesions to display persistent enhancement beyond three months, and such an occurrence should alert one to other possible diagnoses, e.g. granulomatous disease (see Section 4.6).

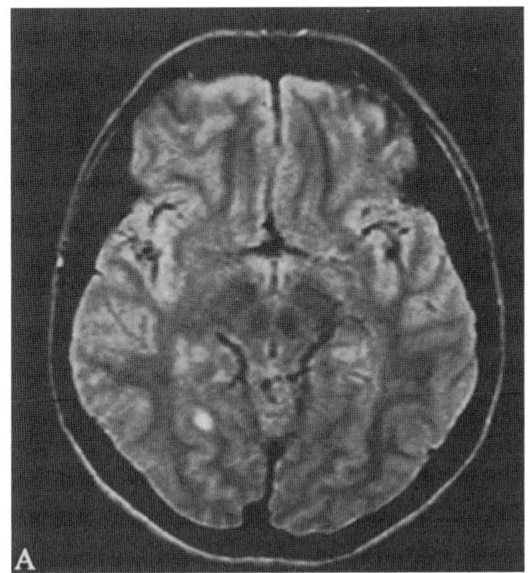
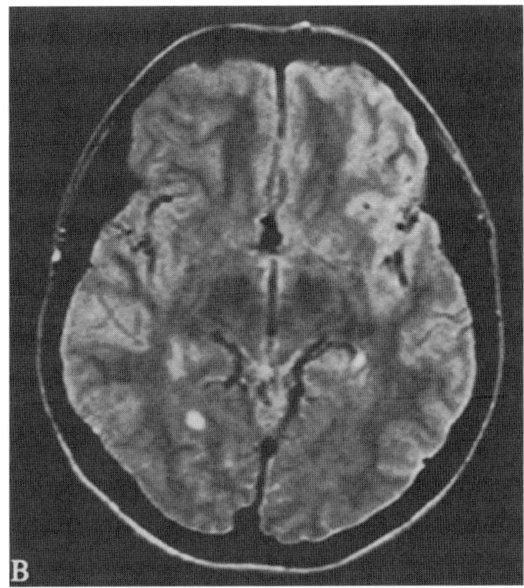
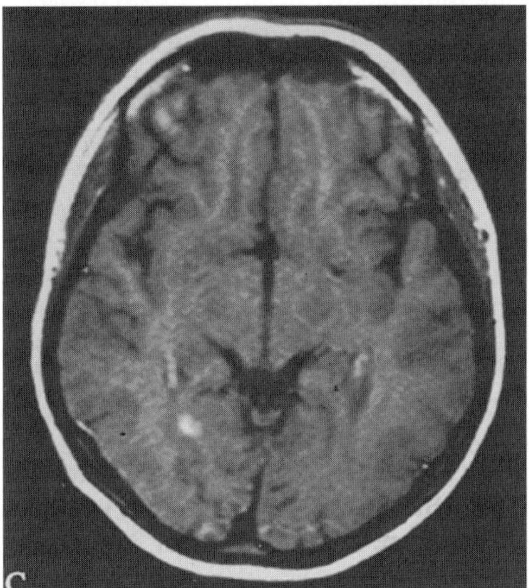

Figure 3.11 *Multiple sclerosis: PD-weighted image reveals a discrete white matter lesion (a) which has not changed in appearance at follow-up one month later (b); however, new enhancement appears on the gadolinium enhanced T1-weighted scan at follow-up (c). (From Miller et al. 1993.)*

3.4 Spinal cord MRI

This is particularly valuable in assessing patients with chronic progressive myelopathy. While multiple sclerosis can produce this syndrome, it is essential to exclude treatable compressive spinal lesions. With regard to the latter, high resolution MRI is the investigation of choice, and when available, it is rarely necessary to resort to myelography, except perhaps when an arteriovenous malformation is suspected, although most of these are detectable with current MRI techniques [Thorpe *et al.* 1994d].

Using multi-array coils and the FSE sequence, we have found one or more intrinsic cord lesions in 75% of patients with clinically definite multiple sclerosis [Kidd *et al.* 1993] (Figure 3.12). Such lesions do not occur in healthy individuals, including older age groups [Thorpe *et al.* 1993]. On sagittal images, the lesions are usually less than 5 mm in length and rarely longer than 1 cm [Campi *et al.* 1995], and most lesions have either a central or posterior location within the cord [Kidd *et al.* 1993]. MRI abnormalities are found more frequently in the cervical than in the thoracic cord, in agreement with previous pathological observations [Oppenheimer 1978]. The C4–6 segments are most commonly involved.

New cord lesions are about one-tenth as frequent as new brain lesions in relapsing-remitting cases [Thorpe *et al.* 1996a], and even less frequent in progressive disease [Kidd *et al.* 1996], but they are more likely to be symptomatic [Thorpe *et al.* 1996a]. Although many new cord lesions display gadolinium enhancement (Figure 3.13), when scanning is performed at monthly intervals, a higher proportion of new lesions do not enhance in the cord compared to the brain [Thorpe *et al.* 1996a]. There may be associated swelling of the cord in new plaques which can last for several months. Prolonged and extensive swelling may suggest a diagnosis of spinal tumour, but clinical and MRI follow-up almost always clarifies the diagnosis without the need for biopsy. Cord atrophy occurs not infrequently, particularly in more disabled patients [Kidd *et al.* 1993].

There are two situations where detection of spinal lesions is of particular diagnostic value: (i) where multiple sclerosis is strongly suspected clinically but brain MRI is normal or shows only minor, non-specific abnormalities; (ii) the older patient in whom brain MRI changes are especially non-specific. In a review of all cases examined in our unit in the last three years, we have identified 20 in whom multiple sclerosis was felt to be the likely diagnosis, but brain MRI was either normal (eight patients) or revealed a small number of small, non-specific, non-periventricular white matter hyperintensities [Thorpe *et al.* 1996b]. The course of the illness was primary progressive in 11, relapsing-remitting in eight and secondary progressive in one. Visual evoked potentials were delayed in 10/18 patients, and CSF oligoclonal bands were present in 13/15 tested, confirming the value of these investigations in this group of patients. Perhaps most helpful of all was spinal MRI, which revealed one or more intrinsic cord lesions in all 20 patients.

3.5   Optic neuritis

Using either STIR or fat-suppressed conventional T2-weighted SE sequences to suppress orbital fat signal, high signal lesions are seen in 80–90% of symptomatic optic nerves in

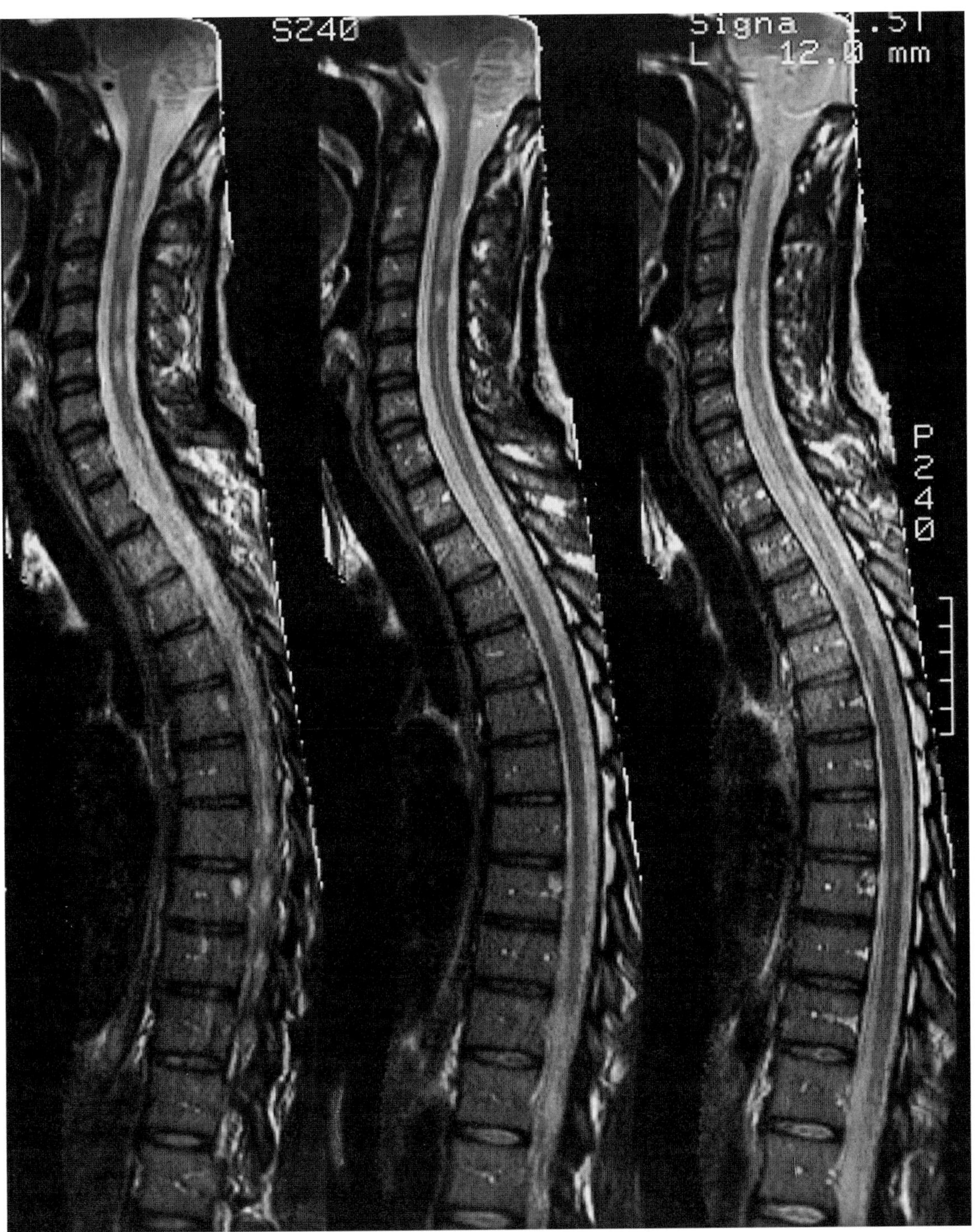

Figure 3.12 *Multiple sclerosis: contiguous, 3 mm thick, sagittal T2-weighted images reveal multiple intrinsic lesions in the cervical and thoracic cord.*

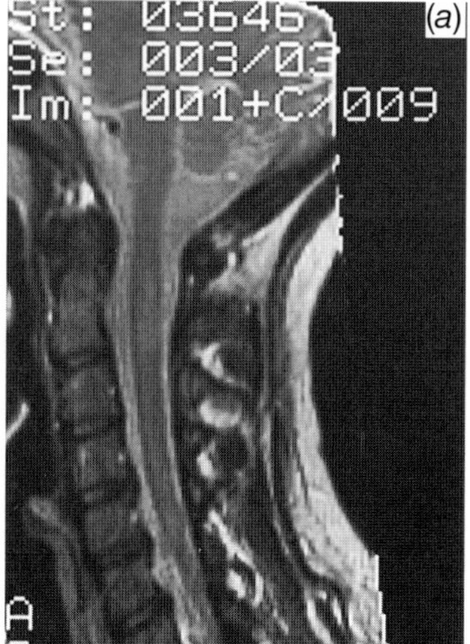

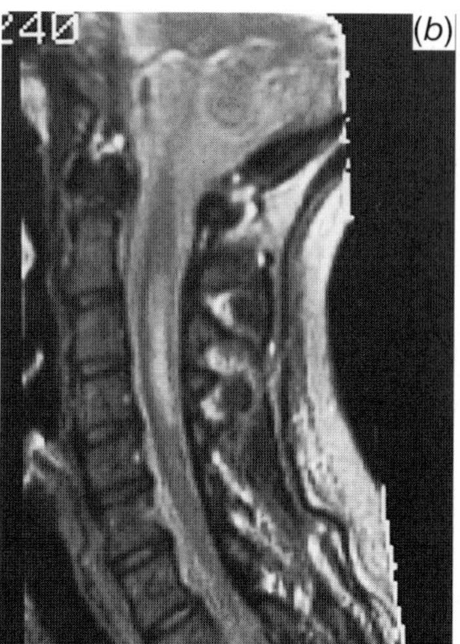

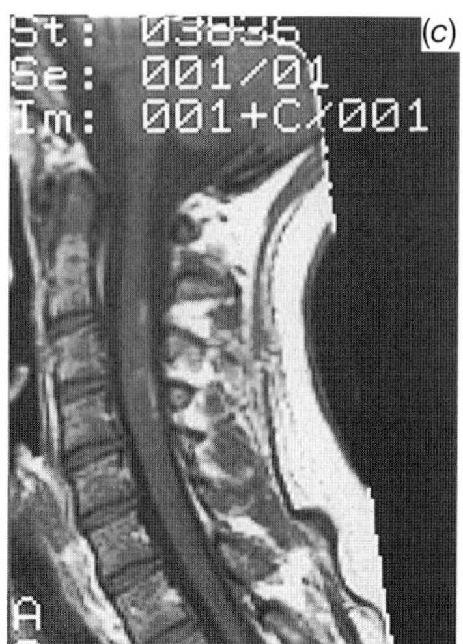

Figure 3.13 *Relapsing-remitting multiple sclerosis in a 27-year-old female: T2-weighted sagittal spinal images (a) baseline and (b) follow-up one month later. There is a large new cervical cord lesion at follow-up, which displays enhancement on the gadolinium enhanced T1-weighted sequence (c). This lesion was associated with a clinical relapse with deafferentation of the left hand. (From Thorpe et al. 1996a.)*

patients with acute optic neuritis [Miller *et al.* 1988b; DH Lee *et al.* 1991] (Figure 3.14). With recent improvements in resolution using fat-suppressed FSE and multi-array receiver coils, nearly 100% of symptomatic optic neuritis lesions are detectable [Gass *et al.* 1995] (Figure 3.15); thus the sensitivity of MRI now equals that of visual evoked potentials.

Lesions most often involve the intraorbital portion of the nerve; the intracanalicular portion of the nerve is involved with moderate frequency, while lesions of the intracranial portion of the nerve and chiasm are seen less often. As elsewhere in the CNS, acute lesions consistently display gadolinium enhancement [Youl *et al.* 1991b; Miller *et al.* 1993a]. Occasionally, the nerve is swollen in the acute phase. We have seen striking swelling of the nerve and chiasm in an 11-year-old girl with acute optic neuritis (Figure 3.16); the swelling increased over several weeks, such that it was felt on radiological grounds that an optic nerve glioma was distinctly possible. However, the child's vision recovered to normal and the swelling resolved over several months.

Signal change within the nerve is apparent from the onset of symptoms in demyelinating optic neuritis – this can be useful in differentiating the condition from anterior ischaemic optic neuropathy. In the latter, the primary lesion is at the optic nerve head, and optic nerve MRI is initially normal; however, signal changes appear within the nerve after several months, probably because of secondary Wallerian degeneration [Gass *et al.* 1995] (Figure 3.17).

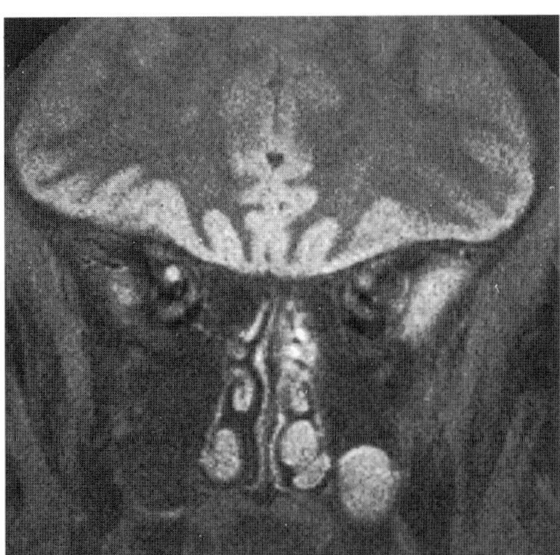

Figure 3.14 *Right optic neuritis: a coronal STIR image through the orbits reveals high signal in the right optic nerve. Note that the resolution of this sequence is not sufficient to distinguish the nerve from its surrounding sheath. (From Miller et al. 1988b.)*

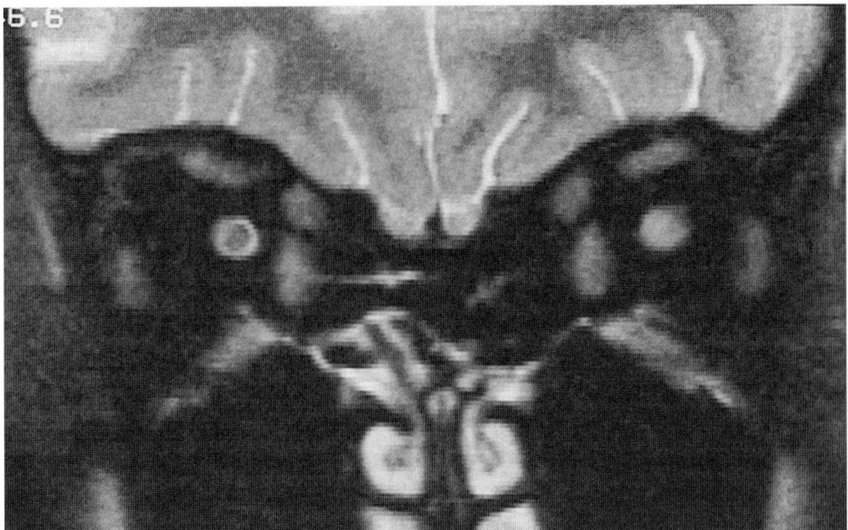

Figure 3.15 *Left optic neuritis: fat-suppressed fast spin echo image reveals swelling and high signal in the left optic nerve. Note the distinction between nerve and sheath on the normal side.*

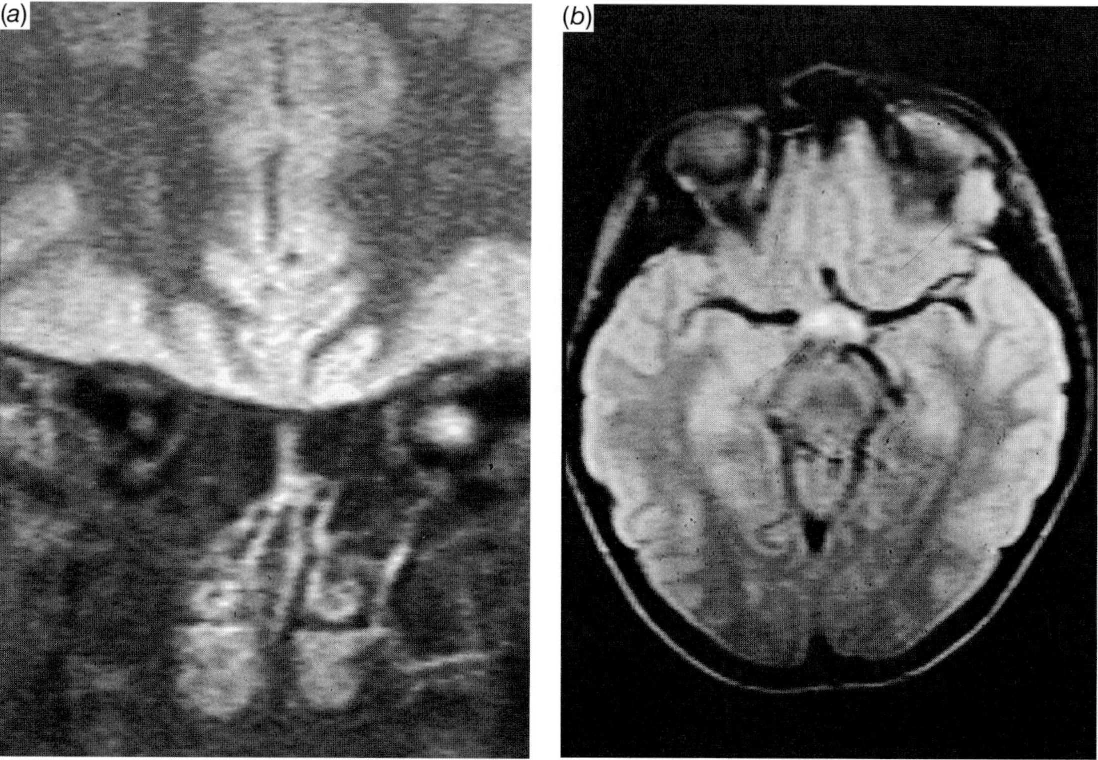

Figure 3.16 *Left optic neuritis in an 11-year-old female: (a) Coronal STIR image during the acute phase of visual loss reveals marked swelling of the intraorbital portion of the left optic nerve. (b) T2-weighted axial MRI one month later reveals high signal in the optic chiasm. By this time intraorbital swelling was less and vision was improving.*

3.6   Special clinical settings

3.6.1   Cognitive dysfunction

Although a frank dementing illness is uncommon, at least in the early stages of the disease, detailed neuropsychological examinations reveal abnormalities in about 50% of multiple sclerosis population cohorts [Ron & Feinstein 1992]. The most common impairments are with attention, memory and speed of thought processes. Many groups have reported a consistent though moderate correlation between the presence of cognitive abnormalities and the global load of brain lesions measured from T2-weighted images [Huber *et al.* 1987; Franklin *et al.* 1988; Rao *et al.* 1989; Anzola *et al.* 1990; Ron *et al.* 1991]. Even the presence of a few white matter lesions at first presentation with optic neuritis is associated with subtle deficits of auditory attention [Callanan *et al.* 1989]. At the

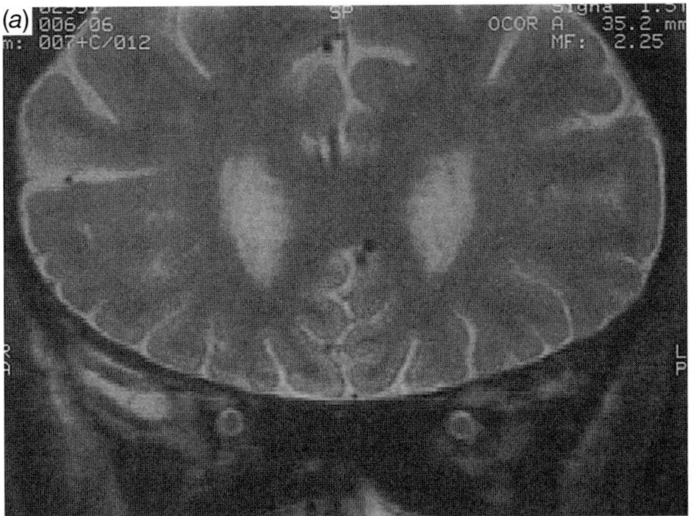

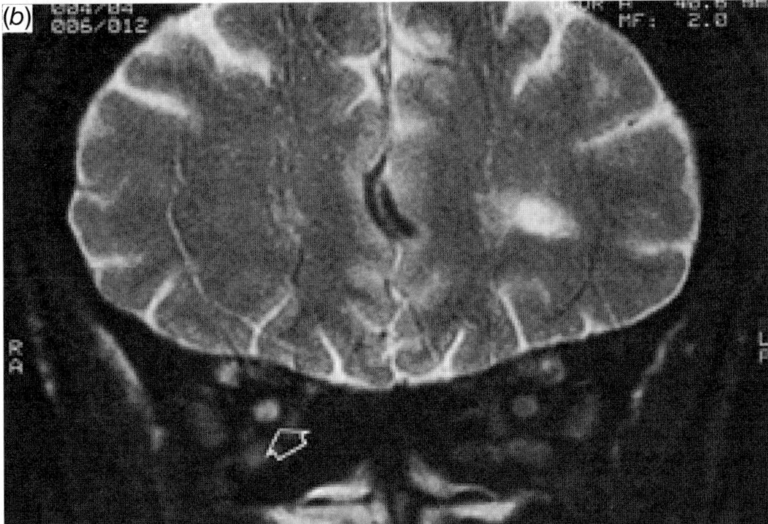

Figure 3.17 *Right anterior ischaemic optic neuropathy: coronal fat-suppressed T2-weighted fast spin echo image shows the right optic nerve appearing normal during the acute phase (a), but a follow-up scan six months later (b) reveals high signal (arrowed). (From Gass et al. 1995.)*

other extreme, patients who have developed a frank dementia generally have MRI or post-mortem evidence of extensive cerebral white matter disease [Bergin 1957], and in addition generalised cerebral atrophy.

Less work has been undertaken to correlate regional imaging abnormalities with specific neuropsychological deficits thought to reflect pathology within a particular brain region. This partly reflects the greater technical difficulties in quantitating regional abnormalities on MRI. Nevertheless, Arnett [1994] has reported that multiple sclerosis patients with frontal lesions demonstrated significantly more abnormalities on a standard conceptual reasoning task which is thought sensitive to frontal lobe function (the Wisconsin Card Sorting Test) when compared to patients without frontal lesions but matched for total brain lesion load. The authors infer that the pattern of cognitive decline in multiple sclerosis is a function of the location of lesions within the cerebrum.

The present data when taken together indicate that while the cerebral hemisphere lesions of multiple sclerosis rarely produce physical symptoms, they have an important functional impact in causing cognitive deficits. In future, higher resolution imaging with thin slices (3 mm or even 1 mm), the use of fast FLAIR (which detects more cortical lesions than conventional PD/T2-weighted SE), and more accurate and reproducible methods for quantifying lesions, should allow a clearer understanding of the relationship between cerebral lesions and cognitive impairments in multiple sclerosis.

3.6.2   Psychiatric illness

Compared to the general (non-multiple sclerosis) population, the incidence of psychiatric morbidity is not increased when patients first present with a clinically isolated syndrome suggestive of multiple sclerosis (e.g. isolated optic neuritis) [Logsdail *et al.* 1988], but it is higher in patients with clinically definite disease [Ron & Logsdail 1989; Feinstein *et al.* 1992a]. The most common psychiatric diagnoses are anxiety and depression, less often hypomania, euphoria or psychotic states. Anxiety and depression do not correlate with either the extent of cerebral abnormalities seen on MRI or with defects of cognitive function [Ron & Logsdail 1989]; rather they relate to social or economic stresses which not infrequently result from the illness.

Two psychiatric manifestations which have been correlated with MRI findings are euphoria and psychosis. Euphoria or elation occurs in about 10% of patients, and these individuals have a higher total brain lesion load and greater cognitive impairment than non-euphoric patients [Ron & Logsdail 1989]. Elation is also more likely to occur during acute relapses [Ron & Logsdail 1989]. It thus seems likely that in multiple sclerosis euphoria is often a manifestation of organic brain disease.

In one study, the presence of a number of psychotic features (thought disorder, flat affect and delusions) were associated with higher temporal lesion loads [Ron & Logsdail 1989]. In a more detailed study of psychosis in multiple sclerosis, Feinstein *et al.* [1992b] demonstrated an excess of temporal horn and trigone lesions in ten patients who had developed a schizophreniform (five) or affective (five) psychosis when compared with ten age and disability matched but non-psychotic multiple sclerosis patients. The authors hypothesised that the location and extent of brain lesions, while not of itself sufficient to cause psychosis, influences the likelihood of a psychosis manifesting in a susceptible individual.

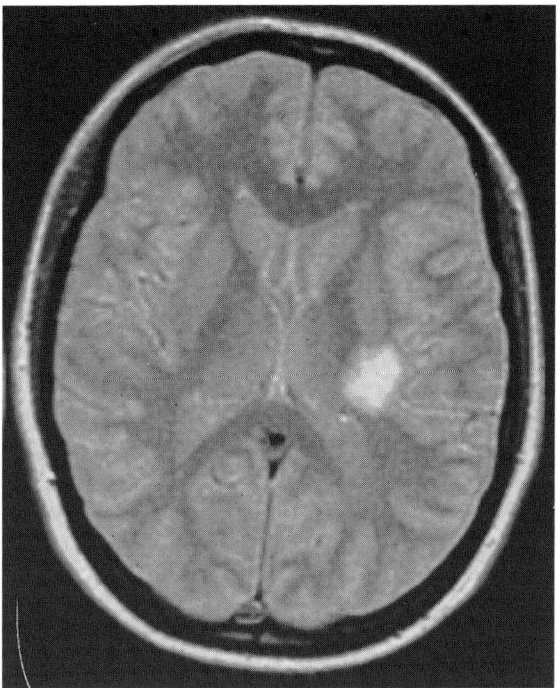

Figure 3.18 *PD-weighted brain MRI in a 31-year-old female presenting with ataxic hemiparesis and hemisensory loss affecting the right side. There is a large lesion involving the posterior limb of the left internal capsule. MRI also revealed other white matter lesions, the CSF contained oligoclonal bands, and clinical recovery occurred over several months, all of which suggested that this was a demyelinating lesion.*

3.6.3   Epilepsy

Seizures occur in about 3% of patients with multiple sclerosis [Matthews 1991]. Not surprisingly, they are often associated with either cortical or subcortical lesions [Thompson *et al.* 1993a; Truyen *et al.* 1994], which may be small or large. Large lesions producing mass effect and involving the cortex are occasionally seen in the context of an acute presentation with a space-occupying lesion and seizures [Youl *et al.* 1991a].

3.6.4   Hemiparesis

Hemiparesis is not unusual in MS, and when MRI is performed at the time of clinical deficit, a lesion appropriately placed in the contralateral internal capsule or cerebral peduncle can usually be demonstrated [Cowan *et al.* 1990] (Figure 3.18 – in addition to

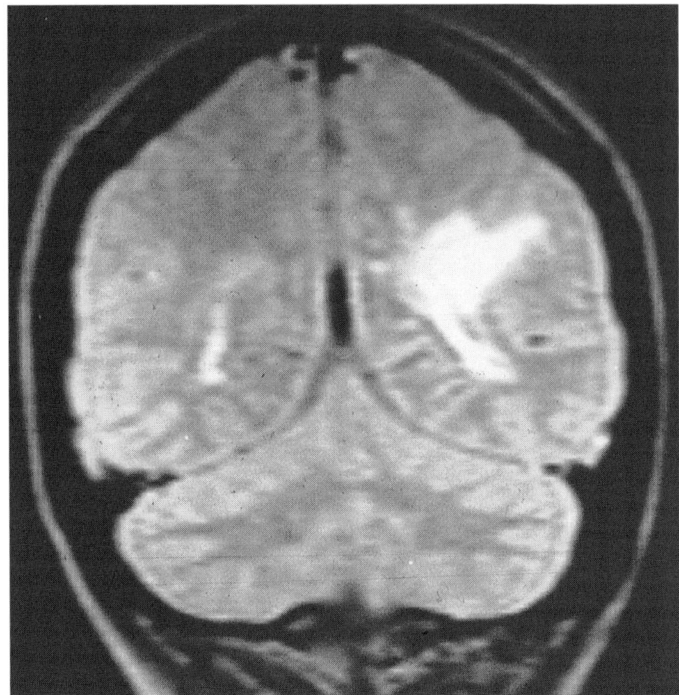

Figure 3.19 *A 33-year-old female with multiple sclerosis and right homonymous hemianopia. Coronal PD-weighted MRI reveals a large lesion involving the left optic radiation. (From Kesselring et al. 1989a.)*

hemiparesis, this patient had hemisensory loss and ataxia in the contralateral limbs). In one patient with hemiparesis sparing the face, MRI revealed a lesion in the anterolateral cord at C1, ipsilateral to the hemiparesis [Miller *et al.* 1987].

3.6.5   Hemianopia

Despite the frequent involvement of the posterior visual pathways by plaques [Ormerod *et al.* 1987], even at first presentation with clinically isolated optic neuritis [Hornabrook *et al.* 1992], symptomatic hemianopias in multiple sclerosis are rare. When they do occur there is invariably a *large* lesion on MRI or CT which involves either the optic radiations or optic tract [Plant *et al.* 1992] (Figure 3.19). These observations suggest that a large proportion of fibres in the posterior visual pathway need to be involved in order to produce a symptomatic field defect.

3.6.6   Involuntary movements

Movement disorders in multiple sclerosis are uncommon. One patient with multiple sclerosis who developed spasmodic torticollis was shown to have a prominent midbrain lesion [Plant *et al.* 1989]; given its location, the authors felt that this lesion may have caused the torticollis. We have seen two patients with both multiple sclerosis and a Parkinsonian syndrome. The MRI appearances were typical of multiple sclerosis; in particular there was no evidence for an abnormal extent of involvement of the basal ganglia. It remains possible that these cases represent the fortuitous association of two relatively common diseases: multiple sclerosis and idiopathic Parkinson's disease.

3.6.7   Paroxysmal symptoms

There are surprisingly few published reports of MRI findings in patients with paroxysmal symptoms in multiple sclerosis, many of which are thought to have a brain stem origin. One patient with tonic spasms was described in whom there was an appropriately placed lesion in the contralateral cerebral peduncle [Rose *et al.* 1993] (Figure 3.20). We have examined several MS patients with trigeminal neuralgia, and have usually found pontine lesions in a location likely to implicate central trigeminal pathways (Figure 3.21).

3.6.8   Spinal cord syndromes

Particularly with the recent improvements in the quality of spinal MRI (multi-array coils, flow compensated SE or FSE) symptomatic cord lesions are readily visualised in a location appropriate to their symptoms and signs. In an early report of a large series with spinal cord syndromes thought to be due to demyelination, Miller [1987a] examined the cord using conventional surface coils and spin echo sequences. Even though image quality was not as good as is now possible, an appropriate correspondence between clinical and MRI findings was apparent, at least in the cervical cord. The findings in three specific clinical syndromes were as follows:

(1) Brown-Sequard syndrome: four young adults presented with an acute, partial, remitting Brown-Sequard syndrome, with a hemiparesis (sparing the face) and contralateral impairment of pain and temperature sensation with a cervical sensory level. In each case, a lesion was visible on the appropriate side in the upper cervical cord (Figure 3.22): there was associated cord swelling in three patients.

(2) 'Useless hand of Oppenheim': five patients presented with a marked proprioceptive deficit in one hand, and all showed lesions in the posterior cervical cord between the cervicomedullary junction and C5 (Figure 3.23). The lesion was ipsilateral to the affected hand in all cases.

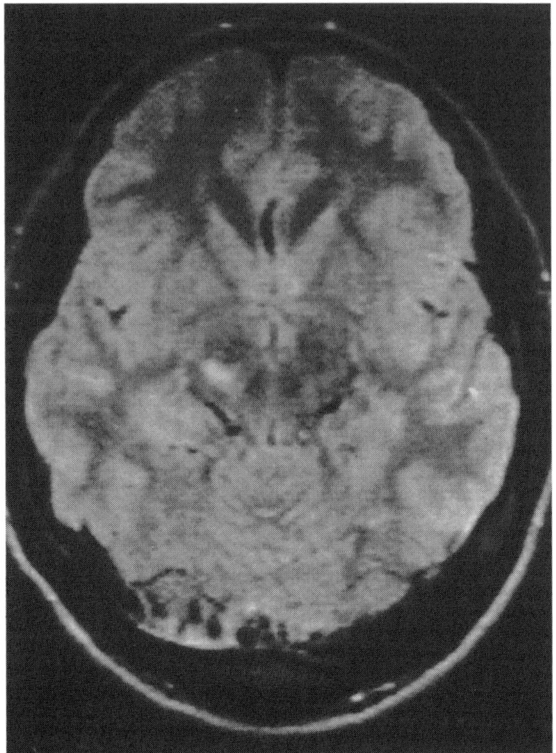

Figure 3.20 *A 27-year-old male with multiple sclerosis and left-sided tonic spasms. PD-weighted scan shows a lesion in the right cerebral peduncle. (From Rose et al. 1993.)*

(3) Lhermitte's sign: 13 patients gave a history of this sign – in 12 there was a lesion visible in the cervical cord, which in 11 cases involved the posterior part of the cord.

3.6.9   Childhood multiple sclerosis

Multiple sclerosis develops with a much lower frequency in children than in adults: only three out of 1000 MS patients have their first symptoms before the age of ten years [Bauer & Hanefeld 1993]. In contrast, the usually monophasic disorder acute disseminated encephalomyelitis (ADEM) is relatively more common in childhood. As both MS and ADEM can produce similar MRI appearances, follow-up is particularly important to enable a clear distinction of the two. Since occasional cases of ADEM can have an early relapse [Miller & Evans 1953; Alcock & Hoffman 1962], we recommend that an interval of at least three to six months elapses before new activity, either clinically or on repeat MRI, is considered likely to indicate multiple sclerosis.

In general, children with multiple sclerosis show the same pattern of MRI abnormal-

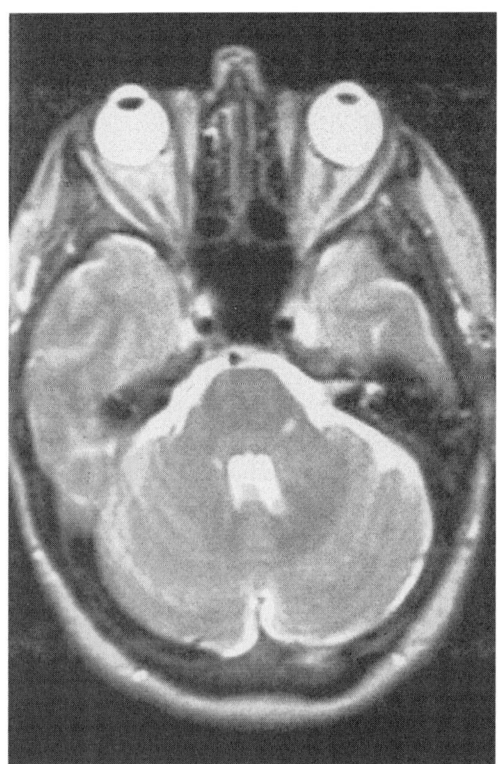

Figure 3.21 *A 48-year-old female with multiple sclerosis and left trigeminal neuralgia. T2-weighted image reveals a left pontine lesion which is in an area likely to implicate left trigeminal sensory fibres.*

ities as occurs in adults. Features which may be more common in children are large, confluent, cerebral white matter lesions, cortical lesions and cerebral atrophy. These findings are concordant with the higher incidence of dementia and seizures reported in some series of childhood multiple sclerosis [Bye *et al.* 1985; Miller *et al.* 1990].

3.6.10 Central and peripheral demyelination

There are rare but well recognised cases in whom both a chronic inflammatory demyelinating peripheral neuropathy and multiple sclerosis co-exist [Thomas *et al.* 1987]. Brain MRI in such patients reveals abnormalities typical of multiple sclerosis. Asymptomatic cerebral white matter abnormalities are also found in about one-third with chronic inflammatory demyelinating polyneuropathy alone [Hawke *et al.* 1990; Ormerod *et al.* 1990]. In some patients with a chronic demyelinating neuropathy, gadolinium enhanced MRI has revealed an enhancing mass in the cauda equina attributable to hypertrophied nerve roots.

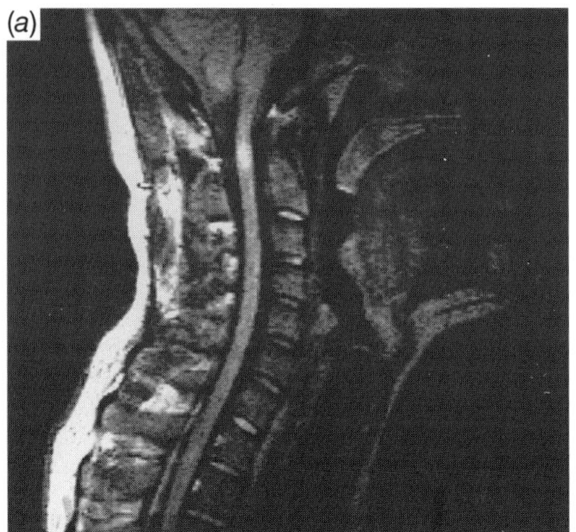

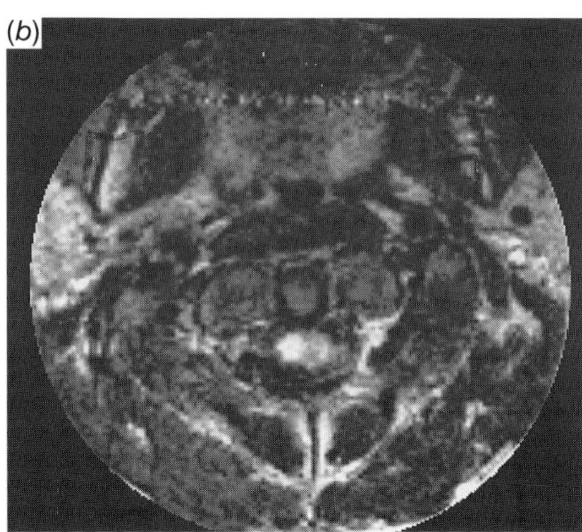

Figure 3.22 *A 25-year-old male with multiple sclerosis and right partial Brown-Sequard syndrome. (a) Sagittal and (b) axial T2-weighted cervical cord images reveal a lesion in the right side of the cord at C2. (From Miller* et al. *1987a, reprinted from* Annals of Neurology *V22, pp. 714–23, by permission of Little, Brown & Co. Inc.)*

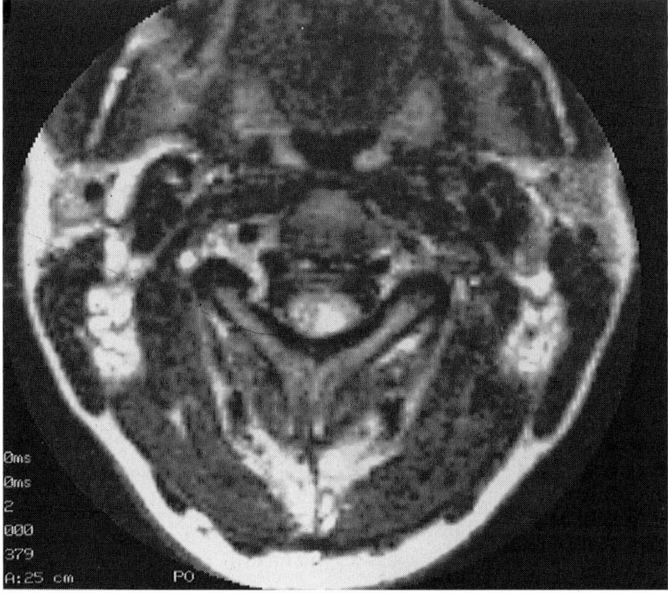

Figure 3.23 *A 36-year-old female with multiple sclerosis and the 'useless hand of Oppenheim'. The patient had deafferentation of the left hand. Axial T2-weighted cervical cord image shows a lesion involving the left posterior quadrant of the cord at C5.*

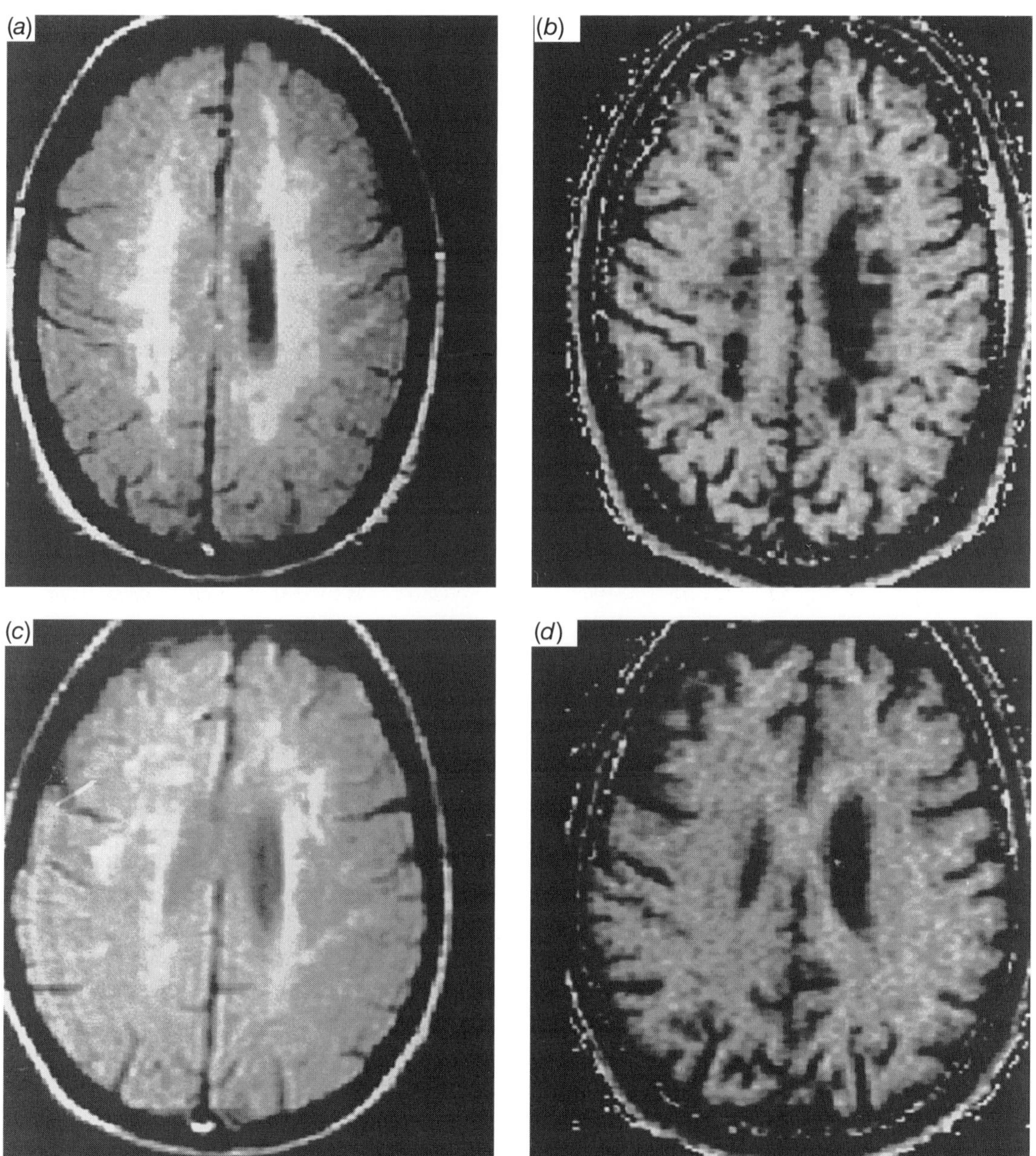

Figure 3.24 *PD-weighted and magnetisation transfer images of white matter lesions in a 31-year-old female with relapsing-remitting multiple sclerosis and marked disability (EDSS=6.5) ((a) and (b) respectively), and an asymptomatic 67-year-old volunteer with presumed small vessel disease ((c) and (d) respectively). Note that while there is extensive white matter abnormality in both cases, MT images show that much of the MS pathology is of lower signal than that seen in small vessel disease, indicating a low MT ratio and greater tissue loss. (From Gass et al. 1994, reprinted from* Annnals of Neurology V36, *pp. 62–7, by permission of Little, Brown & Co. Inc.)*

3.7   New MR techniques to assist diagnosis

Particular emphasis should be placed on developing techniques which are more specific for tissue pathology, for example to distinguish between a plaque, an infarct and a granuloma. Routine PD/T2-weighted and gadolinium enhanced images are relatively non-specific, although the duration of enhancement has some value (see Chapter 4). On unenhanced T1-weighted SE sequences, the cerebral white matter lesions in multiple sclerosis are more often hypointense than those seen in vascular disease [Uhlenbrock & Sehlen 1989]. Greater pathological specificity may be achieved using magnetisation transfer imaging [Dousset *et al.* 1992; Gass *et al.* 1994], and proton magnetic resonance spectroscopy [Arnold *et al.* 1990; Davie *et al.* 1994a], but these techniques are not widely used in diagnostic studies because of the extra time and technical difficulty in acquiring

Table 3.4 *Proton MR spectroscopy abnormalities in different pathologies*

	NAA	Cho	Cr	Lac	Lip	Myo
Acute MS plaques	D	I	N	I	I	I
Chronic MS plaques	D	N	N	N	N	I
Systemic lupus erythematosus	D	N	N	N	N	N
Metachromatic leucodystrophy	D	N	N	I	N	I
Adreno-leucodystrophy-	D	I	N	I	I	N
Canavan's disease	I	D	N	N	N	N
Phenylketonuria	N	N	D	N	N	N
Spinocerebellar degeneration	D	D	N	N	N	N

Note:

NAA = *N*-acetyl aspartate   I = increased
Cho = Choline-containing compounds   D = decreased
Cr = creatine/phosphocreatine   N = normal
Lac = lactate
Lip = lipid
Myo = myoinositol
MS = multiple sclerosis

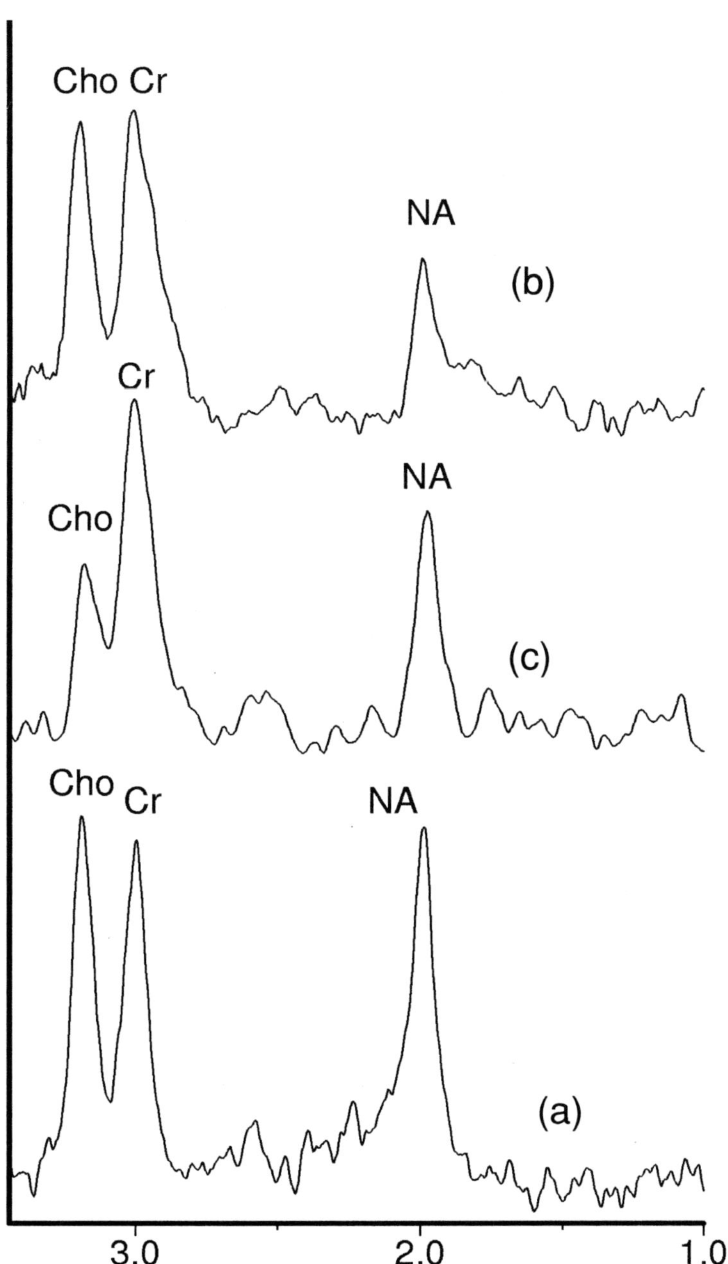

Figure 3.25 *Long echo time (TE 135 ms) proton MR spectroscopy of the cerebellum in (a) a healthy control, (b) an ataxic multiple sclerosis patient and (c) a patient with hereditary spinocerebellar degeneration. The ataxic multiple sclerosis patient has a reduction in N-acetyl aspartate (NA), while the patient with hereditary spinocerebellar degeneration has a reduction in both N-acetyl aspartate and choline-containing compounds (Cho).*

Table 3.5 *MRI and MR spectroscopy findings in multiple sclerosis (MS) and hereditary spinocerebellar degeneration (SCD)*

	MS	SCD
Cerebral white matter lesions	many	few
Cerebellar white matter lesions	frequent	absent
Cerebellar atrophy	mild/none	marked
Cerebellar [NAA]	reduced or normal	reduced
Cerebellar [Cho]	normal	reduced

Note:

NAA = *N*-acetyl aspartate

Cho = Choline-containing compounds

them. In general, multiple sclerosis lesions have a significantly greater reduction in magnetisation transfer ratio when compared with lesions thought likely to be due to small vessel disease [Gass *et al.* 1994; Wong *et al.* 1995] (Figure 3.24). In acute, enhancing multiple sclerosis lesions, proton MR spectroscopy is able to detect abnormal peaks due to mobile lipid protons, which are likely to represent the products of active demyelination [Wolinsky *et al.* 1990; Davie *et al.* 1994a], and a variety of other metabolite abnormalities are seen in different white matter disorders (Table 3.4, Figure 3.25). A consideration of both MRI and spectroscopy findings may help to characterise different disorders (Table 3.5).

3.8 Conclusion

Conventional PD/T2-weighted brain MRI is a very sensitive and useful method for confirming a clinical diagnosis of multiple sclerosis, and sometimes gadolinium enhancement is also valuable. However, low specificity remains a problem with either approach. High resolution spinal MRI can be a very useful adjunct in selected situations, and should always be obtained if the clinical syndrome is confined to the spinal cord, in order not to overlook a compressive lesion. Other MR techniques may improve specificity but their role in routine diagnostic imaging is not yet defined.

4   Differential diagnosis

Jürg Kesselring, David H Miller

4.1   Introduction

While brain MRI is very sensitive in detecting multiple sclerosis lesions, the abnormalities have a low specificity. The causes of white matter lesions are protean (see Table 4.1). While a judicious consideration of the clinical context and the pattern of MRI abnormalities often clarifies the diagnosis, the problem of specificity on conventional PD/T2-weighted images remains a major one. This chapter first discusses the MRI white matter hyperintensities which appear ubiquitously in healthy individuals with aging, and secondly reviews a range of disorders which may be confused clinically or on imaging with multiple sclerosis.

4.2   MRI in healthy persons in various age groups

Multifocal areas of high signal intensity within the cerebral white matter with or without altered signal in the immediate periventricular region may be seen on T2-weighted MRI in neurologically normal subjects [Kesselring *et al.* 1989a]. The incidence of such abnormalities increases with age, and in early studies was reported in more than 30% over the age of 60 years [Brant-Zawadski *et al.* 1985; Zimmerman *et al.* 1986; Drayer 1988]. The white matter abnormalities are more common if there are risk factors for cerebrovascular disease such as hypertension or diabetes [Gerard & Weisberg 1986], and may also be more common in subjects with a history of migraine [Ferbert *et al.* 1991].

High signal intensity around the pole of the frontal horns (caps) is particularly common and is due to an age-related focal loss of ependyma with subependymal gliosis, leading to an increased water content [Sze *et al.* 1986]. Such MRI and histological findings can be considered a normal finding at the frontal poles [Leifer *et al.* 1990], and are sometimes also seen at the occipital poles. More widespread white matter abnormalities on MRI have been correlated histologically to small vessel lipohyalinosis, vascular ectasia and dilated perivascular spaces [Awad *et al.* 1986; Kirkpatrick and Hayman 1987] and, less often, multiple lacunar infarcts compatible with subcortical arteriosclerotic encephalopathy (Binswanger's disease) (cf. Section 4.3).

In order to determine the frequency and extent of asymptomatic MRI abnormalities, we have examined 131 apparently healthy control subjects (91 on a 0.5 T system and 40 at

Table 4.1 *MRI white matter abnormalities* (*From Miller DH & Donald WI*, Clinical Neuroscience, *2, 215–224, 1994. © Wiley-Liss Inc 1994.*)

Condition	MRI features
Multiple sclerosis	Multifocal, asymmetrical, periventricular lesions.
ADEM	Can be identical to MS. Symmetrical cerebral, basal ganglia or cerebellar lesions in some.
Aging	Usually less extensive than MS. Discrete lesions. Little posterior fossa involvement.
Behçets syndrome	Prominent brainstem involvement.
Cerebrovascular disease	Large lesions of arterial territories involving cortex as well as small lesions. Smooth periventricular lesions.
Decompression sickness	Focal subcortical lesions. ?Any difference from healthy controls.
Fat embolism	High signal lesions on T_2-weighted images, high or low signal on T_1-weighted.
HIV encephalitis	Patchy or punctate white matter lesions, commonly involving basal ganglia. Diffuse pattern in AIDS dementia complex.
HTLV1–associated myelopathy	Usually few supratentorial lesions only.
Hydrocephalus	Diffuse smooth periventricular high signal.
Irradiation	Diffuse periventricular and subcortical lesions.
Leucodystrophies	Various patterns of extensive symmetrical white matter abnormalities; atrophy.
Migraine	A few more discrete lesions than age matched controls.
Mitochondrial encephalopathy	Diffuse abnormalities as well as stroke-like lesions.
Motor neurone disease	Symmetrical high signal involving pyramidal tracts, especially internal capsules.
Neurosarcoidosis	Can be identical to MS but large parenchymal lesions, prominent basal involvement and diffuse meningeal enhancement.
Phenylketonuria	Periventricular and subcortical changes.
Progressive multifocal leucoencephalopathy	Large focal lesions.
Subacute sclerosing panencephalitis	Few scattered white matter lesions.
Systemic lupus erythematosus	Mainly subcortical lesions; lesions involving arterial territories.
Trauma	Variable.

Note:

Common causes are shown in bold

Table 4.2 *MRI in normal control subjects*

Age group (years)	Number of subjects		Number with multifocal white matter lesions	
	0.5T	1.5T	0.5T	1.5T
17–49	63	28	1	3
50–59	18	9	4	4
>60	10	3	6	1

Note:

T = tesla

1.5 T) aged 17 to 79 years (Table 4.2). One hundred and eleven of these were neurologically normal and 20 were control subjects with neurological symptoms which did not involve the brain (patients with peripheral neuropathies and cervical spondylosis). Subjects with a history of hypertension, cerebrovascular or cardiovascular disease, or diabetes were excluded.

At all ages, MRI abnormalities were more often seen at 1.5 T than 0.5 T, reflecting the improved resolution and signal-to-noise ratio of the higher field studies (slice thickness was 5 mm for all studies at 1.5 T, but was 10 mm for some of the earlier studies at 0.5 T). In the individuals under the age of 50, four (4.5%) had multifocal white matter abnormalities (2% at 0.5 T and 10% at 1.5 T) and in all these were minor (Figure 4.1).

Of the persons aged 50 to 59 years, eight (30%) had abnormal scans. Seven demonstrated minor abnormalities within the cerebral white matter. One subject, a 51-year-old female, demonstrated gross changes with multiple periventricular and discrete cerebral white matter lesions which were indistinguishable from those seen in patients with multiple sclerosis. The occasional finding of such extensive abnormalities in a normal individual is in keeping with the observation of 'unsuspected multiple sclerosis' at routine post-mortem examination; several large autopsy studies suggest that clinically silent disease occurs with about the same frequency that the disease manifests during life [Gilbert & Sadler 1983; Phadke & Best 1983].

In the 13 subjects aged 60 years or more, seven (54%) had abnormal MRI examinations: three demonstrated minor changes, whereas four showed more marked periventricular and discrete white matter lesions (Figure 4.2). The focal changes within the white matter were essentially indistinguishable from those seen in multiple sclerosis, although the periventricular abnormalities tended to be smooth in outline, in contrast to the characteristic 'lumpy-bumpy' appearance seen in multiple sclerosis. Nevertheless, in this age group, brain MRI is undoubtedly at its least specific. The need for caution arises particularly when multiple sclerosis is suspected but not clinically definite, since cerebral changes may be coincidental – in such circumstances additional support for the diagnosis should be sought by evoked potentials, CSF examination, and spinal MRI.

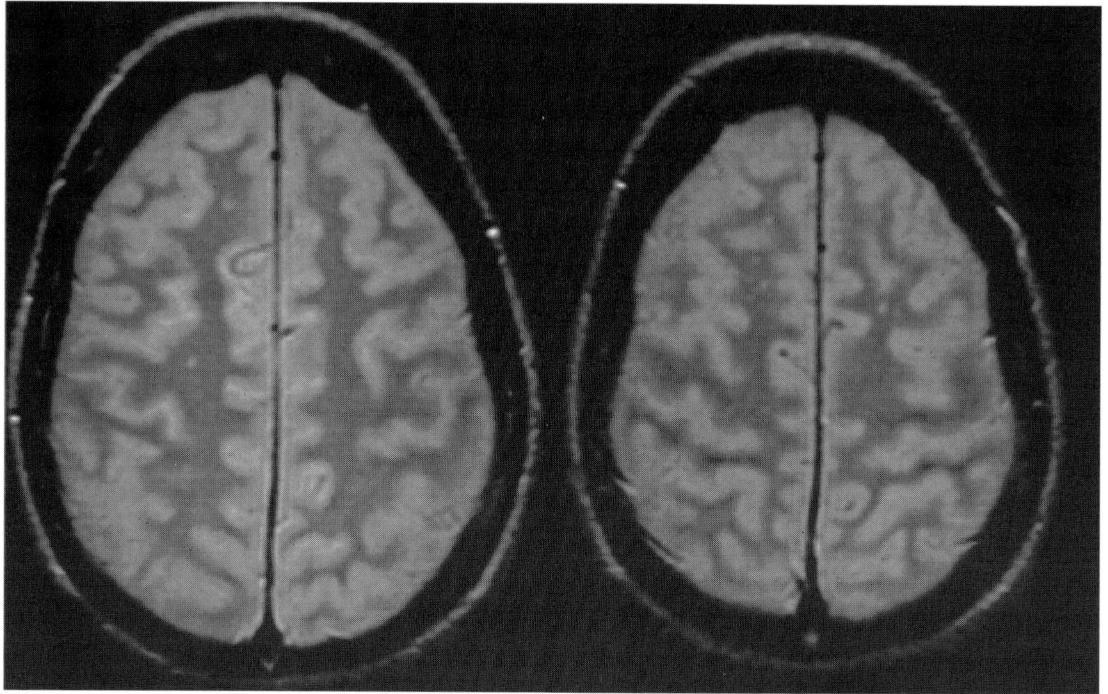

Figure 4.1 *PD-weighted MRI of a 30-year-old normal control, showing a few small subcortical white matter abnormalities.*

Non-specific age-related changes are not such a problem in differential diagnosis of the 90% of multiple sclerosis patients who present before the age of 50 years. In this age group, the incidence of abnormalities is lower (about 10–20% of subjects), and the lesions are usually small, few in number and predominantly subcortical [Fazekas 1989], unlike the predominantly periventricular pattern characteristic of multiple sclerosis.

A number of workers have developed criteria to improve the specificity of MRI patterns for multiple sclerosis [Paty *et al.* 1988; Fazekas *et al.* 1988]. The most extensively evaluated are those of Fazekas. These criteria require the presence of at least three lesions and at least two of the following: a lesion > 5 mm, a periventricular lesion, an infratentorial lesion. Applying these criteria to 1500 consecutive patients undergoing MRI (including 134 with a clinical diagnosis of multiple sclerosis), Offenbacher [1993] reported a specificity for multiple sclerosis of 96% with a sensitivity of 81%. Most false positives were in the over 60 age group.

Because brain MRI is least specific over the age of 50 years, even when the Fazekas criteria are used, spinal MRI is proving diagnostically useful in this age group. In an appropriate clinical context, the presence of intrinsic cord lesions is strong supportive evidence for multiple sclerosis, as such abnormalities do not appear with normal aging in the way that brain lesions do [Thorpe *et al.* 1993]. At all ages, combined spinal and

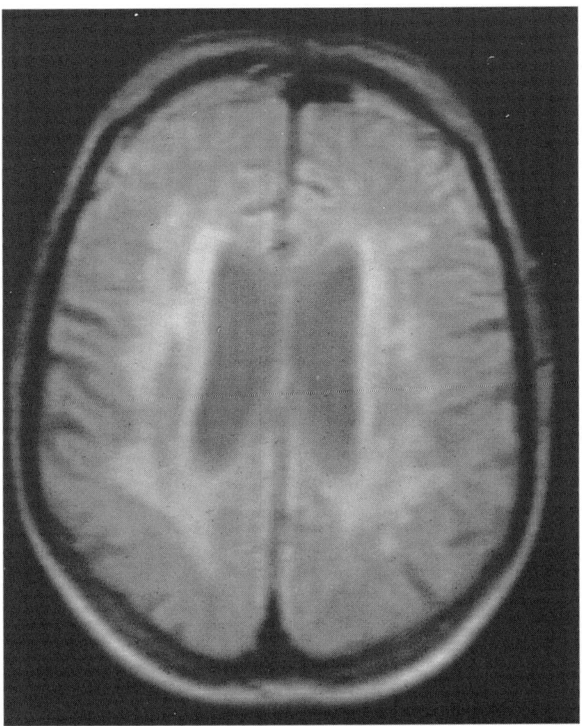

Figure 4.2
PD-weighted MRI of a 64-year-old normal control with extensive white matter abnormalities, most likely due to asymptomatic small vessel disease.

brain MRI is the most helpful paraclinical tool in the differential diagnosis of isolated spinal cord syndromes [Miller *et al.* 1987a].

4.3 Non-inflammatory vascular syndromes

Neither cerebral vascular disease with multiple infarcts nor subacute arteriosclerotic encephalopathy (Binswanger's disease or leucariosis) is frequently confused with multiple sclerosis clinically, in part because the clinical picture is quite different and in part because cerebral vascular disease is more frequent in the older age groups where multiple sclerosis presents uncommonly.

Diffuse periventricular changes and focal lesions are easily detected on MRI in more than half of the patients with clinical evidence of diffuse cerebral vascular disease of both kinds (Ormerod *et al.* 1984; Ormerod *et al.* 1987). It is not always possible to distinguish these changes from those of multiple sclerosis, although the high signal surrounding the ventricles tends to be smoother in the patients with cerebral vascular disease (as for age-

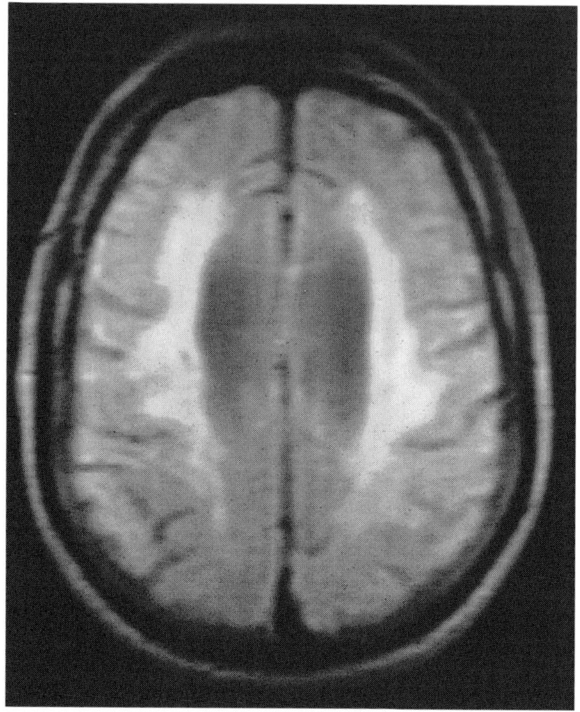

Figure 4.3 *Binswanger's subacute arteriosclerotic encephalopathy with extensive deep white matter abnormalities on PD-weighted MRI.*

related changes in healthy individuals) (Figure 4.2) and, except in subacute arteriosclerotic encephalopathy, the abnormalities are in general less extensive. Nevertheless, a confident distinction on MRI features alone is often not possible.

In subacute arteriosclerotic encephalopathy (Binswanger's disease), which is not a demyelinating disorder, the white matter changes seen on MRI may be as extensive as the ones seen in advanced multiple sclerosis but tend to be rather more marked posteriorly (Figure 4.3). In this condition the arcuate fibres are usually spared, both on MRI and at post-mortem (Révèsz *et al.* 1989). The blood supply to the subcortical U-fibres is from small branches of the cortical vascular tree which may remain intact when there is ischaemia of the deep central white matter, which is believed to be the basis of Binswanger's disease. The U-fibres are frequently involved in multiple sclerosis [Miller 1988].

4.4   Collagen vascular disorders

4.4.1   Systemic lupus erythematosus (SLE)

SLE is a systemic disease of unknown aetiology in which various tissues are damaged by autoantibodies and by the deposition of immune complexes. In approximately half of the patients the CNS is involved clinically. The neurological picture is mostly dominated by psychiatric disorders, organic mental disturbances and seizures, but relapsing-remitting features suggesting multifocal CNS involvement may occur and cause confusion with multiple sclerosis (Lim *et al.* 1988). Notably, optic neuropathy, subacute myelopathy and internuclear ophthalmoplegia may all occur in SLE, as can oligoclonal bands in the CSF [Winfield *et al.* 1983].

The diagnosis of SLE is based on clinical and laboratory criteria (Tan *et al.* 1982). The most common neuropathological finding in SLE is a vasculopathy with hyalinisation of vessel walls, endothelial proliferation and perivascular inflammation [Johnson & Richardson 1968; Ellis & Verity 1979]. A true vasculitis (inflammation of the vessel wall) is seen in only a minority of cases. Multiple microinfarcts are commonly found in the cortex, brain stem and basal ganglia.

On MRI, large cerebral infarcts and multifocal lesions in the cerebral white and grey matter are frequently found [Vermess *et al.* 1983; Aisen *et al.* 1985a; Miller *et al.* 1987b, 1992a] (Figures 4.4–4.6). They occur more often in the presence of manifest cerebral disease but may also be seen in patients without neurological symptoms or signs. The abnormalities are probably secondary to the vasculopathy already described. Multiple periventricular lesions on MRI may resemble those seen in clinically definite multiple sclerosis (cf. Chapter 3), although the lesions in SLE usually predominate in the subcortical white matter. Sometimes, neuropsychiatric syndromes are seen in the presence of normal imaging, suggesting that the vasculopathy is not the sole cause of clinical manifestations.

Gadolinium enhancement of white matter lesions is probably less common in SLE than in multiple sclerosis [Miller *et al.* 1992a]. Enhancement has been reported in a large cortical lesion, the location and shape of which was consistent with recent infarction (blood–brain barrier breakdown with gadolinium enhancement is a characteristic finding in recent infarcts) [Virapongse *et al.* 1986; Imakita *et al.* 1987].

We have seen two patients with lupus myelopathy who had strikingly similar spinal cord findings. In the acute phase, the cord was swollen and displayed abnormal signal over many segments, and gadolinium enhancement was present in the dorsal cord only (Figure 4.7). Swelling and enhancement both resolved within days in association with intensive immunosuppressive treatment. In multiple sclerosis it would be distinctly unusual to see such long cord lesions or such extensive swelling as was seen in these two cases.

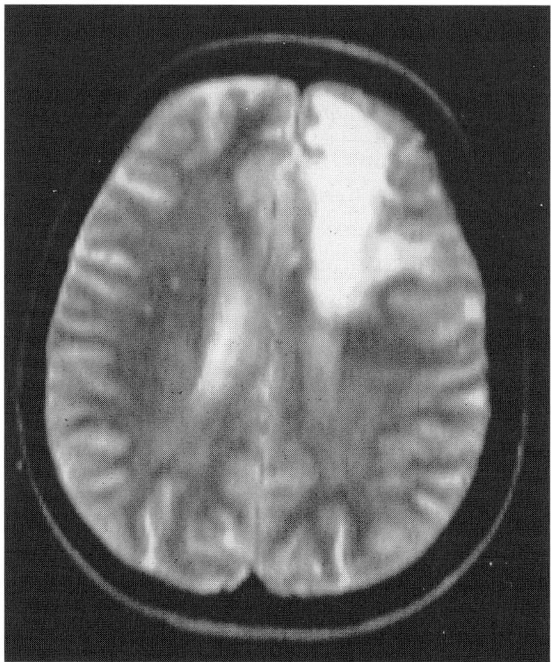

Figure 4.4 *A 25-year-old male with systemic lupus erythematosus. T2-weighted image shows a large area of infarction in the left anterior cerebral artery territory.*

4.4.2   Behçet's disease

Behçet's disease is another systemic vasculitic disorder of unknown cause in which an autoimmune pathogenesis is postulated. The diagnosis is made on clinical grounds. Major diagnostic criteria include recurrent oral and genital ulcers and intraocular inflammation. Minor criteria are erythema nodosum, arthritis and arthralgia, thrombophlebitis and neurological manifestations. Both major and minor criteria are required for a definite diagnosis. Clinical involvement of the nervous system is reported in 4–49% of the cases and most commonly consists of meningoencephalitis, acute or subacute brain stem syndromes or raised intracranial pressure due to cerebral venous thromboses. Neurological syndromes have a tendency to relapse and remit spontaneously and may therefore be confused with multiple sclerosis. Diagnostic confusion is particularly likely with brain stem or spinal cord involvement or with visual symptoms due to intraocular inflammation which may be confused with optic neuritis.

The most common MRI abnormalities seen in Behçet's disease are multifocal cerebral white matter lesions, but these are only few in number (Figure 4.8); extensive confluent periventricular changes were not seen in any of 25 cases of Behçet's syndrome, of whom 15 had clinical involvement of the CNS (Morrissey *et al.* 1993b).

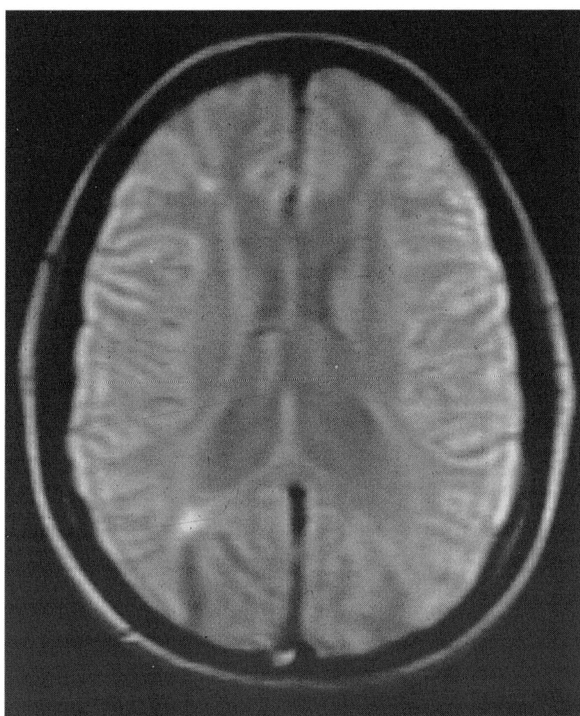

Figure 4.5 *A 41-year-old female with systemic lupus erythematosus and a history of vertebro-basilar transient ischaemic attacks and an optic neuropathy. PD-weighted scan reveals areas of focal occipital cortical atrophy and adjacent white matter signal change consistent with small infarcts. (From Kesselring et al. 1989a.)*

Brain stem lesions are not infrequently found and may be extensive, sometimes with extension into the thalamus and internal capsule [Banna & El-Ramahi 1991; Morrissey *et al.* 1993b] (Figure 4.9). Brain stem lesions without any cerebral white matter changes occur in Behçet's syndrome but would be most unusual in multiple sclerosis (Ormerod *et al.* 1987). Mass lesions in the brain-stem, resembling a brain-stem tumour, have also been reported and may display gadolinium enhancement [Erdem *et al.* 1993a]. They may resolve rapidly following steroid therapy, suggesting that oedema was responsible [Kermode *et al.* 1989a]. Striking atrophy of brain-stem (Figure 4.9) and cerebellum in the absence of cerebral atrophy can be seen in Behçet's syndrome, but again would be unusual in multiple sclerosis. Rarely, MRI abnormalities in the spinal cord and optic nerves have also been reported [Morrissey *et al.* 1993b].

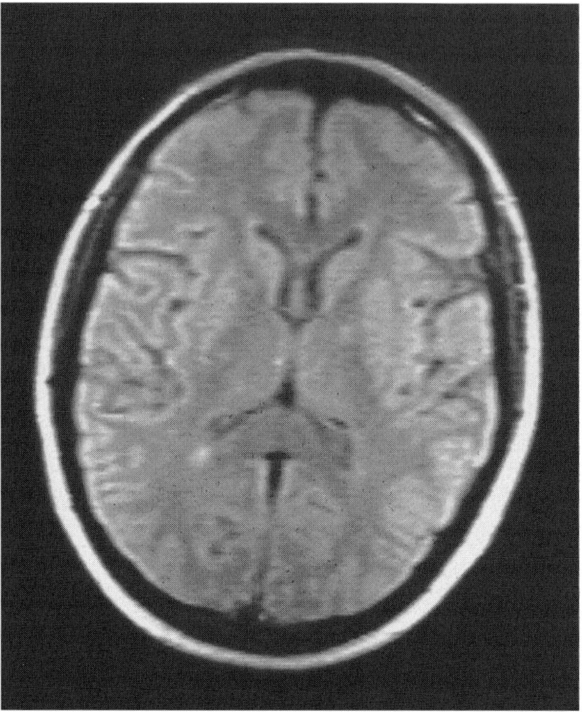

Figure 4.6 *A 33-year-old female with systemic lupus erythematosus and a history of psychosis. PD-weighted scan reveals multiple small white matter lesions.*

4.4.3   Polyarteritis nodosa

In polyarteritis nodosa, the peripheral nervous system is not infrequently involved, the most common clinical picture being a mononeuritis multiplex. Less often, there is central nervous system involvement, and arteritis of medium-sized cerebral arteries can result in ischaemic strokes. There are few reports of MRI findings in polyarteritis, but as might be expected, these have described multifocal lesions of varying size involving either grey or white matter. Such appearances are probably due in part to cerebral infarction consequent upon arteritis, and in part to the small vessel changes described with normal aging, especially if, as applies for many patients with polyarteritis, there is a history of hypertension. A preponderance of cortical lesions was striking in the case described by Miller [1987b] (Figure 4.10).

4.4.4   Isolated angiitis of the central nervous system

Isolated angiitis of the central nervous system is a rare disorder which is unlikely to be confused clinically with MS. The characteristic presentation is with headache and

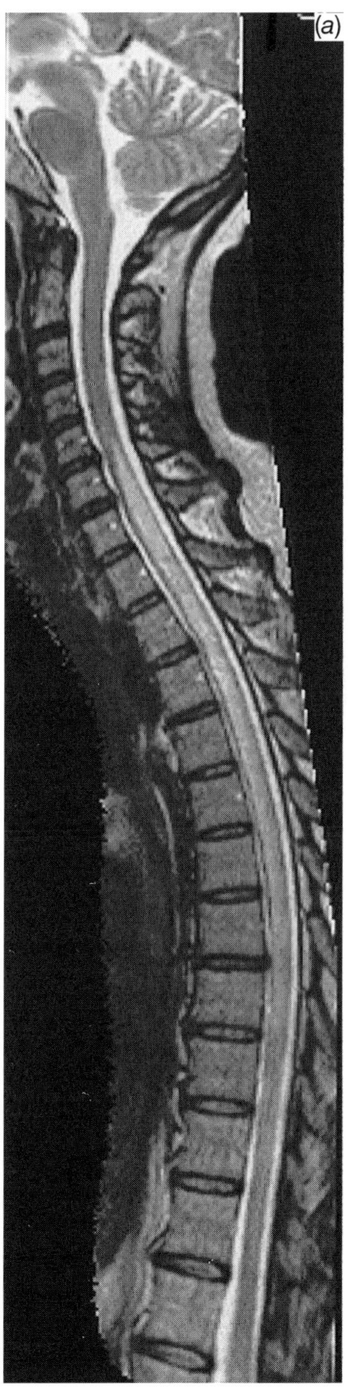

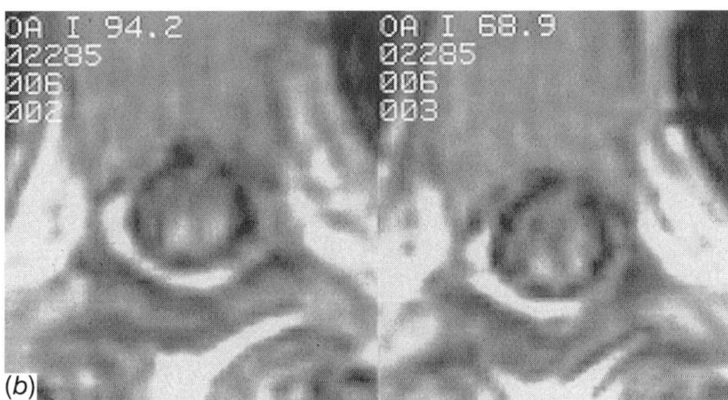

Figure 4.7 *A 44-year-old female with systemic lupus erythematosus. The patient had an acute transverse myelopathy. (a) T2-weighted scan reveals signal change and swelling extending over many segments of the cord; (b) gadolinium enhanced T1-weighted axial image reveals enhancement in the posterior cord.*

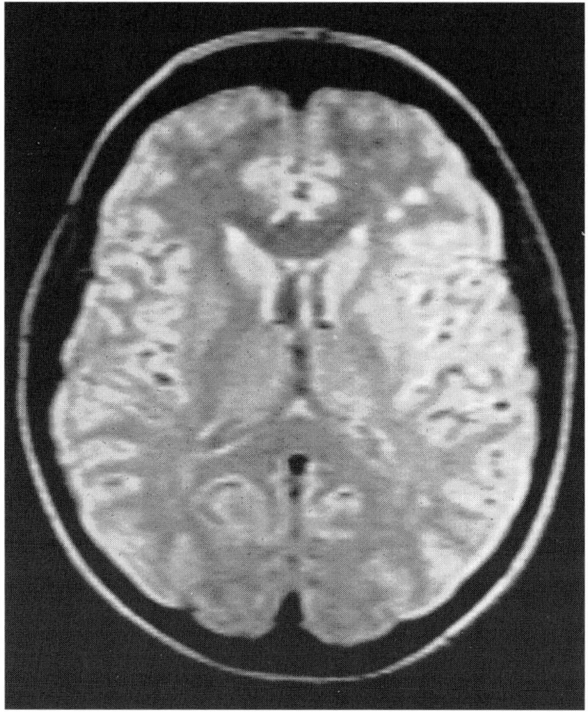

Figure 4.8 *Behçet's disease. PD-weighted brain MRI in a 48-year-old female. There are a few discrete cerebral white matter lesions.*

obtundation along with episodic focal neurological deficits. Diagnosis relies upon demonstration of arteritic involvement of small cerebral arteries, either by finding characteristic segmental narrowing on conventional angiography or by meningeal or brain biopsy. Diagnosis is important since therapy with cyclophosphamide is often effective. MRI abnormalities have included multifocal grey or white matter lesions of varying size, compatible with cerebral infarcts, sometimes with mass effect or gadolinium enhancement [Koo & Massey 1988; Greenan *et al.* 1992; Johnson *et al.* 1989]. One unusual case report described a pattern of multiple small gadolinium enhancing lesions in the brain stem, cerebellum and cerebral white matter, often without corresponding abnormalities on T2-weighted images, in a patient with biopsy proven angiitis [Shoemaker *et al.* 1994]. The appearances were thought to represent the inflammatory changes seen histologically in and around small vessels. We have seen another case of biopsy proven granulomatous angiitis who also had multiple, punctate, gadolinium enhancing lesions and, in addition, extensive T2-weighted white matter abnormalities (Figure 4.11).

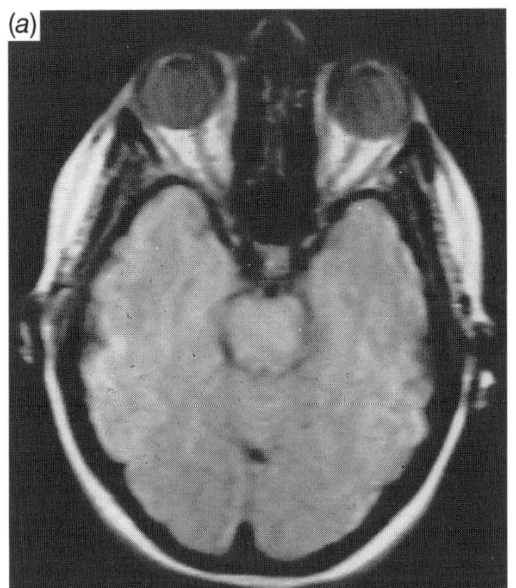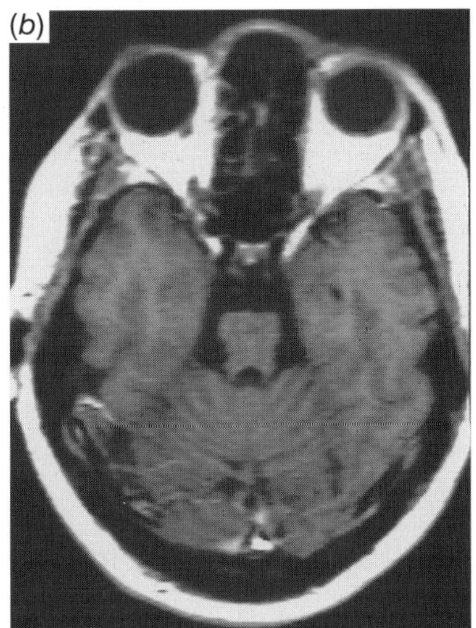

Figure 4.9 *Behçet's disease. Serial MRIs of a female with a brain stem syndrome: (a) during the acute phase (aged 38 years) PD-weighted imaging reveals swelling and high signal in the midbrain; (b) five years later, T1-weighted imaging shows marked midbrain atrophy. The patient had developed progressive neurological deficits in spite of intensive immunosuppressive therapy. (From Morrissey et al. 1993b, by permission of Karger, Basel.)*

4.4.5   Sjögren's syndrome

The most common neurological manifestations of Sjögren's syndrome are a generalised sensory neuropathy in which the primary pathology is probably at the dorsal root ganglion level [Griffin *et al.* 1990], or a trigeminal sensory neuropathy [Kaltreider & Talal 1969]. Central nervous system manifestations occur less often, but include strokes, transient ischaemic attacks, acute or chronic myelopathies, or, rarely, a multiple sclerosis-like picture with multifocal relapsing-remitting disease. The last has been particularly emphasised by one group of investigators [Alexander al 1988]. However, it has been the experience of other investigators who see large numbers of patients with multiple sclerosis that coexistent Sjögren's syndrome is very rare [Noseworthy *et al.* 1989; Miro *et al.* 1990]. That is also the experience of the authors.

There is relatively little information from autopsy material concerning the neuropathology of Sjögren's syndrome manifesting with CNS features. There are isolated reports of small vessel vasculopathy in the brain [Alexander *et al.* 1988] and small vessel vasculitis in the brain [Kaltreider & Talal 1969] or spinal cord [Alexander *et al.* 1982]. In patients with CNS symptoms suggesting either ischaemia or demyelination, Alexander [1988] has reported non-specific multifocal white matter abnormalities. More recently,

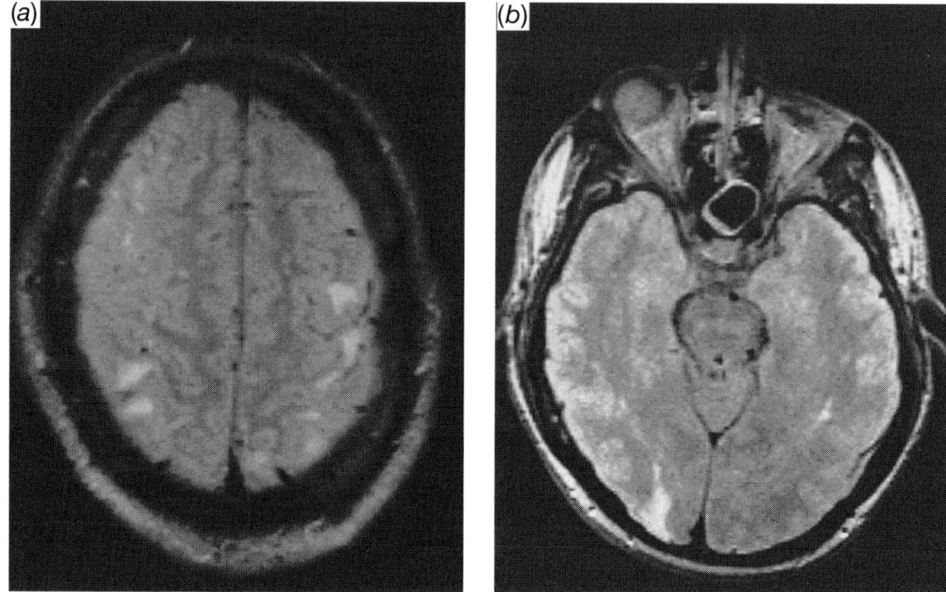

Figure 4.10 *Polyarteritis nodosa. The patient is a 44-year-old male with multi-system involvement including severe retinal vasculitis and an episode of right hemiparesis. PD-weighted scans reveal multiple, small, cortical and subcortical lesions. (From Miller et al. 1987b.)*

Pierot [1993] reported brain MRI findings in 15 patients with Sjögren's syndrome but without clinical CNS involvement. There were multifocal white matter abnormalities in nine and basal ganglia lesions in two; six showed some degree of cerebral atrophy. The white matter lesions were small and mainly subcortical. Some of these changes are likely to be the incidental consequence of normal aging (the patients' age range was from 42–81 years). Nevertheless, the authors felt that there were more abnormalities than could be accounted for by age alone. The general appearance and distribution of the lesions was more in keeping with small vessel disease rather than demyelination.

4.5 Sarcoidosis

The characteristic pathological changes in sarcoidosis consist of non-caseating granulomata. In this systemic disease the central nervous system is involved clinically in approximately 5% of cases. Central nervous system syndromes are either produced by sarcoid tissue present in the meninges or within the brain parenchyma, or by infarction sec-

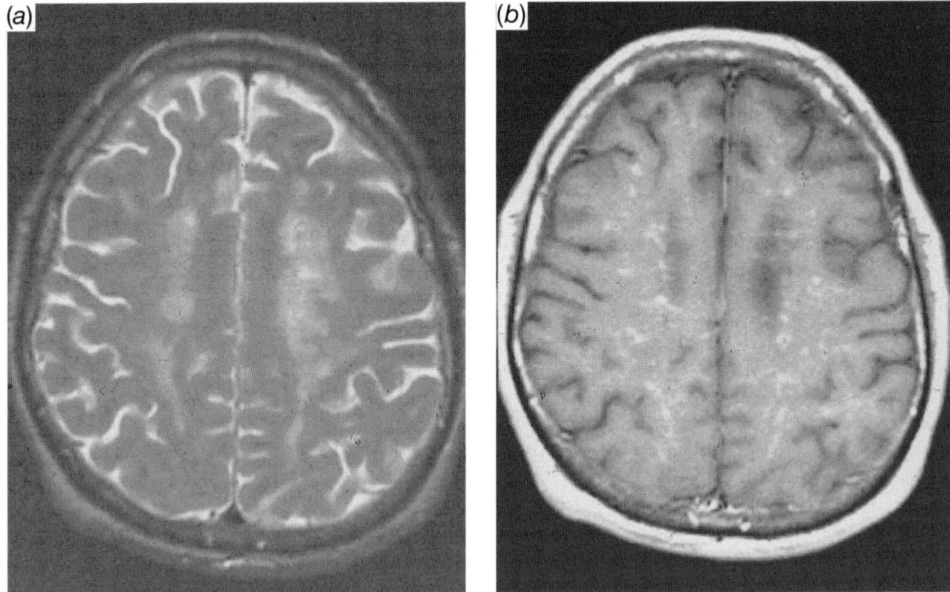

Figure 4.11 *Biopsy proven isolated angiitis of the central nervous system in a 45-year-old male. The patient had a multiphasic disorder with encephalopathy, optic neuropathy and a spastic paraparesis. (a) T2-weighted scan shows extensive periventricular white matter abnormalities. (b) Gadolinium enhanced T1-weighted image reveals multiple, tiny enhancing foci throughout the white matter.*

ondary to occlusion of small blood vessels by granulomata. The most common clinical syndrome is due to diffuse meningeal irritation with a predilection for the basal meninges, which leads to a cranial polyneuritis or hydrocephalus, a chiasmal syndrome, or hypothalamic disturbances, characteristically diabetes insipidus. In addition, spinal cord, optic nerve or brain stem syndromes may also be encountered, and a relapsing-remitting clinical picture similar to multiple sclerosis may be present.

MRI is a sensitive method for detecting lesions within the brain in patients with neurosarcoidosis. Periventricular abnormalities occur in one-third of patients [Miller *et al.* 1988c] (Figure 4.12). These may be due to: (i) subependymal granulomas; (ii) small areas of infarction secondary to granulomatous angiopathy; (iii) hydrocephalus, which characteristically produces a smooth rim of increased signal around the lateral ventricles on SE sequences; (iv) non-specific abnormalities related to aging (cf. Section 4.2); and (v) opportunistic infection, such as progressive multifocal leucoencephalopathy, a rare complication in sarcoidosis patients treated with corticosteroids or other immunosuppressants [Steiger *et al.* 1993]. As in MS, a mixture of enhancing and non-enhancing lesions has been described in sarcoidosis [Seltzer *et al.* 1991] (Figure 4.12). Furthermore, oligoclonal bands may be present in the CSF in both conditions [McLean

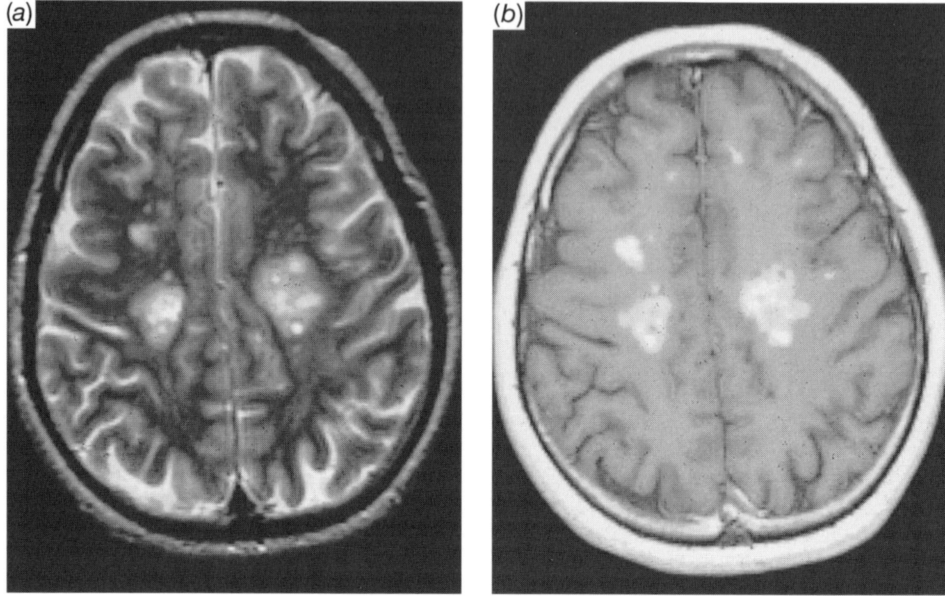

Figure 4.12 *Neurosarcoidosis in a 34-year-old male with spastic paraparesis. (a) T2-weighted and (b) gadolinium enhanced T1-weighted MRI display multifocal periventricular lesions, which display gadolinium enhancement.*

et al. 1995], and the MRI features may not allow a distinction to be made even when quantitative measurements of relaxation times are taken into account [Miller *et al.* 1989a]. Prolongation of relaxation times in normal appearing white matter outside of multiple sclerosis plaques appears to be a real finding and might be explained by an increased water content due to astrocytosis or small disturbances of the blood–brain barrier which are beyond the resolution of the MR system [Kesselring *et al.* 1989b]. However, the range of values within groups of patients with multiple sclerosis and neurosarcoidosis respectively is such that relaxation time measurements of the normal-appearing white matter can not be used to distinguish the two conditions [Miller *et al.* 1989a].

Meningeal involvement (which should not occur in multiple sclerosis) can be shown by gadolinium enhancement of the cranial and spinal meninges in neurosarcoidosis [Seltzer *et al.* 1991; Khaw *et al.* 1991] (Figure 4.13). Enhancement of parenchymal cortical or white matter granulomas also occurs (Figures 4.12 and 4.14), and there is one report of diffuse areas of linear enhancement in the cerebral white matter, the pattern suggesting perivascular involvement [Handler *et al.* 1993]. Persistent enhancement of parenchymal lesions over many months is consistent with granulomatous disease, but is distinctly unusual in multiple sclerosis.

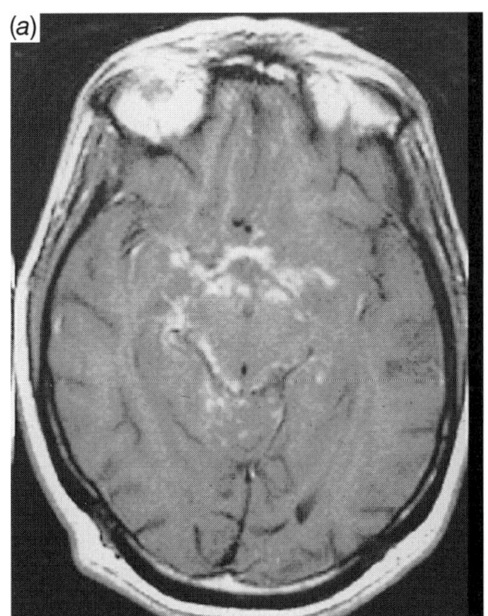
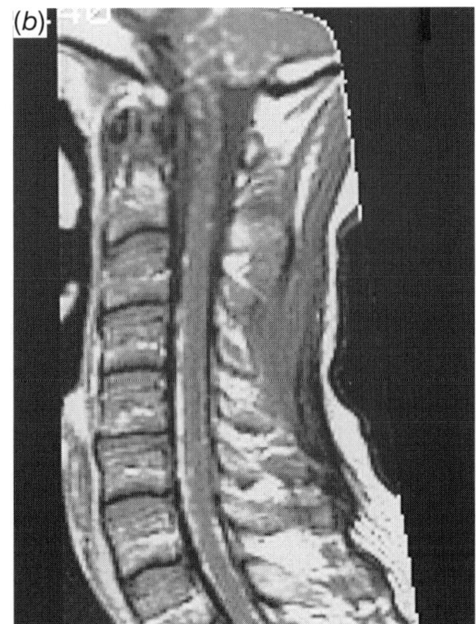

Figure 4.13 *A 33-year-old male with neurosarcoidosis manifesting as optic neuropathy, headache and lassitude. Gadolinium enhanced T1-weighted images (a) axial through the basal cisterns and (b) sagittal through the spinal cord. There is extensive meningeal enhancement in both regions. (From Miller DH & Donald WI* Clinical Neuroscience, 2, 215–224, 1994. © Wiley-Liss Inc 1994.)

4.6 Acute disseminated encephalomyelitis

Post-infectious or acute disseminated encephalomyelitis (ADEM) is an acute inflammatory and demyelinating disease of the central nervous system which develops as an autoimmune response after infections or vaccinations. Symptoms usually begin one to two weeks after the infection or vaccination. Any age group can be affected, but in contrast to multiple sclerosis, it is more common in childhood than in adults.

The main clinical features of ADEM are fever, coma or drowsiness, seizures and multifocal neurological signs. Pathologically there is widespread focal inflammation and demyelination in the central nervous system. Histologically the lesions cannot be differentiated from those in multiple sclerosis, but the clinical course differs in that ADEM is monophasic whereas multiple sclerosis is multiphasic. Problems of differential diagnosis may arise when there is a polysymptomatic presentation in the absence of a preceding infection, and in patients presenting an isolated clinical deficit of a kind seen in both diseases, such as optic neuritis, transverse myelitis or a brain stem syndrome[(Miller *et al.* 1993b]. Several clinical and laboratory differences exist between the two conditions [Kesselring *et al.* 1990]:

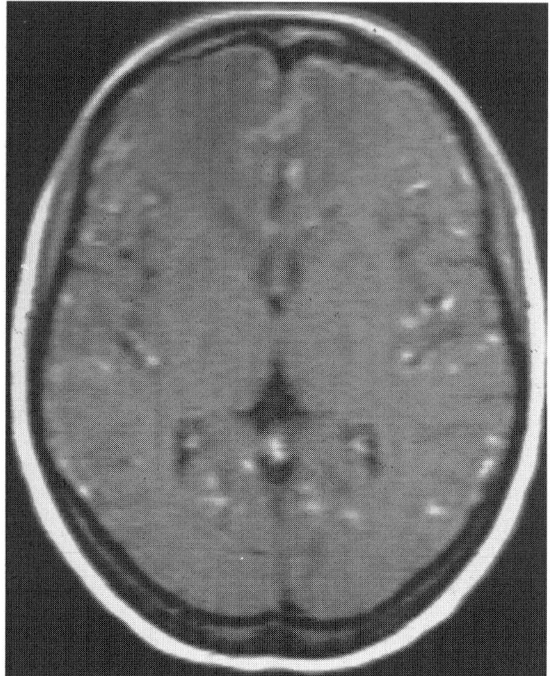

Figure 4.14 *A 35-year-old female with neurosarcoidosis manifesting as headache and obtundation. Gadolinium enhanced T1-weighted scan reveals a large number of enhancing lesions in the cerebral cortex.*

(1) Post-infectious optic neuritis is usually bilateral and symmetrical, whereas optic neuritis in multiple sclerosis is more often unilateral.

(2) Transverse myelitis in multiple sclerosis is often partial, but in ADEM it is often complete and usually associated with areflexia.

(3) The CSF cell count is higher in post-infectious syndromes, and oligoclonal bands are usually absent or occur only transiently during the acute illness (once present, oligoclonal bands in multiple sclerosis usually persist).

(4) On MRI, extensive symmetrical lesions in the cerebellar white matter and the basal ganglia are characteristic of ADEM (and unusual in multiple sclerosis) [Atlas *et al.* 1986; Dunn *et al.* 1986; Kesselring *et al.* 1990] (Figure 4.15 a and b), but only occur in a minority of patients.

In the majority of patients with ADEM, multifocal white matter lesions are indistinguishable from multiple sclerosis [Kesselring *et al.* 1990] (Figures 4.15 c and 4.16). This finding supports the argument that MS should not be diagnosed at presentation in

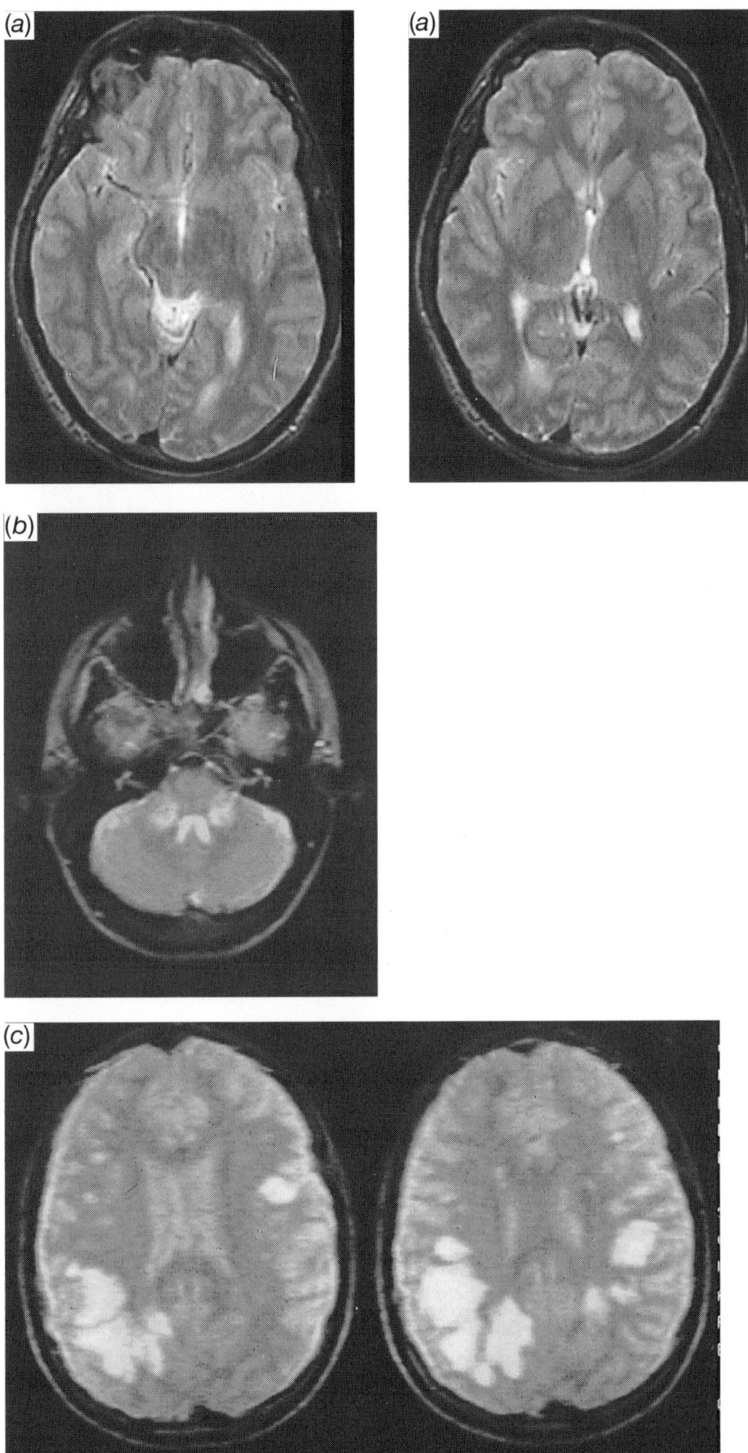

Figure 4.15 *Acute disseminated encephalomyelitis. T2-weighted scans reveal (a) symmetrical occipital white matter lesions in a 30-year-old male; (b) symmetrical middle cerebellar peduncle lesions in a 31-year-old male and (c) extensive, asymmetrical, multifocal white matter lesions predominantly in the posterior hemispheres in an 18-year-old male.*

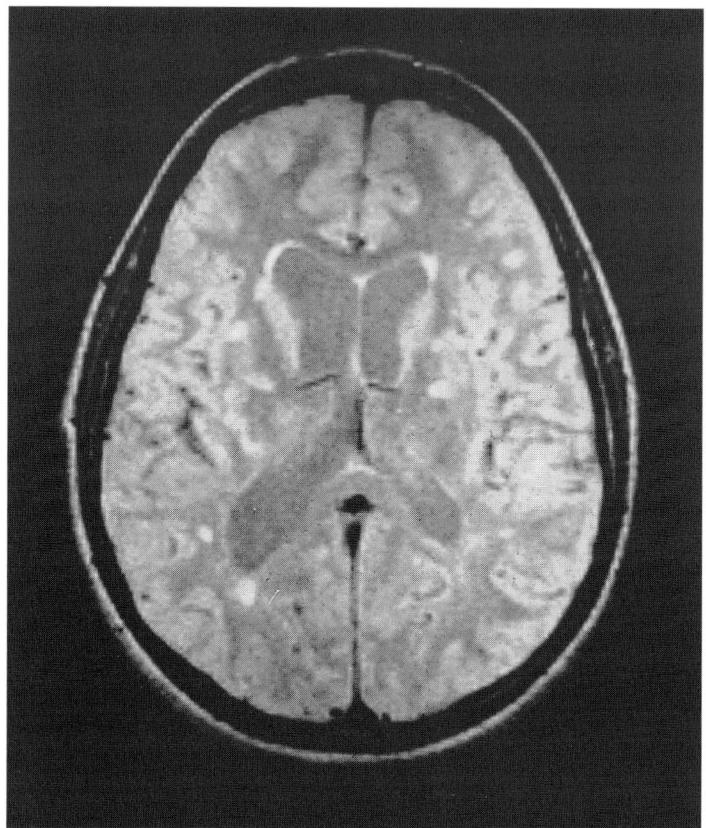

Figure 4.16 *A 19-year-old male with post-mycoplasma acute disseminated encephalomyelitis. PD-weighted MRI shows multifocal, small, asymmetrical periventricular and discrete white matter lesions – the appearances are indistinguishable from multiple sclerosis.*

patients with a single clinical episode and multifocal white matter lesions, since the possibility that they are due to a monophasic illness cannot be excluded [Kesselring *et al.* 1990]. It might be anticipated that the distinction of multiple sclerosis from ADEM on a single scan might be facilitated by inferring the age of the lesions from their capacity to enhance after gadolinium is given. Patients with multiple sclerosis often have both enhancing and non-enhancing lesions at the same time, due to lesions of different ages and states of activity (cf. Chapter 3). In ADEM, which is usually a monophasic illness, it might be expected that all, or at least most, lesions would enhance in the acute phase, while none would do so in the chronic phase. At the present time this hypothesis is unproven, because there is little published data on serial gadolinium enhanced MRI findings in ADEM.

Serial PD/T2-weighted studies greatly facilitate the differentiation of ADEM and MS. New lesions do not develop in ADEM, provided there is a sufficient follow-up interval.

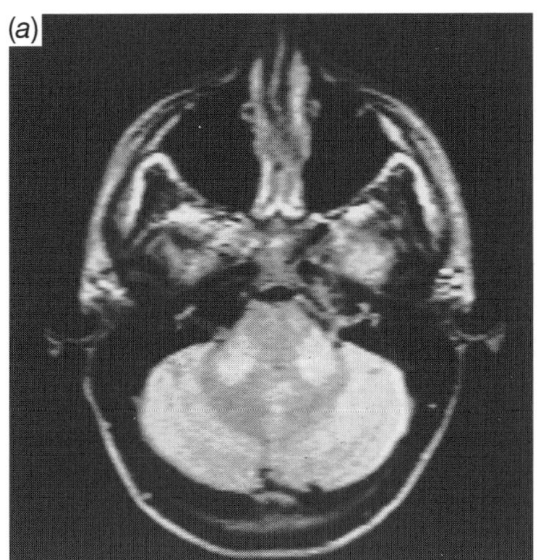 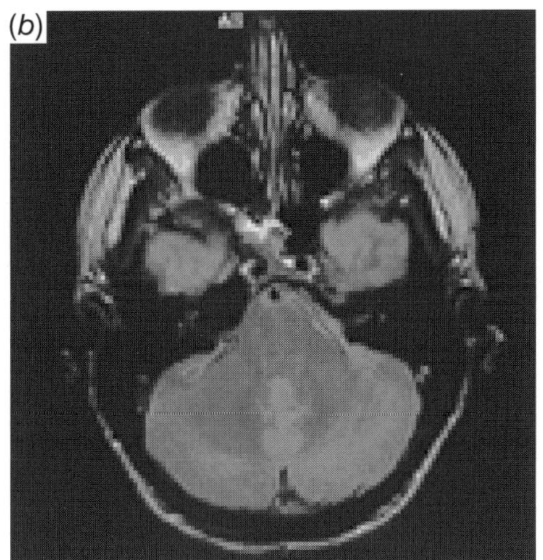

Figure 4.17 *Acute disseminated encephalomyelitis. PD-weighted MRI (a) at first presentation (aged 31 years) reveals lesions in the middle cerebellar peduncles; (b) at follow-up ten years later the lesions had resolved. There had been no new lesions and the patient had had no new clinical episodes. (From Kesselring et al. 1990, by permission of Oxford University Press.)*

However, ADEM may evolve over several weeks. To minimise the risk of confusing MS with a slowly evolving ADEM, we recommend a follow-up interval of not less than three months and preferably at least six months. After such an interval, new lesions occur in many patients with multiple sclerosis. Pre-existing lesions in ADEM often disappear or show marked resolution (Figure 4.17), though this may also occur in multiple sclerosis.

Disseminated brain lesions are not an invariable finding in ADEM [Kesselring *et al.* 1990; Trend *et al.* 1990; Miller *et al.* 1993b]. We have seen a patient who presented with an acute brain stem syndrome, in whom MRI showed a gadolinium enhancing mass in the pons and medulla, but no other lesions [Miller *et al.* 1993b]. Biopsy of the mass revealed multiple small foci of perivascular inflammation and demyelination which was felt to be more characteristic of ADEM than multiple sclerosis, because of the uneven distribution of the areas of demyelination. In support of this diagnosis (and against multiple sclerosis), there were no oligoclonal bands in the CSF and the patient has not had further neurological events after six years of follow-up.

4.7   Devic's neuromyelitis optica

The nosological status of Devic's neuromyelitis optica is controversial. We define it here as a syndrome characterised by a severe, acute transverse myelitis, often with limited recovery, in addition to an acute optic neuropathy which occurs simultaneously or consecutively. There may be a monophasic or multiphasic pattern [O'Riordan *et al.* 1996b]. The main points of clinical distinction from 'typical' multiple sclerosis are the severity of the transverse myelitis and the absence of clinical abnormalities outside of the spinal cord and optic nerves. Nevertheless, occasional cases presenting with a Devic syndrome as defined may subsequently develop features of classical multiple sclerosis [Matthews 1991]. In a few other cases, a specific aetiology is identified, including systemic lupus erythematosus [April & Vansonnenberg 1976], Behçet's syndrome [Motomura *et al.* 1980], and ADEM [Chusid *et al.* 1979]. In many instances, however, the aetiology is unknown. It has been suggested that such patients may have multiple sclerosis, and in some cases that have come to post-mortem, areas of demyelination beyond the spinal cord and optic nerves have been found [Stansbury 1950; Shibasaki & Kuroiwa 1969].

MRI provides the opportunity for assessing the extent of CNS lesions in life, and Mandler [1993] has described eight patients, in all of whom the CSF did not contain oligoclonal bands, while brain MRI was normal in the three who underwent this investigation. We have recently reviewed the records of 12 adult cases who have attended The National Hospital with a diagnosis of Devic's syndrome, of whom 11 underwent MRI examinations [O'Riordan *et al.* 1996b]. Eleven patients were female. Four patients were Asian, two Afro-Caribbean, one Mediterranean, and only five were Caucasian. Severe residual deficits in ambulation and vision were the rule rather than the exception. Brain MRI was normal in 5/11 and showed minor age-related changes considered normal for age in one 60-year-old. Abnormal white matter lesions were seen in five patients; in two of these, both young adults, there was an acute monophasic illness with severe transverse myelitis and bilateral optic neuritis several weeks after a non-specific infective illness. Many of the white matter lesions seen at presentation had disappeared at follow-up after several months and no new lesions were seen. The clinical and MRI findings in these two patients suggest the diagnosis of post-infectious ADEM.

In ten patients there was extensive swelling and signal change on spinal MRI involving many segments in both the cervical and thoracic cord (Figure 4.18). CSF oligoclonal bands were seen in only 2/12 patients. Two patients had a known collagen vascular disorder (one with systemic lupus erythematosus, one with mixed connective tissue disease), and six others had organ-specific autoantibodies.

When Mandler's and our series are considered together, a number of features emerge which are not expected in 'classical' relapsing-remitting multiple sclerosis, namely: (i) a preponderance of non-Caucasians; (ii) poor neurological recovery from the relapses; (iii) a high frequency of normal brain MRI; (iv) a low frequency of CSF oligoclonal bands; (v) unusually extensive spinal cord lesions; and (vi) a high frequency of organ-specific autoantibodies. This suggests that in many cases, Devic's neuromyelitis can be regarded as a clinicopathological entity distinct from multiple sclerosis. Although immunopathogenic mechanisms are likely to be important, the aetiology in these cases remains obscure.

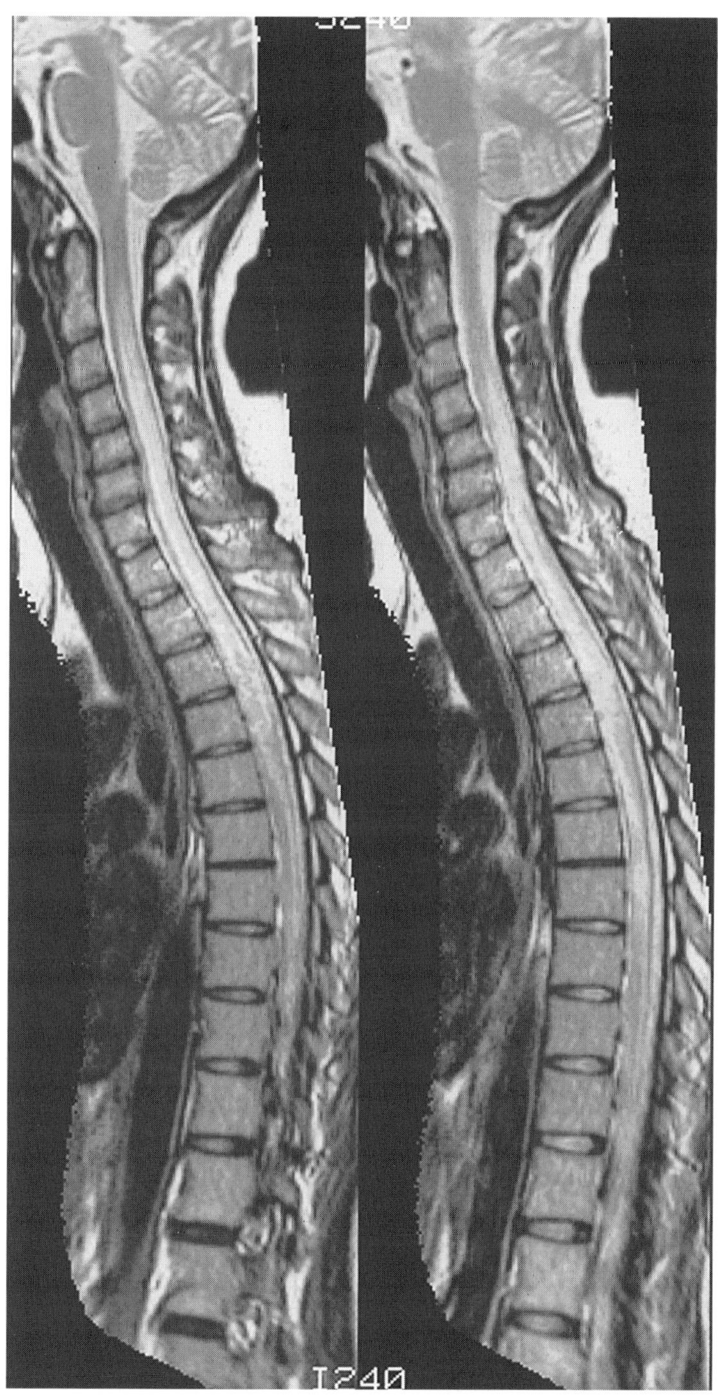

Figure 4.18 *Devic's neuromyelitis optica. During an episode of acute myelopathy, in a 35-year-old Asian female, T2-weighted sagittal spinal MRI reveals signal hyperintensity and swelling extending over many segments.*

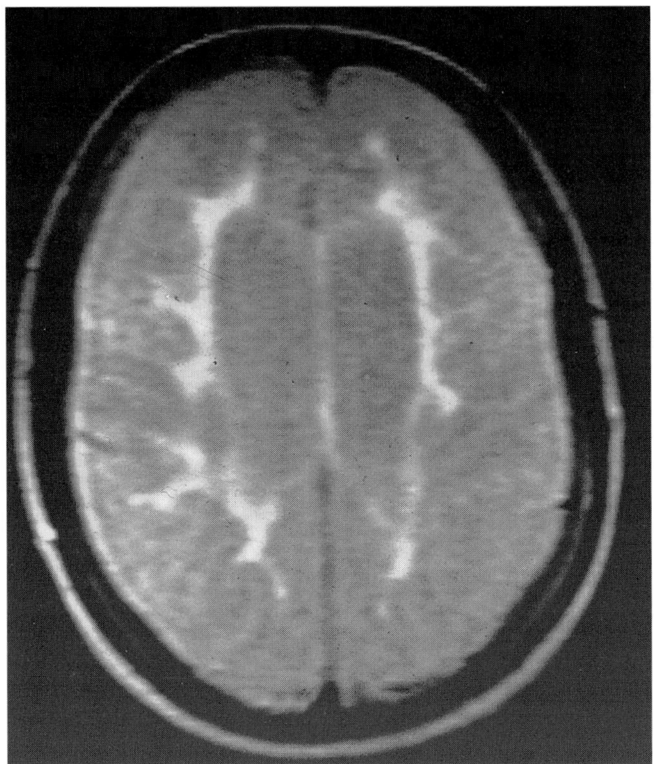

Figure 4.19 *Metachromatic leucodystrophy. PD-weighted brain MRI in a 29-year-old female reveals ventricular enlargement and extensive symmetrical deep white matter abnormalities.*

4.8 Leucodystrophies

Though the various forms of leucodystrophies more often present in childhood, they can do so in adolescence or even in adult life.

4.8.1 Metachromatic leucodystrophy

The adult form of metachromatic leucodystrophy leads over a course of several years to gradual intellectual decline, often accompanied by spastic paraparesis and/or ataxia. During life definitive diagnosis is based on determination of the activity of arylsulfatase A in urine and leucocytes (which is reduced). On MRI widespread, symmetrical, confluent signal changes are found, sparing the U-fibres and sometimes referred to as butterfly configurations (Figure 4.19). The profound loss of white matter leads to

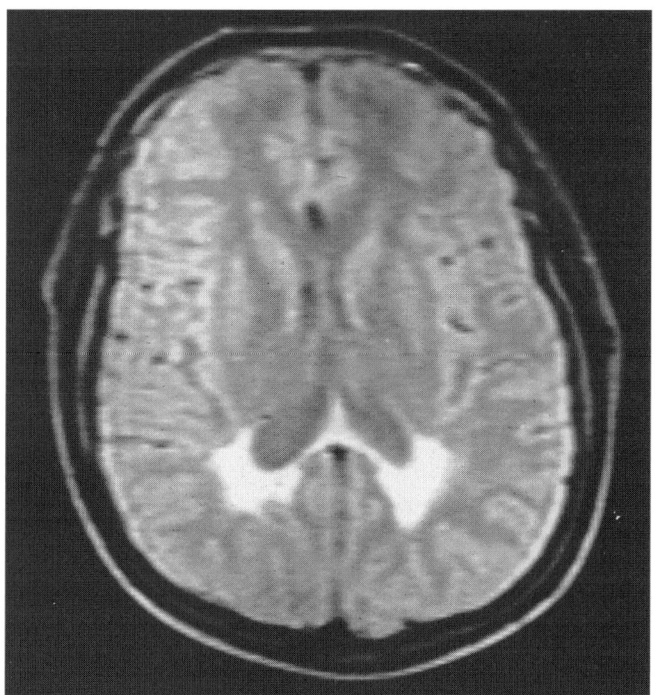

Figure 4.20 *Adrenomyeloneuropathy. PD-weighted brain MRI in a 40-year-old male with progressive spastic paraparesis shows symmetrical parieto-occipital white matter abnormalities. The diagnosis was established by demonstration of abnormal adrenal function and markedly elevated very long chain fatty acids. (From Kesselring et al. 1989a.)*

marked ventricular enlargement. Since there are no inflammatory changes in this condition, there is no gadolinium enhancement.

4.8.2   Adrenomyeloneuropathy

Adrenomyeloneuropathy is an adult variant of the X-linked disorder adrenoleucodystrophy. Its slowly progressive course of spastic paraparesis in young adult males, sometimes with cerebellar ataxia and intellectual deterioration, may easily be misdiagnosed as multiple sclerosis. Clinical clues to the correct diagnosis are evidence of a peripheral neuropathy, or increased skin pigmentation due to adrenal insufficiency. The diagnosis is established by detecting increased plasma levels of ACTH and very long-chain fatty acids.

When present, the MR abnormalities are very characteristic with symmetrical white matter abnormalities in the posterior cerebral hemispheres (Figure 4.20). In some instances, the histological pattern of the lesion is elucidated by gadolinium enhancement: a non-enhancing central zone with complete demyelination and gliosis; a middle zone, inflammatory in nature and with gadolinium enhancement; and an outer, non-enhancing, less demyelinated zone spreading forward [Valk and van der Knaap 1989; van der Knaap & Valk 1991].

4.9   Degenerative ataxic disorders

The degenerative ataxic disorders are a diverse group of diseases some of which have an inherited basis while others appear to arise sporadically and are therefore called idiopathic [Harding 1984]. The clinical picture is varied, with some patients showing an isolated cerebellar syndrome and others having cerebellar ataxia combined with deficits affecting other parts of the nervous system. These patients may demonstrate varying degrees of involvement of the pyramidal tracts, brain stem, spinal cord, cerebral hemispheres and peripheral nerves. Ataxia is frequently part of the clinical picture in multiple sclerosis and the combination of ataxia and spasticity is common. Evoked potentials may show prolonged latencies in both conditions, adding to the diagnostic confusion. These similarities between multiple sclerosis and degenerative ataxic disorders may therefore lead to difficulties in ascertaining the correct diagnosis, particularly in degenerative disorders with no family history, although diagnosis of the latter disorders is now sometimes possible by identification from blood tests of specific genetic mutations.

The most common and characteristic MRI finding in degenerative ataxic syndromes is atrophy of the cerebellum and/or brain stem [Nabatame *et al.* 1988; Wullner *et al.* 1993; Ormerod *et al.* 1994] (Figure 4.21). Most patients with autosomal dominant cerebellar ataxia have both cerebellar and brain stem atrophy, probably reflecting the pathological process of olivopontocerebellar atrophy. Patients with a late onset idiopathic cerebellar syndrome may show either atrophy of the cerebellum alone or atrophy of both the brain stem and cerebellum. The correlation of clinical signs of cerebellar or brain stem involvement with atrophy of the appropriate structure has generally been limited [Ormerod *et al.* 1994]. However, the presence of brain stem atrophy in patients with late onset pure cerebellar syndromes predicts a more rapid progression than if the brain stem is of normal size [Klockgether *et al.* 1990], possibly because some of the patients have multisystem atrophy, a disorder which progresses fairly rapidly.

Heterogeneous patterns of atrophy have been reported in patients with early onset cerebellar ataxia with retained reflexes [Wullner *et al.* 1993; Ormerod *et al.* 1994]. In Friedreich's ataxia, the brain stem and cerebellum are of normal size, apart from some atrophy in the vermis and medulla in advanced cases [Ormerod *et al.* 1994], but spinal cord atrophy is usually evident [Wullner *et al.* 1993]. Not surprisingly, the brain stem and cerebellum appear normal in hereditary spastic paraplegia, since the degenerative changes in this disorder are usually confined to the spinal cord.

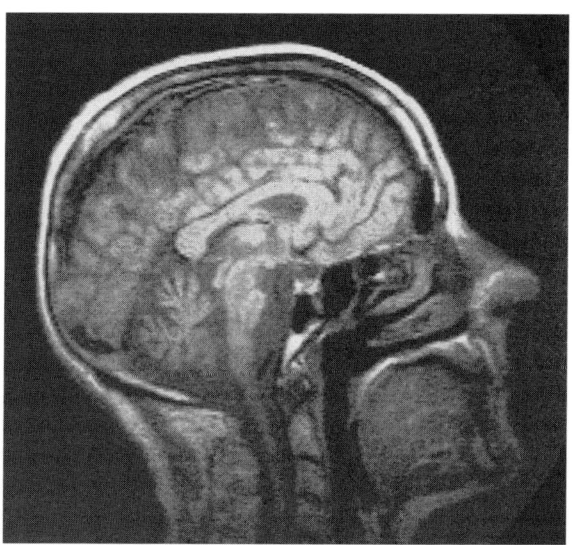

Figure 4.21 *Spinocerebellar degeneration. Sagittal T1-weighted MRI reveals marked atrophy of the cerebellum and brain stem in a 56-year-old female.*

One report has commented on signal abnormalities on T2-weighted images in the pons, middle cerebellar peduncles and cerebellum in patients with a clinical diagnosis of olivopontocerebellar atrophy, perhaps secondary to degeneration of fibre tracts and gliosis [Savoiardo *et al.* 1990].

Ormerod [1994] found that patients with degenerative ataxias had a higher frequency of cerebral white matter lesions than age matched controls. The reason for this was not immediately evident. There was no other clinical evidence for multiple sclerosis and only 1/53 patients had CSF oligoclonal bands (MRI was normal in that patient). The presence of white matter lesions was correlated with the radiological appearance of severe cerebral atrophy. Neuronal fallout and gliosis in the place of axons may account for the white matter lesions, as the fibre tracts connecting the cortical neurones, particularly from the frontal lobes, course the periventricular area. Alternatively, perhaps tissue compliance changes in the presence of atrophy, and perivascular foci of degeneration are thus more likely to occur, such foci being the major pathological substrate of MRI white matter lesions in asymptomatic individuals. Such mechanisms remain speculative, but it is of interest that a similar excess of white matter lesions is seen in another degenerative (and atrophic) disorder, Alzheimer's disease [Scheltens *et al.* 1992].

The frequency and extent of white matter lesions in degenerative ataxias is nevertheless much less than that found in multiple sclerosis. Also, the marked cerebellar and brain-stem atrophy seen in many patients with degenerative ataxia is uncommon other than in advanced cases of multiple sclerosis. Thus, MRI is extremely useful in the distinction of multiple sclerosis from degenerative ataxic disorders.

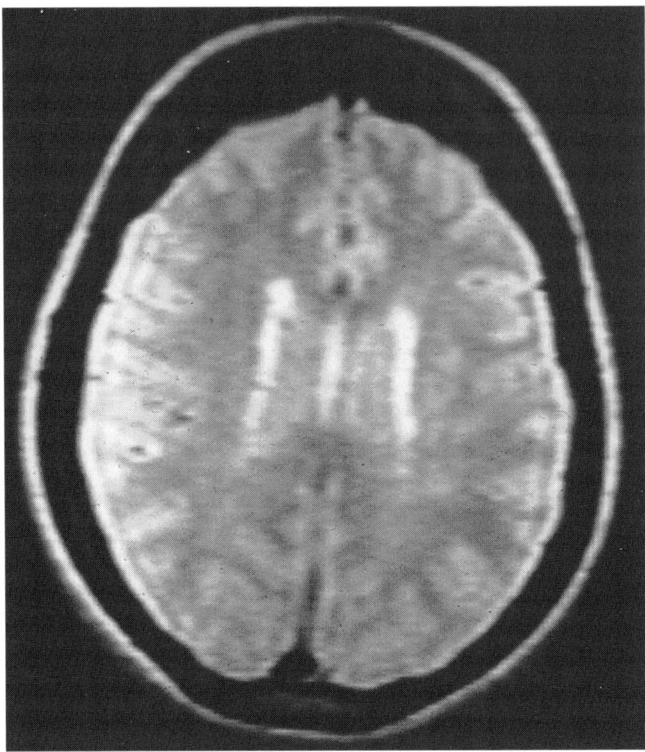

Figure 4.22 *A 48-year-old female with HTLV-1 associated myelopathy. PD-weighted scan shows a few periventricular abnormalities.*

4.10　　HTLV-1 associated myelopathy

The human T cell lymphotropic virus type I (HTLV-1) may produce a chronic progressive paraparesis (also known as tropical spastic paraplegia), in certain geographical regions, most notably the Caribbean. The myelopathy may develop in migrants from the Caribbean to countries where multiple sclerosis is common, some years after migration [Newton *et al.* 1987]. In such a setting, multiple sclerosis is considered in the differential diagnosis, and abnormal evoked potentials and CSF oligoclonal bands can occur in both conditions. Examination of serum for antibodies to HTLV-1 is a crucial diagnostic test.

Brain MRI frequently reveals periventricular and deep white matter lesions in HTLV-1 associated myelopathy (Figure 4.22), but these are rarely extensive, and infratentorial lesions are distinctly uncommon [Cruickshank *et al.* 1989]. Diffuse spinal cord atrophy is invariably present in longstanding cases [Kermode *et al.* 1990c] (Figure 4.23).

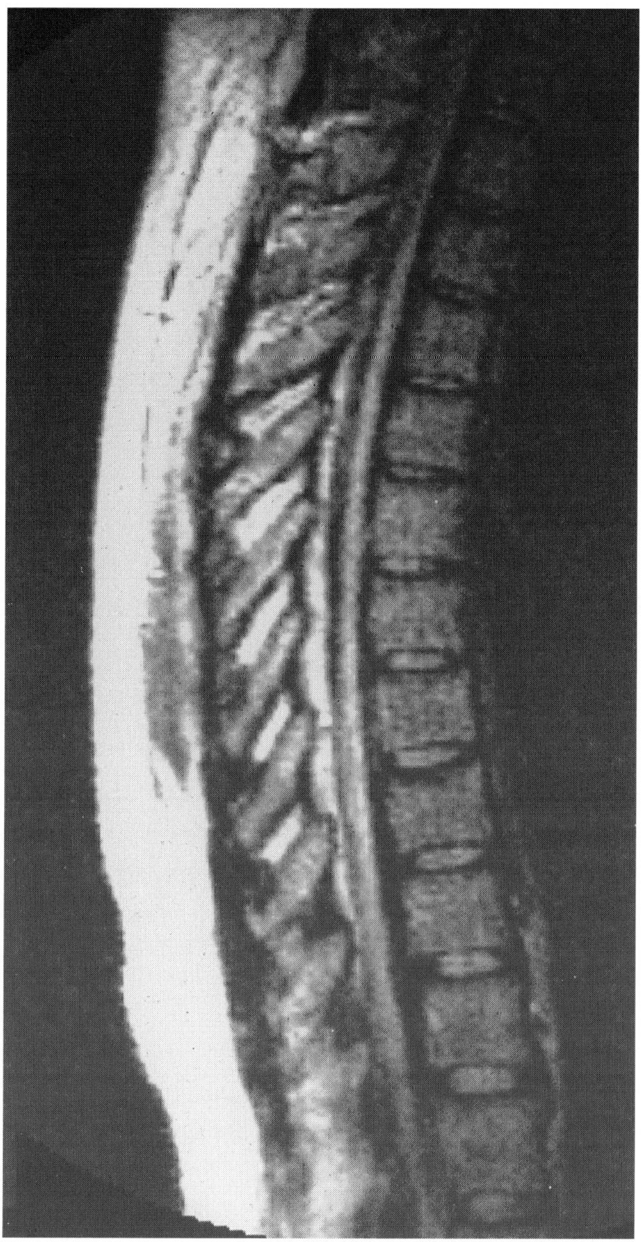

Figure 4.23 *A 48-year-old female with HTLV-1 associated myelopathy. Sagittal PD-weighted spinal MRI shows diffuse cord atrophy. (From Kermode et al. 1990c.)*

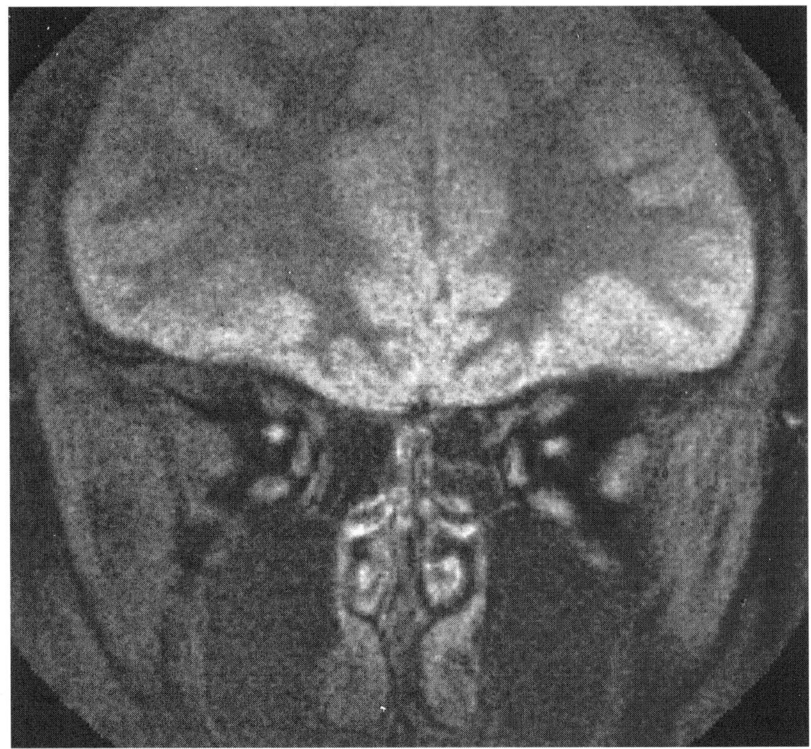

Figure 4.24 *Leber's hereditary optic neuropathy in a 25-year-old male. Coronal STIR images through the orbits. Both optic nerves are abnormally small and display increased signal. (From Kermode et al. 1990b.)*

4.11   Leber's hereditary optic neuropathy

Leber's hereditary optic neuropathy (LHON) is an inherited disorder, characterised by subacute onset of bilateral central visual loss. It can result from any one of several mitochondrial DNA point mutations. Visual loss usually appears in young adults, and 80% of cases are male [Newman *et al.* 1991]. In males, MRI of the brain is usually normal [Kermode *et al.* 1989b]. This is in contrast to clinically isolated acute optic neuritis, in which 50–70% of the patients have multifocal white matter lesions in the brain at presentation. All patients with LHON examined with STIR images, however, showed increased signal in the mid to posterior intra-orbital portions of the optic nerves (Figure 4.24), whereas signal changes in optic neuritis tend to be located more anteriorly [Miller *et al.* 1988b]. In women with LHON, the occurrence of a multiple sclerosis-like illness has been described and corresponding white matter lesions on MRI have been demonstrated [Harding *et al.* 1992] (Figure 4.25).

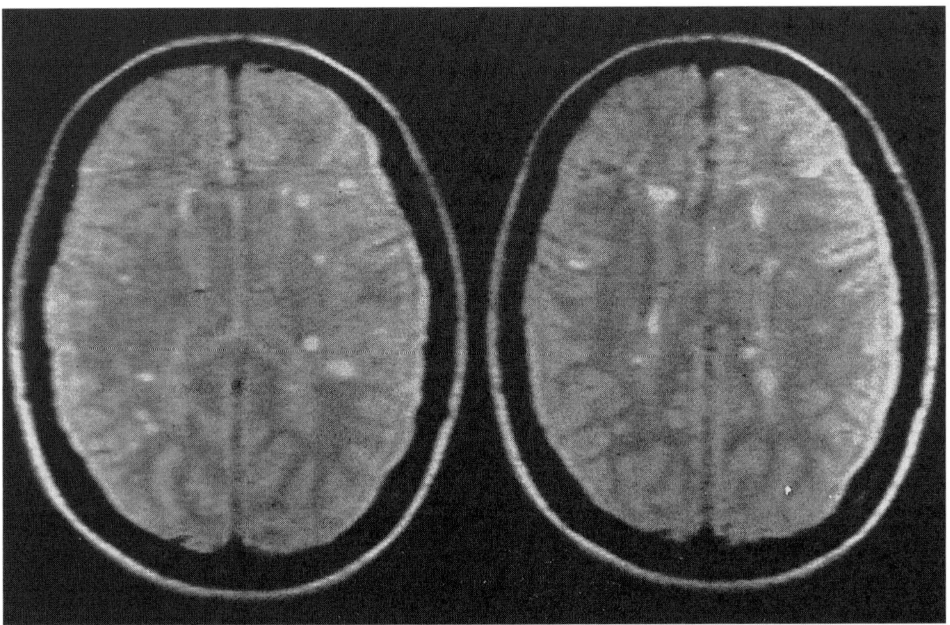

Figure 4.25 *PD-weighted brain MRI of a 40-year-old female with Leber's hereditary optic neuropathy and multiple sclerosis. There are multifocal white matter abnormalities characteristic of demyelination. (From Harding et al. 1992, by permission of Oxford University Press.)*

4.12 Acute intermittent porphyria

In acute intermittent porphyria an inherited deficiency of the enzyme porphobilinogen deaminase leads to overproduction of delta-aminolevulinic acid which is a precursor of haem. Neurological dysfunction, which is a primary feature in this condition, has been attributed to either metabolic derangements or to multifocal ischaemia. During an episode of acute encephalopathy in one patient, MRI revealed multiple, discrete, mainly cortical lesions [King & Bragdon 1991]. These resolved with clinical recovery. The appearances resembled those seen in other cerebral vasculopathies such as SLE and hypertensive encephalopathy. Indirect support for a possible vascular origin of the cerebral lesions seen on MRI are the findings of peripheral vasospasm in the skin and retina during attacks of acute intermittent porphyria, the rise in blood pressure which occurs during cerebral manifestations, and a similarity to malignant hypertension, in which a role of vascular factors in pathogenesis is established.

4.13   Whipple's disease

Whipple's disease is a rare disorder of unknown aetiology in which there is usually multi-organ involvement with the characteristic pathological finding of PAS positive macrophage infiltrates. It is a treatable disorder, most patients responding to anti-bacterial therapy. Multifocal central nervous system involvement may occur. Ordinarily, the clinical and imaging features of Whipple's disease in the central nervous system are quite unlike those of multiple sclerosis. The most common CNS features are dementia, seizures and midbrain syndromes including a characteristic movement disorder, oculomasticatory myorrhythmia. Several MRI case reports have demonstrated large and sometimes multifocal lesions involving both cortex and subcortical white matter, with patchy or ring enhancement with gadolinium [Wroe *et al.* 1991; Erdem *et al.* 1993b]. We have seen one patient who presented with a subacute akinetic rigid syndrome associated with cognitive decline, in whom the initial brain MRI revealed multifocal white matter lesions indistinguishable from those seen in demyelination (Figure 4.26). The CSF was active, and it was thought most likely that the patient had post-infectious acute disseminated encephalomyelitis. However, progressive clinical deterioration ensued over the next month, and repeat MRI revealed extensive new lesions in the caudate nucleus and putamen (Figure 4.26). Brain biopsy in the left frontal region revealed PAS positive macrophages, suggesting a diagnosis of Whipple's disease. The patient was treated with penicillin, streptomycin and cotrimoxazole, and over the next few months there was a partial recovery, although he has been left with significant problems with mobility and cognition. This case emphasises that Whipple's disease can produce an MRI appearance indistinguishable from multiple sclerosis.

4.14   Motor neurone disease

The typical clinical picture of amyotrophic lateral sclerosis, with a mixture of upper and lower motor neurone signs, will not be confused with multiple sclerosis. However, during the early stages in some patients an upper motor neurone syndrome predominates, and at this time the differential diagnosis will include the primary progressive form of multiple sclerosis. Brain MRI is able to visualise degeneration within the corticospinal tracts in about 70% of patients with motor neurone disease; symmetrical hyperintense foci on PD/T2-weighted images are visible in the centrum semiovale, posterior limbs of the internal capsules, and less often in the cerebral peduncles and ventral pons [Goodin *et al.* 1988; Sale Luis *et al.* 1990; Thorpe *et al.* 1994e] (Figure 4.27). Axial spinal cord images may reveal signal abnormalities in the lateral columns [Friedman & Taraglino 1993]; using a gradient echo T2-weighted sequence, Thorpe [1994e] found

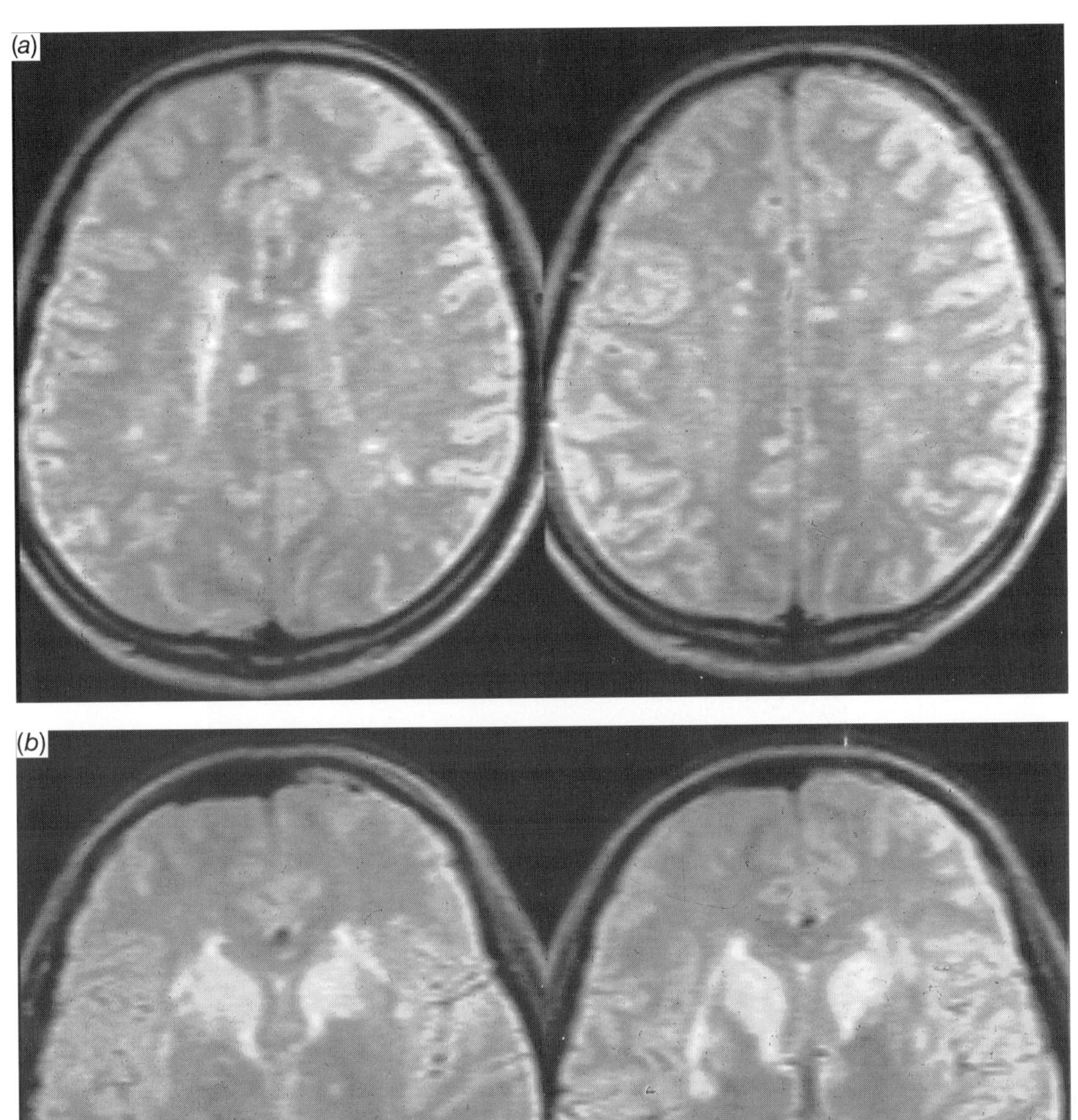

Figure 4.26 *Biopsy proven Whipple's disease in a 38-year-old male. PD-weighted MRI (a) at first presentation reveals multifocal white matter lesions and (b) one month later shows new abnormalities in both caudate nuclei.*

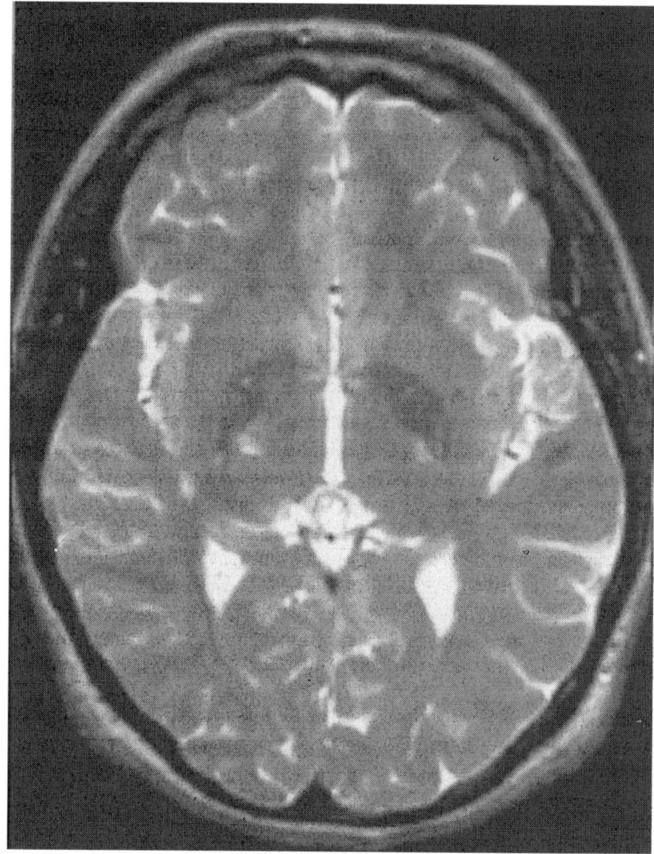

Figure 4.27 *A 38-year-old female with motorneuron disease. T2-weighted brain MRI reveals increased signal in both corticospinal tracts.*

such abnormalities in 8/11 of patients in the cervical cord (Figure 4.28). These appearances are quite unlike multiple sclerosis, and their detection is of value in the differential diagnosis of progressive spastic paraplegia. Such signal changes have not been reported in the brains of subjects with HTLV-1 associated myelopathy or hereditary spastic paraplegia, although an equivalent MRI study of these two disorders in the spinal cord has not yet been reported.

A much less common form of motor neurone disease is primary lateral sclerosis. In this disorder, signs remain confined to the upper motor neurone even after many years. A report of this group of patients identified focal atrophy in the primary motor cortex, detectable on sagittal T1-weighted images [Pringle *et al.* 1992]; signal abnormalities within the pyramidal tracts in the brain have also been described [Marti-Fabregas & Pujol 1990].

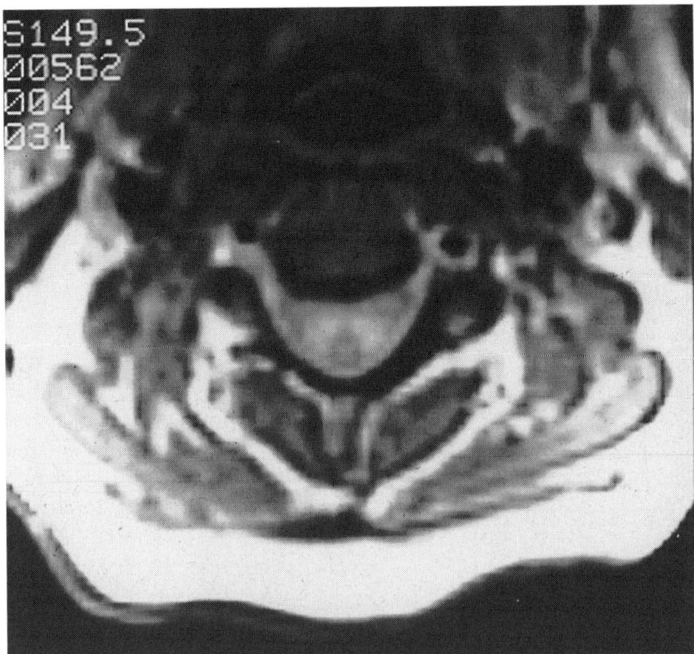

Figure 4.28 *A 40-year-old female with motor neurone disease. Axial T2-weighted gradient echo image through the upper cervical cord. There is increased signal bilaterally in the lateral columns.*

4.15   Subacute combined degeneration of the spinal cord

The characteristic pathological finding in patients with vitamin B_{12} deficiency and neurological impairment is degeneration involving the lateral and posterior columns in the spinal cord. In a case report, MRI signal hyperintensity was seen on axial cervical cord images within the lateral and posterior regions of the cord [Timms *et al.* 1993].

4.16   Wilson's disease

The neurological presentation of Wilson's disease is occasionally misdiagnosed as multiple sclerosis. We have seen a 27-year-old woman who gave a one-year history of steadily progressive ataxia. Upbeating nystagmus was interpreted as being of cerebellar origin. Clinically, multiple sclerosis was suspected. MRI (Figure 4.29) showed areas of low signal

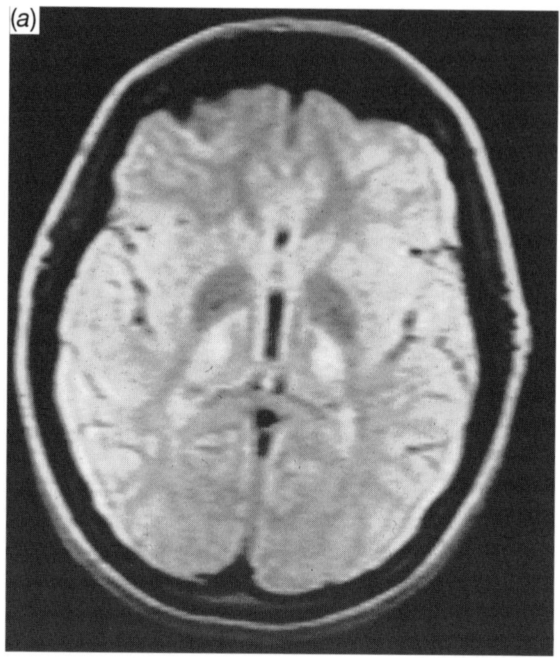

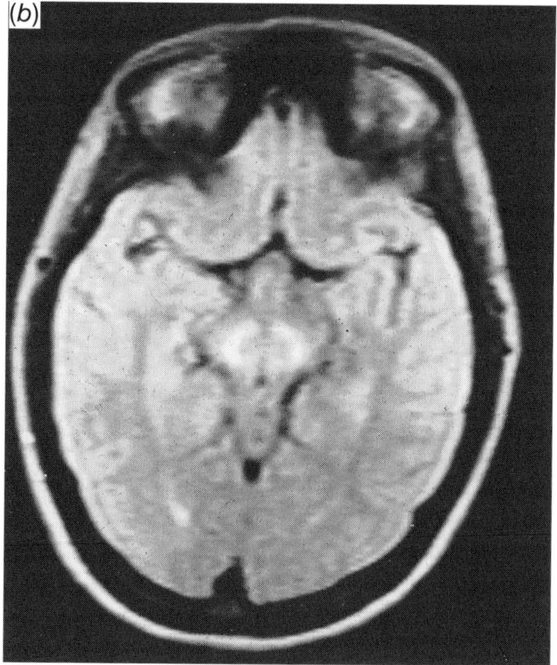

Figure 4.29 *A 27-year-old female with Wilson's disease. T2-weighted MRI reveals (a) low signal in the pallidum consistent with a paramagnetic effect of excessive copper accumulation; (b) increased signal in the substantia nigra.*

anteriorly and of high signal posteriorly in a symmetrical distribution in the lentiform nuclei and the posterior parts of the thalami. On lower axial sections (Figure 4.29) high signal was seen in the substantia nigra and the red nucleus. Wilson's disease was suspected on the basis of these prominent MRI abnormalities, and later confirmed biochemically and by the presence of Kayser-Fleischer corneal rings on both sides. On the basis of the pathology underlying this disease, T2-weighted MRI changes of high signal can be interpreted as oedema, necrosis or gliosis, whereas the symmetrical areas of lower signal intensity might be due to a paramagnetic effect of the copper accumulated in this condition [Aisen *et al.* 1985b; Magalhaes *et al.* 1994].

4.17   Phenylketonuria

Brain MRI abnormalities have been described in adolescents and young adults with phenylketonuria [Thompson *et al.* 1990a; Cleary *et al.* 1994]. Some of these individuals have also exhibited cognitive abnormalities or a mild spastic paraparesis. The MRI findings are characteristically symmetrical, involving periventricular white matter predominantly in the parieto-occipital region [Thompson *et al.* 1990a] (Figure 4.30). The extent of abnormalities correlates with the blood phenylalanine level at the time of imaging [Thompson *et al.* 1993b; Cleary *et al.* 1994], but not with neurological or cognitive impairment (the latter is closely related to phenylalanine control during early childhood [Smith *et al.* 1990]). Rapid regression of MRI abnormalities has been seen when a strict diet has been resumed [Bick *et al.* 1991], suggesting that the underlying pathological process is non-destructive. This conclusion is supported by proton MR spectroscopy evaluation of areas of MRI abnormality, which has revealed a normal concentration of *N*-acetyl aspartate, a neuronal marker, suggesting that axonal integrity has been preserved [Davie *et al.* 1994b].

4.18   Mitochondrial disease

The variety of CNS syndromes due to mitochondrial disease are unlikely to be confused with multiple sclerosis. Imaging abnormalities are also quite different, with a predilection for large, infarct-like lesions [Matthews *et al.* 1991], and cortical or basal ganglia involvement, although diffuse white matter abnormality resembling that seen in a leucodystrophy has been reported in one case presenting as a Kearns-Sayre syndrome variant [Sandhu & Dillon 1991].

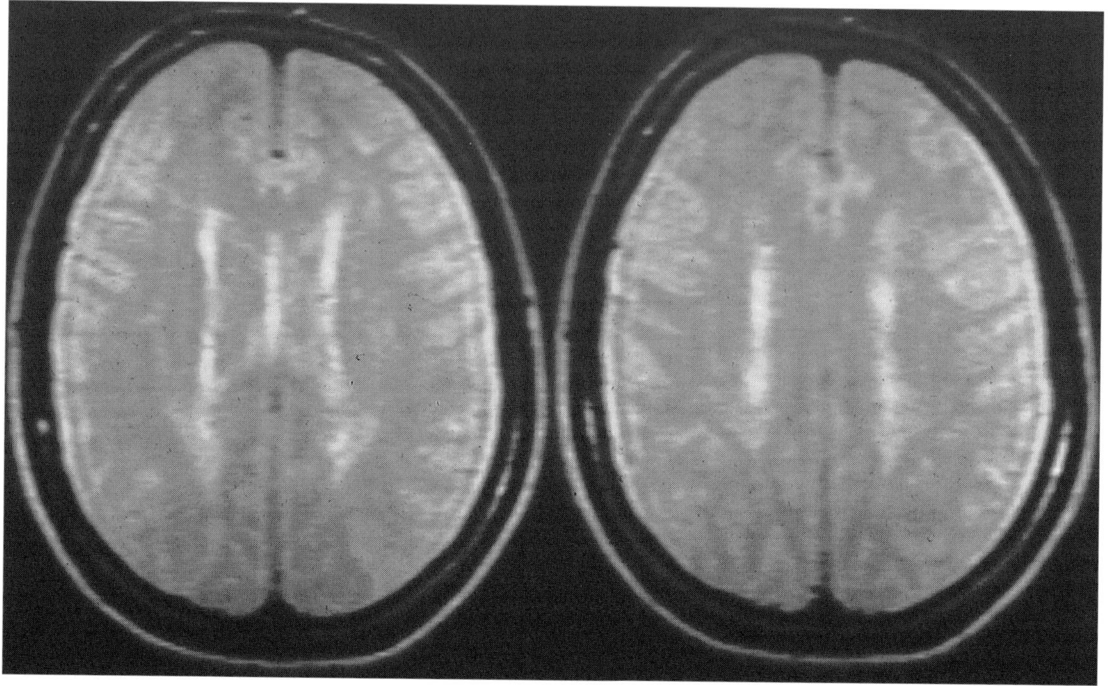

Figure 4.30 *T2-weighted brain MRI in a 34-year-old male with phenylke-tonuria. There are symmetrical, diffuse areas of increased signal in the periventricular white matter; the changes are most obvious posteriorly.*

4.19   Progressive multifocal leucoencephalopathy

This rare and rapidly progressive demyelinating disorder, due to papovavirus-induced destruction of oligodendrocytes, is seen in immunocompromised individuals, most often nowadays in AIDS patients. MRI characteristically reveals large, multifocal abnormalities without mass effect or contrast enhancement [Olsen *et al.* 1988; Hawkins *et al.* 1993], the appearances being dissimilar to multiple sclerosis.

4.20   Subacute sclerosing panencephalitis

This disorder, due to chronic measles virus infection, usually presents in childhood as a progressive illness leading to death within two years, although a minority of cases remit and relapse. Both small and multifocal, and diffuse and confluent white matter abnormalities have been observed on MRI, especially in the parietal or occipital lobes [Miller *et al.* 1990; Winer *et al.* 1991] (Figure 4.31). Atrophy develops in the later stages of the disease [Duda *et al.* 1980].

4.21   HIV encephalitis

An encephalitis attributed directly to the human immunodeficiency virus may result in focal or diffuse white matter abnormalities [Olsen *et al.* 1988; Hawkins *et al.* 1993].

4.22   Radiation- or chemotherapy-induced leucoencephalopathy

White matter abnormalities may occur following cranial irradiation, characteristically limited to the field treated [Curnes *et al.* 1986]. A progressive necrotising leucoen-cephalopathy can develop after treatment for leukaemia or lymphoma with cranial irradiation and/or chemotherapy, most notably methotrexate [Dawson 1992]. MRI reveals extensive white matter abnormalities (Figure 4.32). MRI abnormalities in the cerebral white matter, pons and cerebellum have also been reported in patients with cyclosporin-induced neurotoxicity, which resolved on discontinuing the treatment or reducing the dose [Lane *et al.* 1988; Bird *et al.* 1990]. In patients developing radiation-induced myelopathy, focal cord swelling with gadolinium enhancement has been described [Wang *et al.* 1992].

4.23   Trauma

Closed head injuries may cause white matter abnormalities [Zimmerman *et al.* 1986], but there is a predilection for damage to the frontal and temporal poles; MRI not infre-quently demonstrates focal atrophy along with subcortical white matter signal changes in these regions, an appearance quite unlike multiple sclerosis.

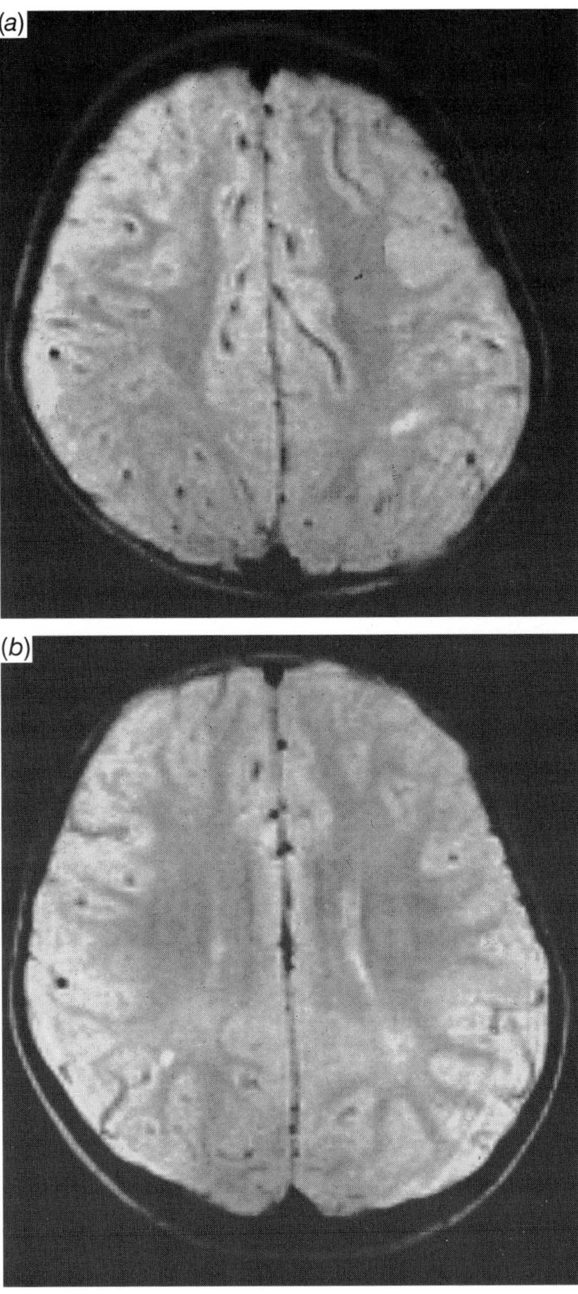

Figure 4.31 *Subacute sclerosing panencephalitis in a 5-year-old male. PD-weighted brain MRI reveals several small foci of increased signal in the parietal white matter. (From Miller et al. 1990.)*

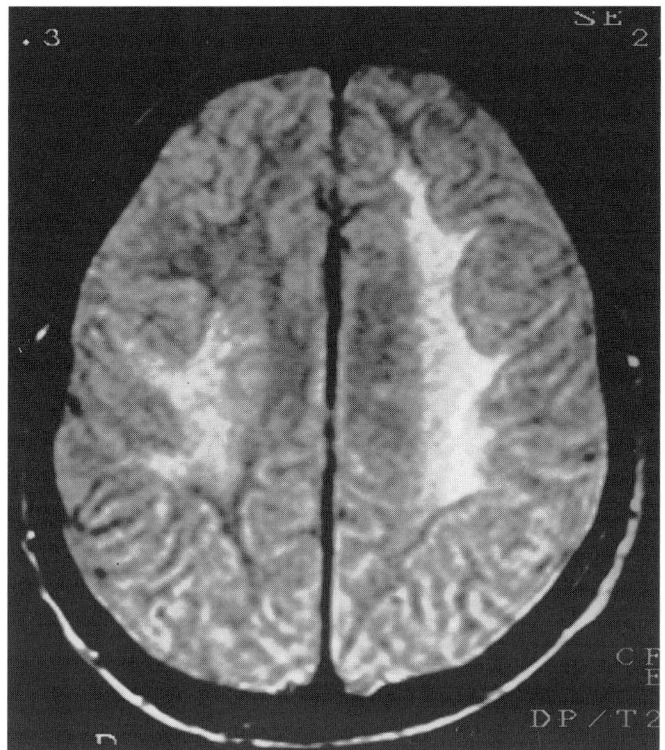

Figure 4.32 *Iatrogenic leucoencephalopathy following cranial irradiation and chemotherapy for cerebral lymphoma in a 43-year-old male. PD-weighted image reveals extensive, diffuse white matter abnormalities.*

4.24   Lyme disease

Lyme disease is due to infection by the tick-borne spirochaete, *Borrelia burgdorferei*. A subacute or chronic meningitis may develop, with CSF pleocytosis and spinal root and/or cranial nerve deficits (especially the facial nerve)[Bateman *et al.* 1987]. A chronic encephalomyelitis with clinical and MRI features similar to multiple sclerosis occurs rarely [Hansen & Lebech 1992]. As with other chronic meningitides, striking gadolinium enhancement of the meninges may be seen (Figure 4.33).

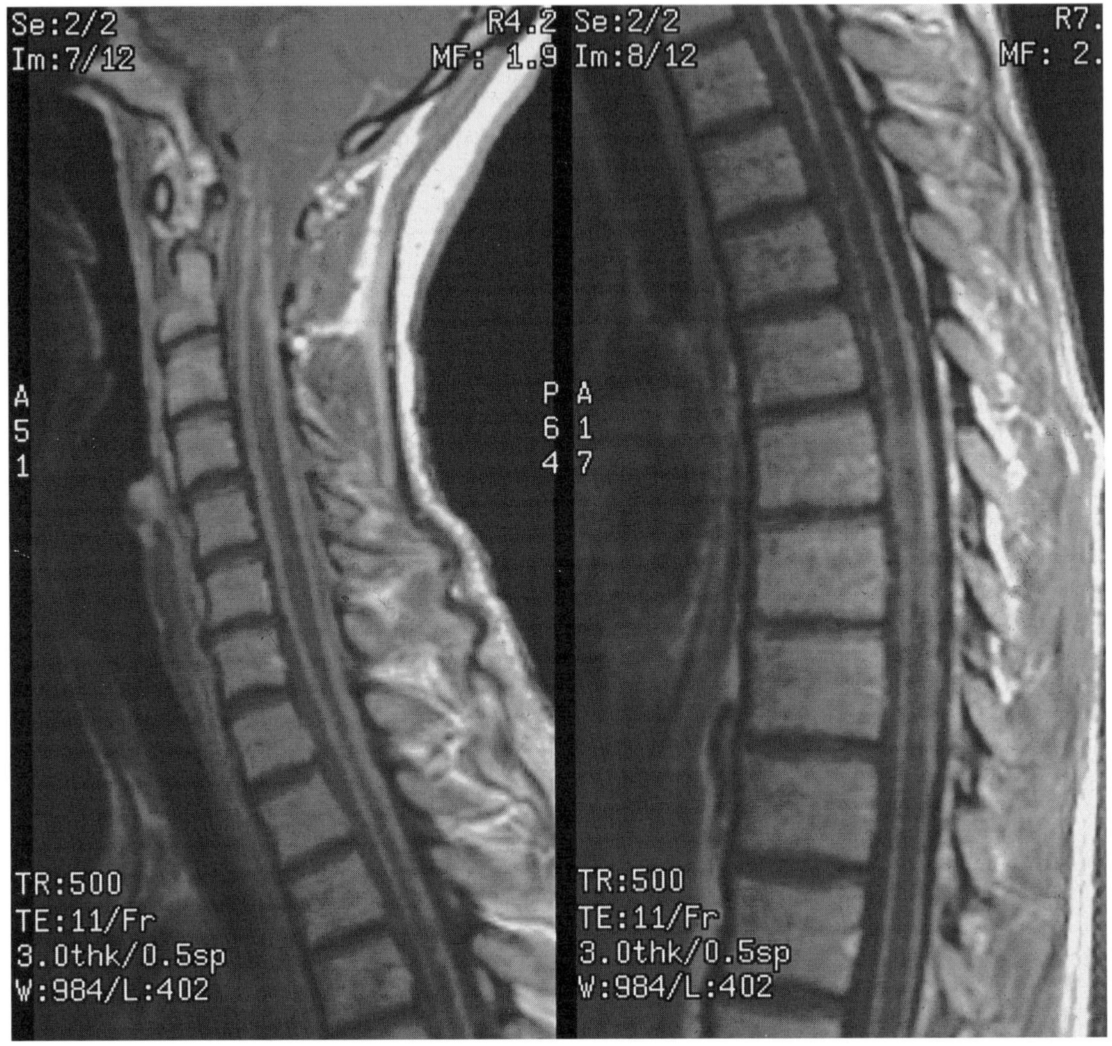

Figure 4.33 *Lyme neuroborreleosis in a 30-year-old female. Gadolinium enhanced T1-weighted spinal MRI reveals florid meningeal enhancement.*

4.25 Structural abnormalities of the brain stem, foramen magnum and spinal cord

Structural abnormalities in the region of the brain stem, foramen magnum and spinal cord not infrequently cause diagnostic difficulties in patients with progressive spasticity and/or ataxia in middle life, and may produce a clinical picture which is readily mistaken

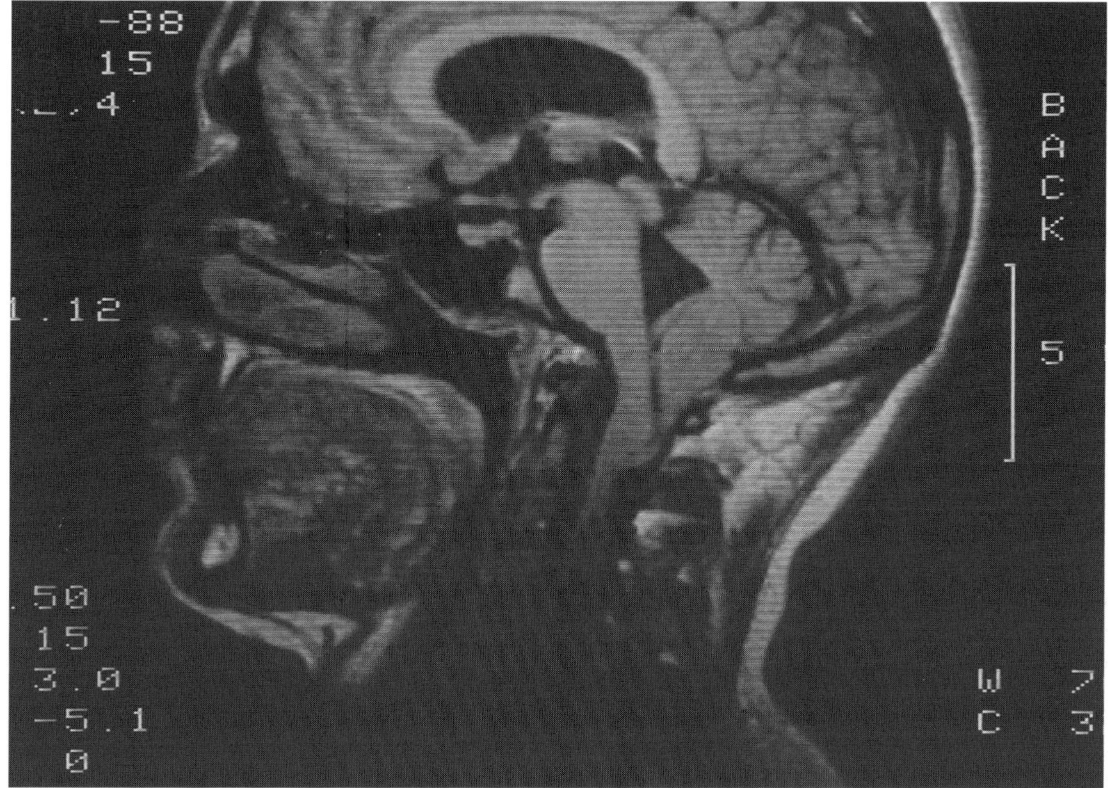

Figure 4.34 *Arnold-Chiari malformation in an 18-year-old male. Sagittal T1-weighted MRI reveals gross cerebellar tonsillar herniation and a syrinx in the upper cervical cord.*

for multiple sclerosis. MRI has now superseded CT/myelography as the investigation of choice in evaluating these regions (Figure 4.34). The advantages of MRI are that it is non-invasive, free of bone hardening artefact, readily depicts soft tissue abnormalities and provides images in multiple planes.

It is beyond the scope of this textbook to review the many structural and often surgically treatable disorders that can occur in the posterior fossa, foramen magnum and spinal cord, and which are readily detected on MRI. These are dealt with comprehensively in standard neuroradiological textbooks. This section will conclude by discussing only one group of disorders: the spinal cord arteriovenous malformations. These are of interest because until recently they have proved difficult to detect on conventional MRI.

4.25.1   Spinal cord arteriovenous malformations

These vascular anomalies most often present in middle-aged males as a chronic progressive or fluctuating myelopathy, involving the thoracic cord [Aminoff & Logue 1974]. Lower motor neurone features are sometimes evident in the legs. Weakness characteristically worsens with exertion, a feature also seen in some patients with multiple sclerosis. The traditional method of diagnosis has been first to perform supine myelography, which demonstrates the large, tortuous draining veins lying on the dorsal surface of the cord in the majority of cases, and secondly spinal angiography. The latter is required for definitive diagnosis and also for therapeutic embolisation. However, it carries a small risk of producing major neurological deficits.

It would be highly desirable to have a reliable non-invasive technique for diagnosis, and also for identification of the level of the fistula, in order to decide who should have angiography, and to determine the level at which the angiography should commence. MRI scanning at high fields shows considerable promise in this context. The abnormal draining veins can be relatively small, yet they may also extend over much of the length of the cord. Therefore, it is important that both resolution and field of view are maximised. We use the multi-array coil to survey the entire cord in a single sagittal image, and a T2-weighted FSE sequence with a 512×512 matrix to provide in-plane resolution of less than 1 mm. In addition, T1-weighted SE sequences are obtained before and after gadolinium enhancement. Using these approaches, Thorpe [1994d] identified abnormalities in 7/7 patients with angiographically proven angiomas (Figure 4.35). The abnormalities included swelling or signal hyperintensity in the cord on T2-weighted images, gadolinium enhancement in or adjacent to the cord, and serpiginous signal voids on the dorsal surface of the cord representing the dilated draining veins. After injection of a rapid bolus of gadolinium DTPA, gradient echo images were obtained at three-second intervals, and transient signal loss was seen as contrast passed through the abnormal vessels 20–30 seconds later [Thorpe *et al.* 1994d]. The initial site of signal loss correlated with the level of the fistula subsequently demonstrated on angiography in five cases. Thus, these MRI techniques are sensitive in the diagnosis of spinal cord angiomas, and dynamic scanning after a contrast bolus helps to demonstrate the level of the fistula, thus facilitating the subsequent procedure of therapeutic embolisation.

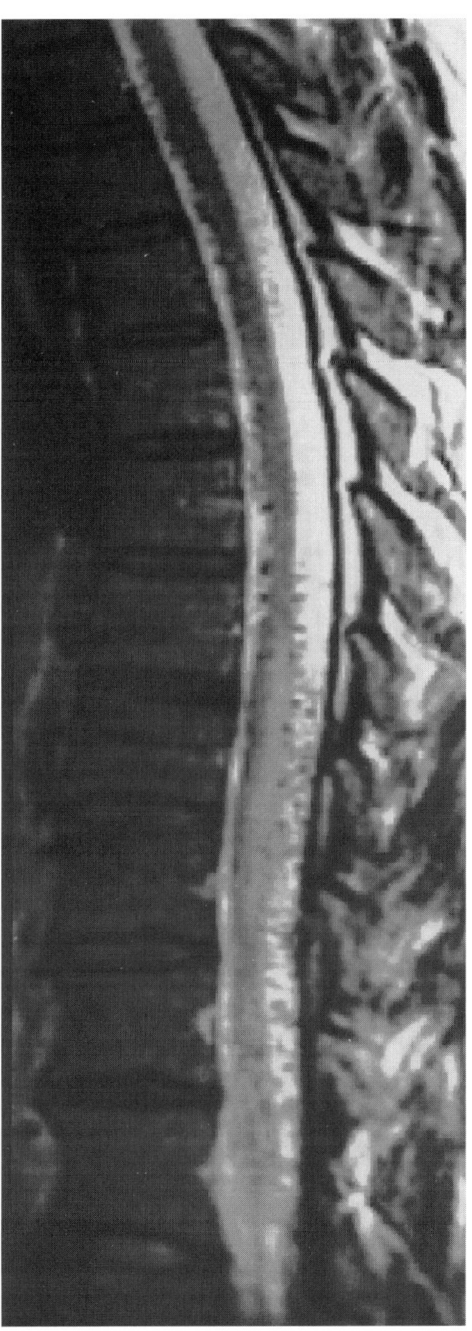

Figure 4.35 *Spinal cord abnormality in a 50-year-old male. Sagittal T2-weighted MRI reveals serpiginous low signal flow voids abutting the dorsal, and to a lesser extent ventral, surfaces of the lumbar cord, and extensive high signal within the cord.*

5   Assigning prognosis

David H Miller

5.1   Introduction

At the time of diagnosis of multiple sclerosis, or even before diagnosis is possible when patients present with a single episode of suspected demyelination, questions regarding prognosis are often foremost for the patient. Unfortunately, clinical features of the early stages of multiple sclerosis are of relatively little prognostic value. A number of studies agree that presentation with optic neuritis or purely sensory symptoms are favourable features [McAlpine 1964; Poser *et al.* 1982], while initial weakness or ataxia is less favourable [Visscher *et al.* 1984; Thompson *et al.* 1986; Phadke 1987]. Nevertheless, the predictive value of such features is weak and of little value in counselling individual patients. Rather more predictive is the patient's disability status five years after the onset of symptoms [Kurtzke *et al.* 1977; Miller *et al.* 1992b], but this observation is hardly surprising since once a substantial disability is established it is unlikely to resolve. What is most needed is a reliable predictor of outcome *before* disability develops; not only would this be of value in counselling patients, it would also enable appropriate selection of patients for trials of new therapies at the earliest stages of the illness.

In the absence of useful clinical prognostic indicators, attention has naturally turned to potential laboratory markers. The HLA antigens and cerebrospinal fluid (CSF) parameters have been most intensively studied. Patients with optic neuritis who are HLA DR2 positive are more likely to progress to clinically definite multiple sclerosis within five years [Compston *et al.* 1978], but with longer follow-up, the increased risk disappears [Francis *et al.* 1987; Sandberg-Wollheim *et al.* 1990]. Numerous reports have established that the presence of CSF oligoclonal IgG bands at presentation with suspected multiple sclerosis confers an increased risk of progression to definite disease over the next few years [Nikolskelainen *et al.* 1981; Moulin *et al.* 1983; Sandberg-Wollheim *et al.* 1990; KH Lee *et al.* 1991]; one study found that oligoclonal IgM bands are even more predictive than IgG bands [Sharief & Thompson 1991]. Nevertheless, the predictive value of oligoclonal bands is moderate rather than marked, and the invasive nature of lumbar puncture makes it unattractive as a routine investigation in many cases with mild, early symptoms, particularly now that MRI is widely used. This chapter will review the status of MRI findings as a prognostic indicator in MS. Several clinical contexts will be considered: (i) MRI abnormalities in healthy individuals with or without relatives with multiple sclerosis; (ii) MRI at presentation with a clinically isolated syndrome and the risk for (a) progression to clinically definite multiple sclerosis and (b) disability; (iii) MRI in established multiple sclerosis and the risk for future disability.

5.2   MRI abnormalities in healthy individuals

It is not uncommon to encounter a brain MRI study showing multifocal white matter lesions in an otherwise healthy individual who may have been studied as a healthy control in a research project, or perhaps who underwent MRI for the evaluation of minor, non-specific neurological symptoms, e.g. headache or dizziness. How should such abnormalities be interpreted? First, the MRI findings should be seen in the light of the patient's age and the radiological pattern – a few small subcortical foci of signal change are a frequent and non-specific finding in older adults and not uncommon in younger adults [Fazekas 1989; Ferbert *et al.* 1991; Thorpe *et al.* 1994f]. Such a pattern is not characteristic of multiple sclerosis, and probably reflects small vessel disease, at least in older age groups, in whom direct pathological verification has been obtained at autopsy [Awad *et al.* 1986]. In older individuals, small vessel disease can produce more extensive white matter changes, including confluent periventricular abnormalities similar to those seen in some MS patients. However, a pattern of multifocal, asymmetrical, predominantly periventricular lesions, some with a rounded or oval shape, and perhaps accompanied by callosal, brain-stem or cerebellar lesions in young adults is most likely due to multiple sclerosis. This 'classical' MRI pattern is rarely seen in healthy young adults, but that it is occasionally seen should not cause surprise: several large post-mortem series have identified unsuspected multiple sclerosis (not diagnosed in life) with a frequency varying from 1 in 500 to 1 in 1000 [Gilbert & Sadler 1983; Phadke & Best 1983] suggesting that asymptomatic multiple sclerosis occurs as often as the disease manifests clinically during life. At this time, it is not known whether healthy individuals with MRI findings typical of MS will develop symptoms of the disease. Given this uncertainty, and the fact that even characteristic MRI patterns are not entirely specific, a diagnosis of multiple sclerosis should not be based on imaging alone.

5.3   MRI in healthy relatives of patients with multiple sclerosis

The likelihood of multiple sclerosis developing in first degree relatives of patients with the disease is significantly higher than the prevalence for the general population. The risk

Table 5.1 *Frequency of 'MS-like'* cerebral white matter abnormalities in asymptomatic co-twins of twins with multiple sclerosis*

	Monozygotic	Dizygotic
Alperovich *et al* 1992	3/13	6/29
Sadovnick *et al* 1993	4/21	1/11
Thorpe *et al* 1994f	2/15	3/33
Total	9/49(18.4%)	10/73(13.7%)

Note:

* 'MS-like' defined using the criteria of Paty (Alperovich) or Fazekas (Sadovnick and Thorpe).

for a first degree relative has been studied most closely by Sadovnick and colleagues [1988] in Canada, where the population prevalence is 1 in 800. Sadovnick has estimated that multiple sclerosis will develop in 2–3% of non-twin siblings and 3–5% of children of patients (with the exception that father–son concordance is extremely rare). In twins with multiple sclerosis, the two largest population-based surveys have reported occurrence of the disease in approximately 5% of dizygotic and 25% of monozygotic co-twins [Ebers *et al.* 1986; Mumford *et al.* 1994]. It has been reported that multifocal multiple sclerosis-like abnormalities occur on brain MRI in about 10% of healthy non-twin siblings in families with two or more cases of multiple sclerosis [Lynch *et al.* 1990; Tienari *et al.* 1992] and 10–20% of healthy co-twins; notably, the incidence is no higher in monozygotic than dizygotic twins [Alperovich *et al.* 1992; Sadovnick *et al.* 1993; Thorpe *et al.* 1994f]. In this respect, three large national twin studies were remarkably consistent in their findings (see Table 5.1). Only with long-term clinical follow-up will the risk of these asymptomatic abnormalities for the development of clinically manifest MS be determined.

5.4   MRI in clinically isolated syndromes: risk for developing multiple sclerosis

5.4.1   Introduction

In over 90% of patients who subsequently develop multiple sclerosis, the first clinical manifestation is with an acute episode of neurological disturbance which characteristically remits, in part or whole, over a period of weeks to months. The initial episode usually implicates either the spinal cord, brain stem, or optic nerves. The eventual rate of conversion to definite multiple sclerosis has been studied most thoroughly in optic neuritis, where several prospective long-term clinical follow-up studies have suggested that 30–70% will develop the disease, with rather higher figures apparent in the United Kingdom than in the United States [Bradley & Whitty 1968; Cohen *et al.* 1979; Perkin & Rose 1979; Landy 1983; Francis *et al.* 1987; Rizzo & Lessell 1988; Sandberg-Wollheim *et al.* 1990]. Until recently, there was very little follow-up data available on patients presenting with an isolated syndrome of the spinal cord or brain stem. Lipton and Teasdall [1973] reported that only one of 29 patients presenting with a complete transverse myelitis subsequently developed multiple sclerosis over more than five years of follow-up. However, a complete transverse myelitis with loss of all function below the lesion is unusual in multiple sclerosis; a partial syndrome is more common.

The prognosis following an acute partial spinal cord syndrome or brain stem syndrome has been more difficult to define than in the case of optic neuritis. This difficulty arises because the clinical syndromes are more heterogeneous, and have a wider differential diagnosis than acute optic neuritis. With the improved diagnostic precision when using MRI at presentation, it has recently been possible to identify appropriate cohorts with these syndromes, in whom demyelination is considered likely. In such a cohort, Morrissey *et al.* [1993a] have recently described the rate of conversion to multiple sclerosis after a mean follow-up of around five years: 24/44 (56%) who had presented with optic neuritis (mean follow-up 66 months), 8/17 (47%) with a brain stem syndrome (mean follow-up 70 months), and 11/28 (39%) with a spinal cord syndrome (mean follow-up 56 months). Allowing for slight differences in the length of follow-up, it appears that the overall risk for developing multiple sclerosis is similar for all three syndromes. This section now deals with MRI findings at presentation with such syndromes and their predictive value for the future development of clinically definite MS.

5.4.2   Conventional PD/T2-weighted brain MRI

In the last decade, many groups have reported brain MRI findings in patients at presentation with isolated syndromes suggestive of multiple sclerosis. Optic neuritis has been most extensively studied. There is a consistent agreement in that about 50–70% of individuals demonstrate clinically silent cerebral white matter lesions on MRI at presentation [Ormerod *et al.* 1986a; Jacobs *et al.* 1986; Stadt *et al.* 1990; Frederiksen *et al.* 1991; Martinelli *et al.* 1991] (Figure 5.1). The lesions are usually multiple and their appearances indistinguishable from those seen in established multiple sclerosis. Excluding cases in whom MRI has revealed an alternative diagnosis, a similar proportion of patients presenting with isolated syndromes of the spinal cord and brain stem also manifest asymptomatic cerebral white matter lesions [Ormerod *et al.* 1986b; Miller *et al.* 1987a; Ford *et al.* 1992].

The presence of such lesions does not allow an immediate diagnosis of multiple sclerosis, since the criterion of dissemination in time is not yet fulfilled – it is conceivable

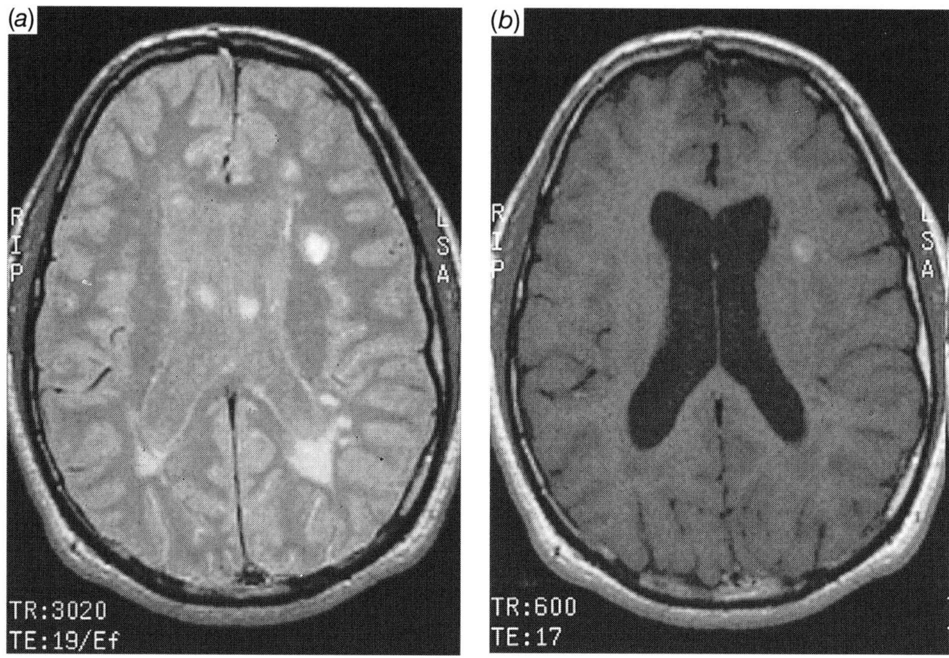

Figure 5.1 *Clinically isolated optic neuritis. (a) PD-weighted MRI reveals multifocal white matter abnormalities indistinguishable from those seen in established multiple sclerosis. (b) Gadolinium enhanced T1-weighted MRI reveals enhancement of one of the lesions.*

that some of these patients have the multifocal yet monophasic demyelinating disorder acute disseminated encephalomyelitis (ADEM). In adult life, ADEM is rare and multiple sclerosis is common, so it is likely that the lesions are most often due to multiple sclerosis. A critical issue is to determine the frequency with which the clinically manifest disease expresses itself subsequently, and whether the MRI abnormalities can predict future clinical events.

A number of follow-up studies, ranging from one to five years, have consistently reported a higher rate of progression to multiple sclerosis in those with MRI abnormalities at presentation compared with those with normal scan (Table 5.2). The earliest report was from Miller and co-workers at The National Hospital in London, who reported their findings after a mean follow-up of 12 months in 53 patients presenting with isolated optic neuritis [Miller *et al.* 1988d]. New symptoms and/or signs allowing a diagnosis of clinically definite or probable multiple sclerosis (using the Poser criteria [Poser *et al.* 1983]) were seen in 12/34 (36%) patients with abnormal brain MRI at presentation, but in none of 19 with a normal scan. A higher incidence of patients manifesting new MRI lesions was also noted in the group with an abnormal initial scan (12/34 versus 3/19). The same research team also reported their follow-up findings after a mean

Table 5.2 *Clinically isolated syndromes: brain MRI at presentation and risk for subsequent progression to multiple sclerosis*

Study	Duration of follow-up (months)	Progression to MS†	
		Abnormal MRI	Normal MRI
Martinelli *et al* 1991	32	7/21 (33%)	0/22
Frederiksen *et al* 1991	11	7/31 (23%)	0/19
KH Lee *et al* 1991[+]	24	52/118 (44%)	3/66 (5%)
Jacobs *et al* 1991	48	6/23 (26%)	3/25 (12%)
Ford *et al* 1992	39	11/12 (93%)	1/3
Morrissey *et al* 1993a	64	37/57 (65%)	1/32 (3%)
Beck *et al* 1993	24	16/56 (31%)	2/62 (3%)*
Soderstrom *et al* 1994	24	14/38 (37%)	3/22 (14%)
Tas *et al* 1995	14	16/34 (47%)	1/23 (4%)*
Campi *et al* 1995	18	8/11 (73%)	0/19
Total		174/401 (43%)	14/293 (5%)

Note:

† Clinically or laboratory supported definite multiple sclerosis

[+] Includes cases of clinically probable multiple sclerosis and chronic progressive myelopathy

* Includes minor abnormalities, all small or non-periventricular

of 16 months in 56 patients who had presented with an isolated syndrome of the spinal cord or brain stem [Miller *et al.* 1989b]. New clinical relapses allowing a diagnosis of clinically probable or definite multiple sclerosis were seen in 17/35 (48%) with an abnormal initial scan and in only 1/21 (5%) with a normal scan. Fredriksen [1991] and Martinelli [1991] reported similar outcomes in their cohorts of patients with optic neuritis: after respective mean follow-up of 11 and 32 months, clinically definite multiple sclerosis had developed in 7/31 (23%) and 7/21 (33%) with abnormal MRI but in none of 41 patients with a normal initial scan.

More recently, Morrissey performed a five-year follow-up of the same cohort of National Hospital patients studied by Miller after 12–16 months [Morrissey *et al.* 1993a]. By this time, progression to clinically definite multiple sclerosis had occurred in 37/57 (65%) with an abnormal MRI and in only 1/32 (3%) with a normal scan. The outcome was similar for each subgroup of patients. Thus for optic neuritis patients, multiple sclerosis developed in 23/28 with an abnormal MRI and 1/16 without disseminated lesions; the corresponding outcomes for those with a spinal cord syndrome were 10/17 and 1/11, and for those with a brain stem syndrome 8/12 and 0/5.

Ford [1992] examined 15 patients with an isolated partial myelitis. Brain MRI was abnormal in 12 and normal in three; at follow-up after a mean of 38 months, 11/12 with MRI abnormalities had developed clinically or laboratory supported definite multiple sclerosis, compared with only 1/3 without lesions.

The study of Beck *et al.* [1993] is important as it was a particularly large study of patients who had been recruited into the North American Optic Neuritis Treatment Trial. The primary aim of this study was to ascertain whether or not a course of steroids, either high dose intravenous methylprednisolone(IVMP) followed by oral prednisolone or oral prednisolone alone, improved visual outcome in comparison with placebo. The study concluded that although the speed of recovery is hastened by IVMP followed by oral prednisolone [Beck *et al.* 1992], the final visual outcome is not affected [Beck & Cleary 1993]. An unexpected observation was that the rate of progression to multiple sclerosis after two years was halved in the group treated by IVMP [Beck *et al.* 1993], but there was no difference in progression rate with longer follow-up [Beck 1995]. Most patients had brain MRI scans at entry, but because of the apparent modifying effect of IVMP on progression to MS during the first two years, evaluation of the predictive value of MRI is best ascertained by concentrating on the placebo group. In this group, clinically definite multiple sclerosis had developed after two years of follow-up in only 2/62 (3%) with either a normal brain MRI or grade 1 abnormalities (defined as either small or non-periventricular abnormalities). In contrast, 16/51 (31%) with more extensive MRI abnormalities had developed MS.

Both Morrissey's and Beck's studies have extended the observations in showing that the number or grade of MRI abnormalities also influences the risk for developing multiple sclerosis. Thus in the London cohort, progression to multiple sclerosis was seen in 13/24 (54%) with one to three lesions and in 28/33 (85%) with four or more lesions; in the placebo arm of the US trial, multiple sclerosis developed after two years in 2/12 (17%) with grade 2 MRI abnormalities (one periventricular or ovoid lesion at least 3 mm in size) and in 14/39 (36%) with grade 3 or 4 MRI abnormalities (two or more periventricular or ovoid lesions at least 3 mm in size).

KH Lee and colleagues [1991] reported their two-year follow-up findings on a group of 200 patients in whom multiple sclerosis was suspected at presentation but could not be classified as definite. This cohort was more heterogeneous than those in the studies already mentioned: it included not only those with an isolated acute syndrome such as optic neuritis, but also patients with chronic progressive myelopathy or those with clinically probable multiple sclerosis. Nevertheless, the follow-up findings are remarkably consistent with the series of Morrissey and Beck. After two years, 16 were proved to have an alternative diagnosis. Of the remaining 184 patients, 55 had developed clinically definite multiple sclerosis by having 'clinical relapses, appropriate clinical progression or both'. Clinically definite disease developed in 46/94 (48%) with the initial MRI classified as 'strongly suggestive of multiple sclerosis' (four lesions present, all non-periventricular, or three lesions present and at least one periventricular), 6/24 (25%) with one to three lesions, none of which were periventricular, and in only 3/66 (5%) with normal MRI.

The study of Jacobs *et al.* [1991] is notable, in that MRI findings did not confirm an altered risk for developing multiple sclerosis. Patients with isolated optic neuritis were followed up for a mean of four years. As reported in all other studies, there was a low frequency of progression to multiple sclerosis in those with normal MRI at presentation: at follow-up only 3/25 (12%) had developed MS. However, only 6/23 (25%) with abnormal MRI had converted to multiple sclerosis in the same period. In seeking an explanation for this discrepancy, it is relevant to note that the range of follow-up in Jacobs' series was extremely variable, ranging between two months and 15.5 years from the onset of optic neuritis. The inclusion of cases who are first scanned several years after the onset of optic neuritis introduces the bias that cases were excluded in whom clinical conversion to multiple sclerosis had already taken place; on the other hand, cases who have been followed up for only a few months will naturally exhibit a lower rate of clinical conversion.

Three more recent studies show a clearly increased risk of conversion to multiple sclerosis if MRI abnormalities are present:

(1) After a follow-up mean of 24 months in 60 patients who had presented with isolated optic neuritis, Soderstrom *et al.* [1994] found conversion to multiple sclerosis in 14/38 (37%) with MRI abnormalities and 3/19 (16%) with a normal scan.

(2) Of 30 patients presenting with an isolated transverse myelitis who were followed up after a mean of 18 months, progression to multiple sclerosis was seen in 8/11 (73%) with MRI abnormalities and none of 19 with a normal scan [Campi *et al.* 1995]. In this study, it was also notable that the multiple sclerosis cases usually had small cord lesions, less than one vertebral segment in length; in contrast, much longer lesions were seen in many patients with a monophasic transverse myelitis.

(3) In the third study, follow-up after 14 months in 57 patients who had presented with a clinically isolated syndrome revealed that multiple sclerosis had developed in 16/34 (47%) with MRI abnormalities fulfilling the Paty criteria (as defined in KH Lee *et al.* [1991]) but in only 1/23 (4%) with a normal scan or minor abnormalities not satisfying the Paty criteria [Tas *et al.* 1995].

When the results of all the currently published studies are considered as a whole, the evidence is compelling that brain MRI findings at first presentation with a clinical syndrome compatible with multiple sclerosis are highly predictive of the risk of subsequent conversion to definite disease in the next one to five years. This information is of practical importance in counselling individual patients, and will be useful in selecting appropriate patients for trials of therapy aimed at preventing the conversion from suspected to definite multiple sclerosis – indeed, it is already being used in this manner. For those patients presenting with a normal MRI, an optimistic prognosis can be given – only about 5% of these individuals will develop definite multiple sclerosis in the next five years. Of course, much longer follow-up is needed to elucidate the final risk for this patient cohort. We have recently started a 10-year follow-up of some of the original cohort seen at The National Hospital, Queen Square – to date 24 patients with a normal initial scan have been reviewed, and of these 3 (13%) have developed clinically definite multiple sclerosis [O'Riordan *et al.* 1996a].

5.4.3   Gadolinium enhancement

There is less published experience concerning the findings of gadolinium enhanced MRI at presentation with a clinically isolated syndrome suggestive of multiple sclerosis. Miller and colleagues [1987c] described their experience of ten patients with isolated optic neuritis who underwent both PD/T2-weighted and gadolinium enhanced brain MRI. Six patients had multiple PD/T2 abnormalities, in three of whom some but not all of the lesions displayed gadolinium enhancement, while in three none of the lesions enhanced. Christiansen [1992] performed the same MRI assessment in 19 patients at presentation with isolated optic neuritis. The MRI examinations were obtained a mean of 12 days after the onset of visual loss. There were multiple PD/T2 white matter lesions in 14(73%); in 7/19(37%) all the PD/T2 lesions were non-enhancing, while in 7/19(37%), some but not all lesions enhanced. Finally, Youl [1992] studied 18 patients within 14 days of the onset of optic neuritis. There were PD/T2 abnormalities in 11; enhancement of some lesions was seen in six.

Taking these three studies together, it appears that patients with optic neuritis can be divided into three groups of roughly equal size according to brain MRI findings at presentation: one third have completely normal imaging, another third have multiple non-enhancing PD/T2 lesions, and one third have a mixture of enhancing and non-enhancing lesions (Figure 5.1). It could be postulated that a mixture of enhancing and non-enhancing lesions indicates multiphasic disease and by inference is strong evidence in favour of a diagnosis of multiple sclerosis rather than ADEM. However, if the scan is obtained within one month of the onset of visual symptoms and all the brain lesions are non-enhancing, it is also likely that multiphasic disease exists, since most non-enhancing lesions are likely to be older than one month. The practical issue of importance here is whether or not enhancement is associated with an altered risk for future progression to multiple sclerosis.

Barkhof [1994] has addressed this issue by follow-up of a cohort of 67 patients who had undergone PD/T2-weighted and gadolinium enhanced MRI within a median of four weeks of presenting with a clinically isolated syndrome suggestive of multiple sclerosis. After a median follow-up of 14 months, 22 (34%) had developed clinically definite disease. Multiple sclerosis had developed in 21/45 (47%) with MRI abnormalities typical of the disease on PD/T2-weighted images (four lesions all non-periventricular or three lesions, one of which is periventricular), and in only 1/22 (5%) with lesser degrees of abnormality or a normal scan. One or more gadolinium enhancing lesions were seen in 18 patients, of whom 14 (78%) developed multiple sclerosis at follow-up. However, eight patients without gadolinium enhancing lesions had also developed the disease, indicating that enhancement is less sensitive than 'classical' PD/T2-weighted abnormalities in identifying patients who will develop multiple sclerosis, although it is more specific and carries a higher risk of progression, at least over the first year of follow-up.

Based on the data currently available, it is clear that PD/T2-weighted images provide powerful prognostic information in patients presenting with clinically isolated syndromes. The additional value of gadolinium enhancement is that it detects a subset who are particularly likely to progress to multiple sclerosis within one year; longer follow-up is needed to ascertain whether this difference is maintained.

5.5 MRI in clinically isolated syndromes: risk for disability

To date, there has been much less data concerning MRI and the subsequent risk for disability. This is hardly surprising, since very few patients become severely disabled within the first five years from disease onset. The experience of the National Hospital cohort is the most informative source of data at the present time. After five years, only 8% had developed a severe disability (EDSS $\geq$ 6) but 20% had at least moderate disability (EDSS $\geq$ 3). The likelihood of obtaining a moderate disability did correlate significantly with the initial number of PD/T2-weighted MRI lesions [Morrissey *et al.* 1993a] and with the total lesion load [Filippi *et al.* 1994a], the latter being measured using a semi-automated thresholding technique for segmenting lesions [Wicks *et al.* 1992]. No patient with no or one lesion at presentation had an EDSS greater than or equal to three after five years; however 17% with two to three lesions did, as did 30% with four to ten lesions and 56% with more than ten lesions [Morrissey *et al.* 1993a]. The quantified initial lesion load correlated moderately with the EDSS after five years ($r = 0.62$, $p < 0.0001$) and with the increase in lesion load over the five years ($r = 0.61$, $p < 0.0001$) [Filippi *et al.* 1994a] (see also Table 5.3, and Figures 5.2 and 5.3).

These data suggest an important predictive value of MRI for subsequent neurological impairment and disability when obtained at or near the clinical onset of the disease. Nevertheless, further studies are needed, both from other centres and also with longer follow-up of the National Hospital cohort. This is especially needed to ascertain the relationship between initial MRI findings and the more severe locomotor disabilities (e.g. inability to walk unaided or inability to walk at all), which for most patients develop only after ten to 15 years or longer from the onset of symptoms.

5.6 MRI in established multiple sclerosis: risk for disability

5.6.1 Conventional PD/T2-weighted brain MRI

In contrast to clinically isolated syndromes, little if any correlation has to date emerged between conventional PD/T2-weighted MRI findings in established multiple sclerosis and the patient's current, evolving or future disability status. Indeed, Thompson [1990b] has noted paradoxically that the small group of patients who have progressive disease

Table 5.3 *Clinically isolated syndromes: five-year follow-up (Filippi et al 1994a)*

	Group A	Group B	Group C
Progression to MS*	19/21 (90%)	17/31 (55%)	2/32 (6%)
Clinically definite	18 (86%)	15 (48%)	1 (3%)
Clinically probable	1 (4%)	2 (7%)	1 (3%)
EDSS $\geq$ 3**	11/21 (52%)	7/31 (23%)	0/32 (0%)
Increased lesion† load $\geq$ 1cm³	18/21 (86%)	11/31 (35%)	2/32 (6%)

Note:

Group A – initial lesion load > 1.23 cm³

Group B – initial MR abnormal, lesion load < 1.23 cm³

Group C – initial MR normal

* A vs B p < 0.01; A vs C p < 0.001; B vs C p < 0.001

** A vs B p < 0.05; A vs C p < 0.001; B vs C p < 0.005

† A vs B p < 0.001; A vs C p < 0.001; B vs C p < 0.005

(All statistical comparisons performed using chi-squared test)

MS = multiple sclerosis

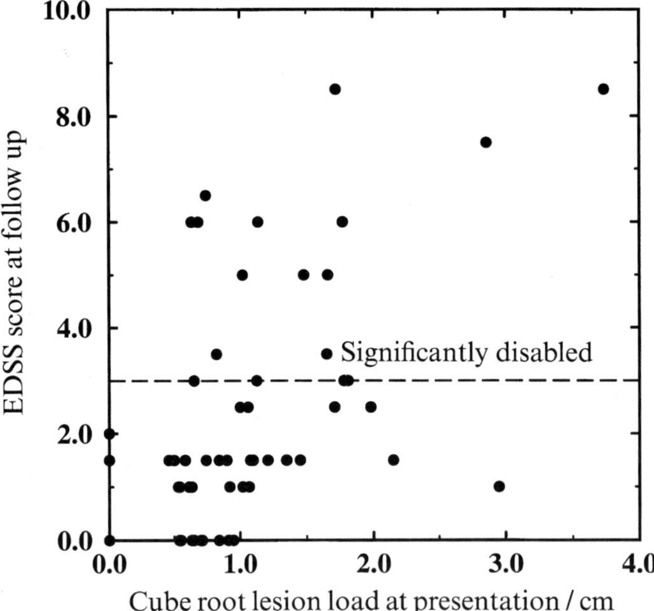

Figure 5.2 *Correlation between T2 lesion load at presentation with a clinically isolated syndrome and disability (EDSS) five years later. (From Filippi et al. 1994a.)*

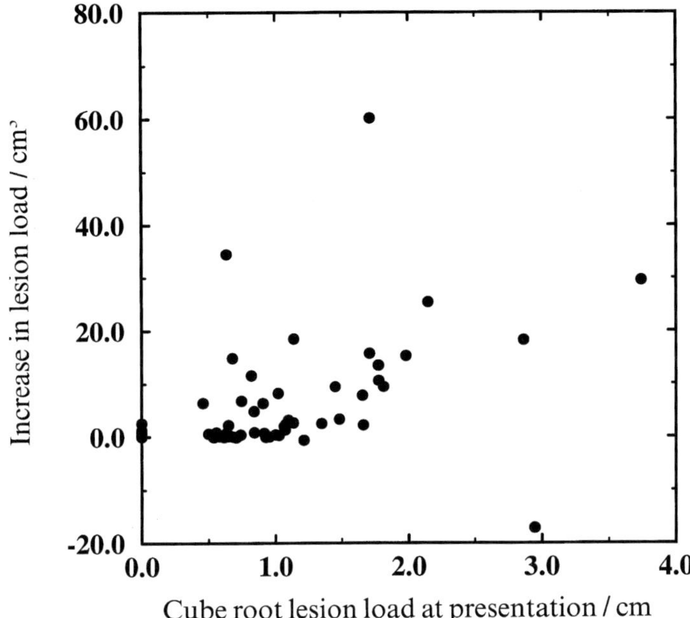

Figure 5.3 *Correlation between T2 lesion load at presentation with a clinically isolated syndrome and change in T2 lesion load over the next five years. (From Filippi et al. 1994a.)*

from onset (primary progressive multiple sclerosis), and who accumulate major disabilities, actually have a smaller brain lesion load than patients with benign disease.

Several methodological factors may contribute to the poor correlations seen in many studies. While a lack of relationship between brain MRI lesion load and locomotor disability is not too surprising, since the majority of brain lesions do not involve motor tracts, it might be expected that the more lesions there are, the more by chance will affect such pathways and thereby cause disability. However, a large sample size might be required to demonstrate a statistical association, and many studies may have failed in this regard because only relatively small numbers of patients were surveyed.

A lack of relationship between changes on MRI and EDSS in short-term follow-up studies (e.g. 6–12 months) is also not too surprising, since in general disability alters little over such periods. Furthermore, the number of patients in such reported studies has also been small and probably insufficient to recognise a correlation. Also, the techniques for measuring lesion load have often been relatively crude – now that computerised techniques are available for accurate outlining of lesions, this deficiency should not arise in future studies.

In order to overcome the problem of small sample size and limited follow-up, four centres have recently pooled their data on 281 patients who had had both a T2-weighted brain MRI scan and an EDSS assessment on two occasions separated by an interval of two to three years [Filippi *et al.* 1995d]. A weak but statistically significant correlation did indeed emerge between a change in EDSS on the one hand and the number of new and enlarging T2-weighted lesions on the other ($r = 0.13$, $p = 0.04$). That a correlation existed at all is noteworthy, given the highly heterogeneous nature of the data: the field strength of the scanners used ranged from 0.15 T to 1.5 T, slice thickness from 5 mm to 10 mm, multiple raters were used for both the MRI and EDSS evaluations and patients were heterogeneous with respect to the disease course, disease duration, and the use of immunomodulatory therapies during the observation period. A stronger subgroup correlation emerged when only untreated patients with relapsing-remitting disease were analysed ($r = 0.30$, $p = 0.02$).

The North American Trial of interferon β-1b in relapsing-remitting multiple sclerosis provided another opportunity to examine the relationship between PD/T2-weighted brain MRI and EDSS in a large cohort over a period of several years. Although there was a modest correlation between lesion load and EDSS at entry and exit, there was not a significant association between changes in the two parameters over the first two to three years [Paty *et al.* 1993]. However, a correlation did emerge in the smaller group of patients who continued to be followed up for a fourth year ($r = 0.23$, $p < 0.05$; [The IFNB Study Group 1995] Table 7.3).

Overall, these studies suggest that there is a significant relationship between long-term changes on conventional PD/T2-weighted brain MRI and EDSS in established multiple sclerosis, but in comparison with clinically isolated syndrome cohorts, it is relatively weak. Probably a stronger relationship will emerge in a large cohort which is clinically highly homogeneous (e.g. with a narrowly defined disease duration and EDSS at entry to a study), and in whom MRI data is collected in a uniform manner for each patient, ideally on the same scanner. Nevertheless it seems likely that even with such methodological improvements, correlations between the total load of conventional MRI abnormalities in the brain and disability will be moderate rather than strong. Three other MR strategies are now considered which might be expected to yield stronger correlations with disability: (i) quantitation of lesions of locomotor pathways in the brain; (ii) spinal cord MRI; (iii) MR techniques to improve pathological specificity.

5.6.2   Quantitation of lesions of locomotor pathways in the brain

Naturally, lesions directly implicating pyramidal pathways may contribute to spastic paraparesis and those in the cerebellum, cerebellar peduncles or brain stem may contribute to ataxia. There is surprisingly little published work in which lesions have been classified and quantitated within such structures. However, Koopmans [1989b] and Filippi [1994b] have demonstrated a higher infratentorial lesion load in patients with chronic or secondary progressive multiple sclerosis in comparison with those with benign disease, while Baumhefner [1990] has reported a correlation between brain-stem lesion area and clinical deficits measured on the Kurtzke scale. These associations were modest, and were obtained using relatively low resolution MRI systems. The fact that there is a better correlation between the length of the MRI detected optic nerve lesion and visual outcome following an attack of optic neuritis [Miller *et al.* 1988b; Thorpe *et al.* 1995] suggests that stronger associations between MRI and disability will indeed emerge when the extent to which lesions involve the relevant locomotor pathways can be more accurately quantified. Resolution will greatly improve with the expected widespread availability of 3D fast spin echo sequences in the near future. These should allow 1 mm thick slices. Nevertheless, given the pathological observation that lesions tend to be orientated in relation to venules rather than nerve fibre tracts [Lumsden 1970; Fog 1965], it would not be too surprising if the correlations between MRI lesions and disability remain modest even with better resolution.

5.6.3   Spinal cord MRI

Spinal cord disease accounts for much of the locomotor disability in multiple sclerosis. Therefore, a recent study of 80 patients using multi-array coils and T2-weighted fast spin echo (technique described in Chapter 2), was both surprising and disappointing in that it revealed no association whatever between the number and extent of cord lesions seen on sagittal images and EDSS [Kidd *et al.* 1993]. Better resolution of lesions in relation to motor pathways is now needed using axial imaging or 3D fast spin echo.

5.6.4   MR techniques to improve pathological specificity

An important, and perhaps the most important, explanation for the limited relationship bewteen conventional PD/T2-weighted MRI abnormalities and functional deficit is pathophysiological heterogeneity of lesions which all appear the same on the conventional image. As discussed in detail in Chapter 6, a PD/T2-weighted MRI while highly sensitive to multiple sclerosis plaques, has a low pathological specificity. All the cardinal pathological features of MS lesions – oedema, inflammation, demyelination, gliosis and axonal loss – will result directly or indirectly in an increase in water content and thus signal hyperintensity on a PD/T2-weighted image. However, the functional consequences of these features are different. Inflammation is likely to contribute to acute, reversible deficits (see Chapter 6). In causing conduction block, demyelination also contributes to acute deficits, and perhaps to chronic disability, although conduction may be restored in persistently demyelinated axons [Bostock & Sears 1978; Black *et al.* 1991; Moll *et al.* 1991]. Axonal loss, if substantial, will cause persistent, irreversible disabilities. Thus it might be hoped that a stronger correlation with clinical status will emerge when MR techniques are employed which specifically identify the pathological features thought to underlie the functional deficits, namely inflammation and demyelination in acute relapse, and axonal loss and (possibly) persistent demyelination in chronic disability.

5.6.4.1   *Gadolinium enhancement and acute relapse*

Beyond reasonable doubt gadolinium enhancement in multiple sclerosis lesions indicates the presence of an active inflammatory process – two studies on post-mortem or biopsy tissues suggest this [Katz *et al.* 1993; Rodriguez *et al.* 1993]. The association of gadolinium enhancement and inflammation has also been documented in studies in chronic relapsing experimental allergic encephalomyelitis [Hawkins *et al.* 1990a]. Gadolinium enhancing lesions are more commonly seen during clinical relapses [Grossman *et al.* 1986; Miller *et al.* 1988a; Bastianello *et al.* 1990; Harris *et al.* 1991; Thompson *et al.* 1991]. Enhancement is a regular feature of new MRI lesions, and generally lasts two to six weeks, similar to the duration of relapses (although the majority of enhancing cerebral lesions are symptomatic). In acute optic neuritis, enhancement of the symptomatic lesion is associated with acute visual loss and conduction block (the latter measured on visual evoked potentials); cessation of enhancement coincides with recovery of vision and restoration of conduction [Youl *et al.* 1991b]. In conclusion, new gadolinium enhancing lesions appear likely to produce acute reversible clinical deficits when strategically placed.

5.6.4.2   *Gadolinium enhancement and long-term disability*

A crucial question is whether the amount of MRI activity in a short duration follow-up study – for example the number of new enhancing lesions on monthly MRI over six months – is predictive of disability status several years later? A positive association would lend strong justification to the present widespread use of MRI to perform an initial evaluation of the efficacy of new treatments in short-term studies. However, at this time, the predictive value of short-term MRI activity is not fully elucidated because clinical follow-up studies of a sufficient duration and including adequate patient numbers have not been performed. Nevertheless, current observations suggest that a significant association will emerge. Firstly, at the National Institutes of Health in Washington, nine patients with relapsing-remitting MS have been followed with monthly scanning for up to three years [Smith *et al.* 1993]. A close relationship between clinical relapse and the number and area of gadolinium enhancing brain lesions has been noted; a non-significant trend has also appeared for disability (due to relapse) to increase more in patients with large enhancing lesion numbers or area. Secondly, another study followed 18 patients for one year with frequent scanning (weekly to monthly) and clinical (monthly) assessment [Khoury *et al.* 1994]; a positive correlation, albeit of low magnitude, was found between the cumulative number of new MRI lesions and deterioration in disability. Thirdly, Paty [1992a] noted a weak relationship between the number of new lesions seen on PD/T2-weighted MRI (gadolinium enhancement was not undertaken) performed at two- to four-week intervals for six months, and clinical status four years later in a group of 24 patients (Table 5.4). Finally, in 11 secondary progressive patients who underwent monthly gadolinium enhanced scanning for six months, those who had the greatest increase in disability five years later had significantly more enhancing lesions during the initial study [Losseff *et al.* 1995a].

All these observations are very preliminary; longer follow-up in larger cohorts is

Table 5.4 *Clinical outcome on 24 multiple sclerosis patients in the original UBC (Vancouver) serial studies (about four years' follow-up)*

	Clinically worse	Clinically Stable
Number of patients	7	17
Average no. active lesions during study	9.9 (2–26)	3.4 (0–13)
Average no. new lesions	3.1 (1–6)	1.7 (0–5)
Average no. reactive lesions	6.8 (0–20)	1.6 (0–9)

Table 5.5 *Putative MR markers of demyelination and axonal loss in multiple sclerosis*

Technique	Marker
Unenhanced T1–weighted spin echo	Hypointensity
Magnetisation transfer imaging	Low MT ratio
Multi-echo T2-weighted spin echo	(i) Loss of very short T2 component
	(ii) Appearance of long T2 component
Proton MR spectroscopy	(i) Lipid peaks
	(ii) Reduced NAA
Diffusion imaging	Increased diffusion coefficient and loss of anisotropy
Spinal cord cross-sectional area	Cord atrophy
Corpus callosum area	White matter atrophy

Note:

(From Miller *et al.* 1996, reprinted from *Annals of Neurology* V39, pp. 6–16, by permission of Little, Brown & Co. Inc.)

required to define properly the relationship between short-term MRI activity and long-term disability in established multiple sclerosis.

5.6.4.3 *MR markers of axonal loss/demyelination and chronic disability*

There are at least seven putative MR markers for the tissue disruption and destruction which results from axonal loss and/or demyelination (Table 5.5). Several recent studies have revealed stronger correlations between disability and these putative markers than between disability and conventional T2-weighted MRI findings.

Firstly, Gass [1994] found that magnetisation transfer ratio abnormalities of cerebral lesions correlated more strongly with disability ($r = -0.44$) than with conventional PD/T2 lesion load ($r = 0.33$). Secondly, Kidd [1993] examined the relationship between spinal cord MRI and disability. While there was no relationship of disability with either the number or load of lesions seen on the conventional T2-weighted cord image, those patients with atrophy, as measured from axial gradient echo images through the spinal cord at four levels (C5, T2, T7, and T11), had significantly more disability than those with a normally sized cord. Atrophy reflects tissue loss and by inference demyelination and/or axonal degeneration.

Thirdly, Davie [1995] has used proton spectroscopy to study the concentration of *N*-acetyl aspartate (NAA), a neuronal marker, in the cerebellum of MS patients with and without ataxia. The concentration of NAA in non-ataxic patients was normal when compared with healthy controls, but was significantly less in the ataxic group. Autosomal dominant cerebellar ataxia, a pathological control group in which neuronal loss in the Purkinje cell layer is known to occur, was found to have a low concentration of NAA similar to that in the ataxic multiple sclerosis patients.

Fourthly, Filippi [1994b] found a higher incidence of chronic lesions with biexponential T2 decay in patients with secondary progressive MS compared with a benign cohort. Biexponentiality in chronic lesions is probably due to an expanded extracellular space [Barnes *et al.* 1991], and this in turn may develop when there is extensive axonal loss.

Finally, van Walderveen [1995] obtained baseline and two-year follow-up T2-weighted brain MRI scans in 49 multiple sclerosis patients plus additional gadolinium enhanced T1-weighted scans in 19. The total load of T2 hyperintense lesions and non-enhancing T1 hypointense lesions was measured on each occasion using a computer assisted seed growing technique, and disability was recorded using the EDSS scale. There was a weak and non-significant association ($r = 0.19$) between change in T2 lesion load and change in disability; however, the correlation between change in T1 lesion load and disability was much stronger ($r = 0.76$) and statistically significant. A strong correlation exists between lesion hypointensity on T1-weighted images and low magnetisation transfer ratios of the lesions [Hiehle *et al.* 1995; Loevner *et al.* 1995]; thus, hypointense lesions on T1-weighted images probably have substantial amounts of tissue loss.

These promising but preliminary observations suggesting a stronger relationship between putative MR markers of demyelination and axonal loss on the one hand and disability on the other, now need to be extended by follow-up studies in order to determine the longitudinal relationship between the putative markers and clinical change. In parallel, experimental studies are needed in order to consolidate the hypothesis that these parameters are indeed reliable in demonstrating demyelination and axonal loss. Further techniques, most notably diffusion imaging [Larsson *et al.* 1992; Horsfield *et al.* 1994], measurement of the short T2 component of myelin using multi-echo sequences [MacKay *et al.* 1994], and accurate quantitation of progressive cerebral atrophy [Losseff *et al.* 1996b] may also prove useful as markers of tissue destruction. In particular, with the acquisition of echo planar imaging systems, the evaluation of diffusion imaging and its relationship to clinical status in multiple sclerosis will be well worth while. Such work is important, as it offers the prospect of identifying objective and quantifiable laboratory markers which predict the future clinical course and in particular the evolution of disability.

6   Pathogenesis and mechanisms of disability

Alan J Thompson

6.1   MR/pathology correlates

The pathological characteristics of the multiple sclerosis lesion seen at post-mortem have been well documented and include demyelination, relative preservation of axons, gliosis and inflammation [Carswell 1838; Charcot 1868; Dawson 1916; Adams 1989]. Because of the inaccessibility of the central nervous system to histological study during life it has not been possible until recently to document the dynamics of the disease process. This is now being achieved through the application of serial MRI.

The first study which addressed the relationship between pathology and MRI findings in multiple sclerosis, carried out in 1984, showed a very close correlation between the pattern of pathological change and MRI abnormalities demonstrated on a 0.15 tesla machine with 10 mm slice thickness [Stewart *et al.* 1984]. Images from the fixed brain tissue of a single case showed a pattern of abnormality identical to that already described in the patient population and involved the periventricular area and brain stem. These findings were supported by a second study using a 0.5 tesla machine in 1987 [Ormerod *et al.* 1987] which looked at six formalin fixed histologically proven cases and again showed an excellent correlation between pathological change and MRI, allowing for the fact that the MR signal represents an average over a 10 mm slice whereas histology is only 30 μm thick, and therefore the configuration of lesions was not identical. The authors suggested that the signal in acute lesions was likely to result mainly from oedema while in chronic lesions gliosis might be responsible. It was felt that demyelination *per se* was unlikely to make a major contribution to the MR signal.

A further study carried out on the unfixed whole brain tissue of 17 multiple sclerosis cases and six controls showed a reasonable correlation between pathological lesions and MRI abnormality [Newcombe *et al.* 1991]. In five cases the area of MRI abnormality appeared greater than obvious pathological change. Pathological abnormalities in the cerebral grey matter and brain stem were often not detected on MRI. Furthermore, abnormalities were detected in the spinal cord on both MRI and histological examination (in three cases MRI abnormalities and histological plaques were restricted to the cord).

Finally, microscopic abnormalities, such as small foci of perivascular inflammation or myelin breakdown products, or astrocyte hyperplasia, are well recognised at post-mortem in multiple sclerosis [Allen *et al.* 1981]. In vivo MR studies using a number of different quantitative techniques have reported abnormalities in the normal appearing white matter [Miller *et al.* 1989a; Dousset *et al.* 1992; Barbosa *et al.* 1994; Husted *et al.* 1994b]. The extent to which these 'normal' white matter abnormalities contribute to clinical dysfunction in multiple sclerosis is at present unclear.

In summary there are a number of distinct components to the pathological evolution of lesions in multiple sclerosis:

(1) A disturbance of the blood–brain barrier.

(2) An inflammatory process which is usually perivascular and may be associated with oedema.

(3) Demyelination which usually, though not inevitably, follows inflammation.

(4) Gliosis which develops during or following demyelination.

(5) Axonal loss which is likely to result in irreversible disability and may be associated with an expanded extracellular space.

It is important to appreciate that the high signal areas seen on PD/T2-weighted MRI scans give no indication of the underlying pathological process, and each of the processes may contribute to a greater or lesser extent. Furthermore, the clinical sequelae of each of these processes may differ considerably, particularly in relation to the crucial issue of the development of disability.

It is possible to learn more of the individual processes through other MRI techniques. The significance of enhancement with the contrast agent gadolinium diethylenetri-amine pentacetic acid (Gd-DTPA) has been studied both in chronic relapsing experi-mental allergic encephalomyelitis (CREAE) and, more recently, in multiple sclerosis [Katz *et al.* 1993]. The findings suggest that gadolinium enhancement indicates increased permeability or leakage of the blood–brain barrier in association with inflammation. This interpretation is supported by a single case study of a patient who died of another cause ten days after gadolinium enhanced MRI [Katz *et al.* 1993]. Enhancing lesions showed intense perivascular inflammation whereas non-enhancing lesions did not.

Information regarding other pathological processes may be acquired from more recently developed imaging techniques (discussed in Chapter 2). The detection of active demyelination requires the demonstration of myelin degradation products or lipid. A number of MR techniques, notably echo difference imaging [Hawkins *et al.* 1990b] have been applied but have met with only limited success because of a poor signal-to-noise ratio. A more promising technique is MR spectroscopy which with short echo times can demonstrate lipid peaks in the acute lesion [Davie *et al.* 1994a].

It is particularly important to be able to demonstrate destructive lesions which are associated with loss of tissue integrity and axons (see also Section 5.6.4.3). T2 magnetisation decay curves may give some indication of the expansion of extracelluar space present within a lesion, an indirect measure of axonal loss [Barnes *et al.* 1991], and loss of the short T2 component found in normal white matter may indicate demyelination [MacKay *et al.* 1994]. A more promising technique is magnetisation transfer imaging [Dousset *et al.* 1992], which reflects signal from bound protons and thereby gives an index of tissue destruction. A further technique which may give similar information is the volume of low signal lesions seen on a T1-weighted scan [van Walderveen *et al.* 1995]. Spectroscopy may also give an indication of axonal function through measurement of one of the metabolite peaks, *N*-acetyl aspartate (NAA). A number of studies have shown convincingly that in the acute lesion this peak may be much reduced but with time recovers often back towards normal [Davie *et al.* 1994a; Arnold *et al.* 1994]. Persistent reduction in chronic lesions is seen and in such a context is likely to indicate axonal loss. Finally diffusion imaging, which gives an indication of the size and orientation of extracellular space and by inference the extent of tissue disruption, may contribute useful information with regard to axonal loss [Larsson *et al.* 1992].

6.2   MR studies in experimental allergic encephalomyelitis

Experimental allergic encephalomyelitis (EAE) and, more particularly, the chronic relapsing form (CREAE), is considered to be a useful animal model for multiple sclerosis. Although the underlying pathogenesis is significantly different there are important histological similarities between the lesions seen in multiple sclerosis and those seen in CREAE in guinea pigs [Lassman 1983]. In EAE, MRI abnormalities have been documented on T2-weighted scans in primates [Stewart *et al.* 1991] and dogs, and also in guinea pigs, particularly if thin slices are used [Grossman *et al.* 1987]. CREAE is characterised by an initial acute episode of paralysis with weight loss developing ten to 14 days after inoculation. Most animals recover and enter a chronic phase of disease some six weeks later. This chronic phase may be either relapsing-remitting with good recovery or progressive: with time the progressive course usually dominates. Hawkins studied the nature and mechanism of enhancement with gadolinium DTPA in the guinea pig [Hawkins *et al.* 1990a] and showed that enhancing lesions were present at the time of clinical relapse. The duration of enhancement was very short in acute EAE, usually less than five days, but it ranged from five days to greater than five weeks in CREAE. Hawkins demonstrated that not all lesions showing enhancement were visible on the T2-weighted image, particularly if the duration of enhancement was less than four weeks. When animals were perfused at this stage, gadolinium nitrate or other blood–brain barrier markers were present in the perivenular spaces and extended for a short distance into the parenchyma between the perivascular inflammatory cells which were invariably present in enhancing lesions.

Further studies were carried out to elucidate the mechanism of increased permeability of the blood–brain barrier [Hawkins *et al.* 1992]. This did not appear to be due to opening of the tight junctions between adjacent endothelial cells. A constant feature was the presence of vesicles in the cytoplasm of endothelial cells within the lesion, which using energy dispersive X-ray microanalysis were shown to contain gadolinium. Perfusion with dinitrophenol shortly before injecting gadolinium nitrate completely prevented the appearance of gadolinium in the cytoplasm and in the extravascular space, suggesting that pathological permeability of the venules in the EAE lesion is to an important extent mediated by an energy dependent process.

6.3   Early lesions in multiple sclerosis

The first observation made about the early lesion in multiple sclerosis was that it tended to have a waxing and waning course with a tendency to increase in size over the first two to four weeks, remain unchanged for a further two- to four-week period and then reduce in size [Isaac *et al.* 1988]. Following the introduction of Gd-DTPA, serial MRI studies have demonstrated a consistent pattern of events in the evolution of the new lesion. The first detectable abnormality is a focal increase in permeability of the blood–brain barrier which is followed in a matter of days by the appearance of abnormal signal on the unenhanced PD/T2-weighted scan (or the PD/T2 abnormality appears at the same time as the blood–brain barrier leak) [Kermode *et al.* 1990a]. When such areas of enhancement are strategically placed (such as at the root entry zone of the 8th nerve) they have been shown to precede clinical symptoms, though this may be associated with an electrophysiological abnormality [Barratt *et al.* 1988] (Figure 6.1). Enhancement with Gd-DTPA usually lasts from two weeks to three months but for the majority of lesions it is between two and six weeks, and over 95% have ceased enhancing by eight weeks [Thompson *et al.* 1991; Harris *et al.* 1991, Lai *et al.* 1996] (Figure 6.2). At this stage the area of abnormal signal on the unenhanced scan progressively diminishes in size leaving a small residual lesion which sometimes corresponds with the original area of enhancement. It has been reported that a number of lesions may disappear completely, though this is probably only between five and ten per cent. Higher percentages may relate to such MR parameters as the magnetic field of the imager or slice thickness. It is of interest that soon after a new lesion appears, the peak of enhancement following injection of a bolus of Gd-DTPA is reached at about 15 minutes, a time similar to that seen in the choroid plexus in which there is no comparable blood–brain barrier. As the lesion ages the time to peak enhancement increases, suggesting gradual repair of the permeability defect [Kermode *et al.* 1990b]

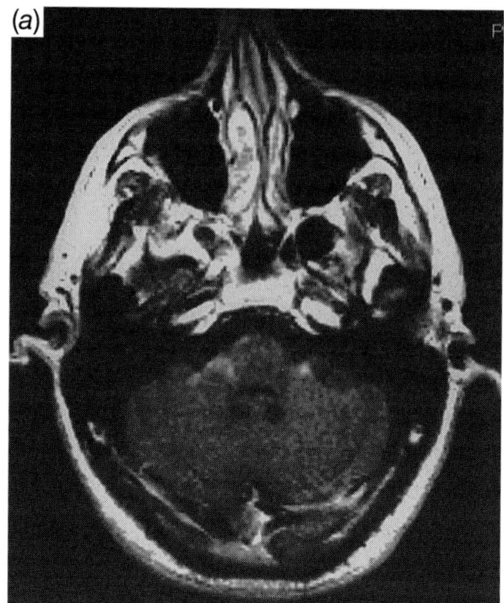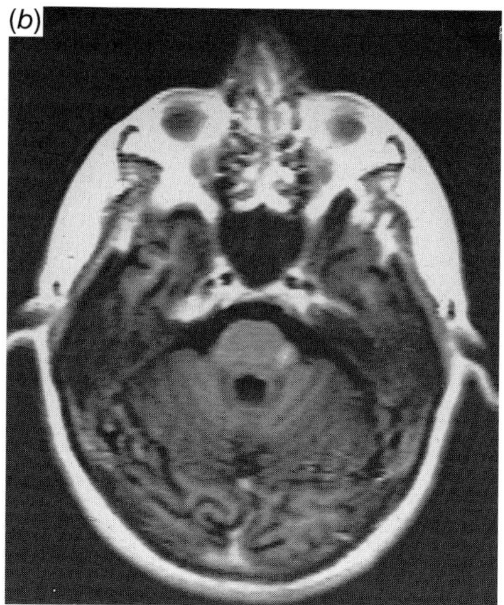

Figure 6.1 *(a) Gadolinium enhanced T1-weighted MRI in a 45-year-old male with clinically definite multiple sclerosis presenting with acute right-sided hearing loss. There is an enhancing lesion in the right lateral pons. Note also a small enhancing lesion in a similar location on the left. (b) Follow-up scan one month later reveals more extensive enhancement in the left lateral pons; the patient had developed acute left-sided hearing loss between the two scans.*

6.4   The relationship between PD/T2-weighted abnormality, gadolinium enhancement and clinical activity

Gadolinium enhancement is seen in the majority of new lesions (with the notable exception of the primary progressive group – see Section 6.6.4) and it also occurs with reactivation of old lesions, either at the edge, producing a ring enhancement (Figure 6.2) or within the lesion (Figure 3.11).

In a recent study by Miller and Barkhof it has been shown that a much higher proportion of MRI activity may be detected using Gd-DTPA than using PD/T2-weighted MRI [Miller *et al.* 1993c]. In a monthly study of 25 patients with relapsing-remitting or secondary progressive multiple sclerosis, carried out over three months, 22 new lesions were seen on both gadolinium enhanced and PD/T2-weighted scans, while 48 were seen on gadolinium enhanced scans alone and 16 on PD/T2-weighted scans alone. It has also been shown that using larger doses of Gd-DTPA such as triple dose (0.3 mmol/kg), will allow the detection of even more activity [Wolansky *et al.* 1994, Filippi *et al.* 1996b].

The vast majority of acute relapses (though not all) are associated with new enhancing lesions on MRI and a good correlation has been demonstrated in a number of studies

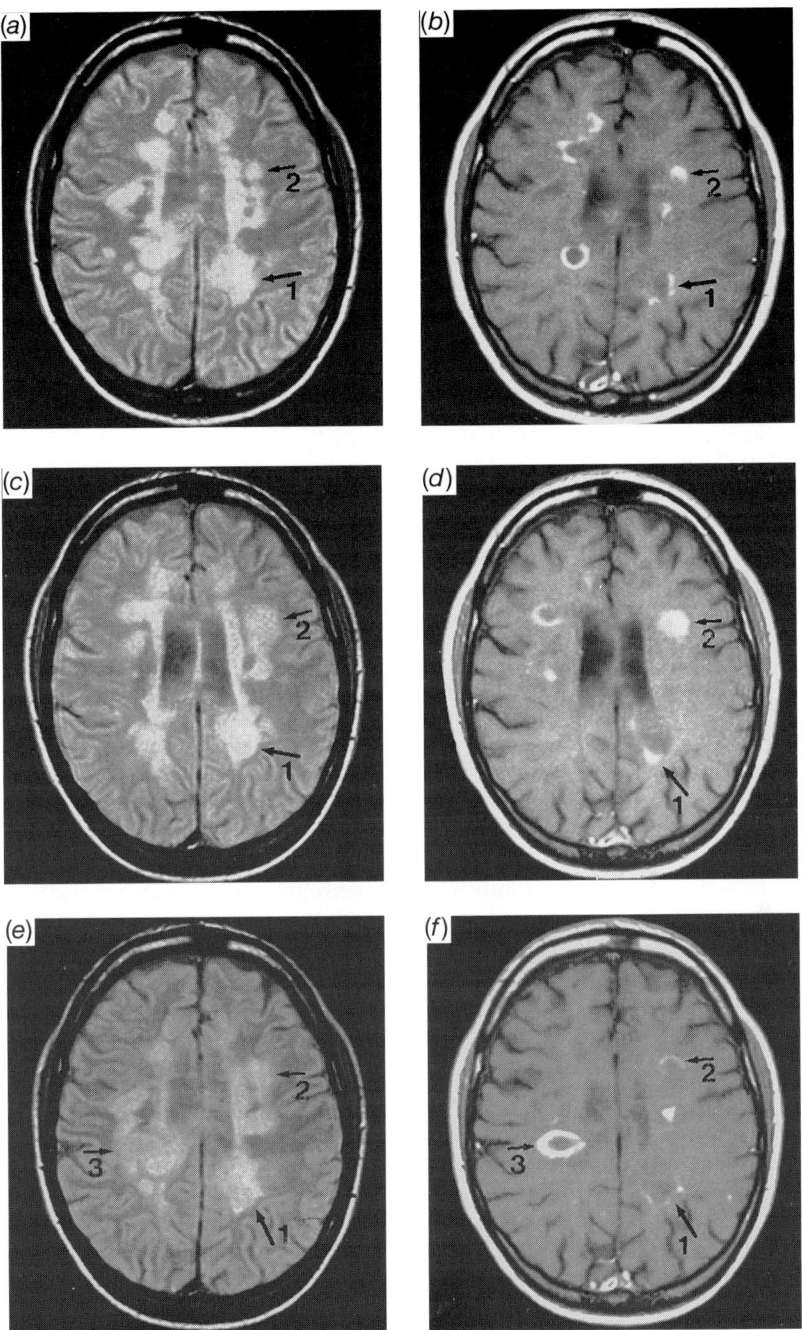

Figure 6.2 *Multiple sclerosis. Serial monthly PD-weighted [(a), (c) and (e)] and gadolinium enhanced T1-weighted [(b), (d) and (f)] MRI scans. New areas of abnormality on the PD scan are accompanied by enhancement which may be homogeneous (lesion 2) or ring-shaped (lesion 3).*

[Grossman *et al.* 1986; Smith *et al.* 1993; Thompson *et al.* 1992; Stone *et al.* 1995b, Thorpe *et al.* 1996a]. Monosymptomatic relapses are frequently associated with multiple new areas of activity on MRI and serial studies have shown that new MRI lesions frequently occur when the patient has no new symptoms, although MRI activity is greater during relapse than remission. Overall the frequency of new MRI lesions is approximately ten times higher than the frequency of clinical relapse. In a study of 12 patients with secondary progressive multiple sclerosis over six months, a total of 109 new lesions (18.2 lesions per patient per annum) were seen but only 17 clinical relapses occurred [Thompson *et al.* 1991] (Figure 3.9).

6.5 MRI and clinical subgroups

Having established the nature of the acute lesion in multiple sclerosis and its relationship to clinical activity, the next question is, how does MRI behave in the subgroups of patients defined according to the pattern of their clinical activity? Any such studies must take account of the fact that not all patients fall within tightly defined populations and some may move between groups [Goodkin *et al.* 1990]. There is also considerable variation among investigators in the use and definition of terms, though consensus definitions have been proposed recently [Lublin & Reingold 1996].

The vast majority of patients have an initial relapsing and remitting course to their condition. After a variable period of time, usually between five and ten years, approximately two-thirds of these patients will enter a progressive stage of the disease which may or may not be associated with superimposed relapses (secondary progressive multiple sclerosis). Of those who do not enter this progressive phase, many remain relatively unimpaired at ten years; these may be classified as having benign multiple sclerosis provided their disability is 3 or less on Kurtzke's Expanded Disability Status Scale (EDSS) [Kurtzke 1983]. This scale ranges from zero (normal) to 10 (death) and is heavily biased towards mobility. Patients at level 3 have minimal disability and are completely independent in their mobility and activities of daily living. A small but important group of patients are those who never have a relapsing-remitting component to their illness but who are progressive from onset (primary progressive multiple sclerosis). These constitute between five and ten per cent of the multiple sclerosis population, they tend to have an older age of onset and it is suggested that they have a worse prognosis in relation to the development of disability, in keeping with the suggestion that one of the main determinants for the development of disability is onset of the progressive phase of the disease [Runmarker & Andersen 1993].

A cross-sectional PD/T2-weighted study of 43 multiple sclerosis patients involved three of these subgroups (primary progressive, secondary progressive and benign) [Thompson *et al.* 1990b]. Surprisingly, patients with benign disease often had quite

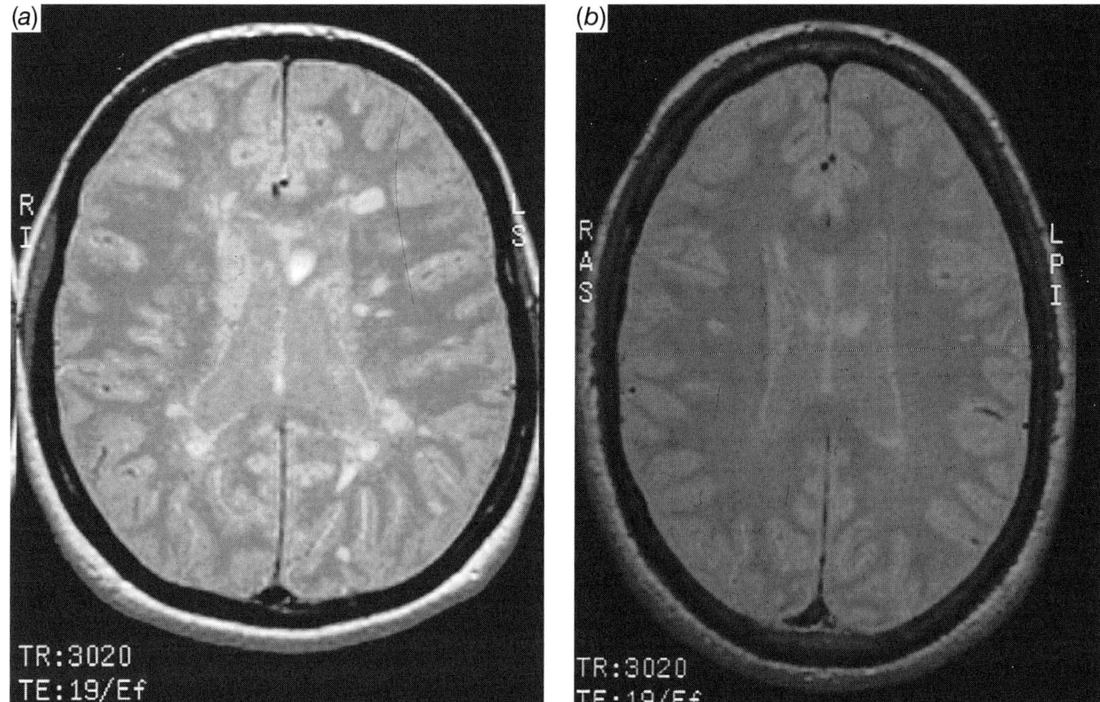

Figure 6.3 *PD-weighted brain MRI in (a) benign and (b) primary progressive multiple sclerosis. There is a much larger lesion load in the patient with benign disease. The lesions in the primary progressive multiple sclerosis patient are all small.*

extensive areas of high signal on their MRI (Figure 6.3) despite having minimal disability, and there was no significant difference between the lesion load in the benign group and that of the significantly more disabled secondary progressive group. An important caveat to the second finding is the inadequate evaluation of cognitive function contained within the EDSS.

It has been suggested that patients with benign multiple sclerosis have fewer lesions in such potentially disabling areas as the brain stem and the cerebellum, and that lesions that are present in those areas have never been associated with clinical symptoms [Koopmans *et al.* 1989b]. A more recent study comparing 13 patients with benign multiple sclerosis with 13 with secondary progressive disease found a significantly higher total lesion load in the secondary progressive group and, in particular, more marked infratentorial involvement when compared with the benign group [Filippi *et al.* 1995e]. However, there was no difference between the two groups in the number or extent of enhancing lesions.

Compared with benign and secondary progressive groups, patients with primary progressive disease tend to have fewer lesions on MRI and those lesions which are present tend to be small (85% were less than 5 mm in diameter) [Thompson *et al.* 1990b] (Figure

6.3). This paucity of abnormality was seen in patients who were severely disabled (EDSS greater than 6.5). It is therefore clear that the relationship between disability (as measured by the EDSS) and the extent and site of MRI lesions on cranial scanning is far from straightforward.

One possible explanation for this lack of relationship is that the above studies take no account of the spinal cord – an area presumed to be responsible for much of the disability in multiple sclerosis. More recently this omission has been rectified, at least in part, by advances in imaging techniques and hardware which have allowed faster and more accurate imaging of the spinal cord [Thorpe *et al.* 1993]. In a cross-sectional study of 80 patients, 20 in each of the four clinical subgroups (early relapsing-remitting, benign, primary and secondary progressive), using multi-array coils and fast spin echo, lesions were demonstrated in 75% of patients [Kidd *et al.* 1993]. However, there was an equal distribution of spinal cord lesions in all the clinical subgroups, and again no relationship between combined brain and cord lesion load and disability was seen.

This study documented for the first time the presence of spinal cord atrophy, which is presumed to result from axonal loss. This was measured on axial slices, acquired at four vertebral levels (C5, T2, T7, T11) by a gradient echo sequence (5-mm slices, TR 400 ms, TE 15 ms, flip angle 15 degrees). Cross-sectional area was calculated by a manual outlining technique. Atrophy was defined as a cross-sectional area less than twice the standard deviation of the mean for a normal population [Thorpe *et al.* 1993]. It was detected in 40% of patients but no significant difference in the frequency of atrophy between the clinical subgroups was demonstrated, though atrophy was evident in a slightly higher proportion of patients with primary progressive disease. Of particular importance was the finding of a significant association between the presence of cord atrophy and disability in the group as a whole ($p = 0.05$), suggesting the possible role of axonal loss in its development.

6.6   Serial MRI studies in clinical subgroups

Insight into the dynamics of the individual subgroups is best acquired from longitudinal studies with frequent MRI scans.

6.6.1   Relapsing-remitting multiple sclerosis

All of the many studies which have been carried out in this subgroup [Isaac *et al.* 1988; Willoughby *et al.* 1989; Harris *et al.* 1991, Thompson *et al.* 1992; Barkhof *et al.* 1992b;

Smith *et al.* 1993; Kidd *et al.* 1994; Frank *et al.* 1994; Thorpe *et al.* 1996a] confirmed that MRI activity as evidenced by new, enlarging or enhancing lesions occurs more frequently than clinical activity. An annual rate of MRI activity of 18 new lesions per year has been described [Thompson *et al.* 1992]. There is a suggestion by McFarland *et al.* [1992] that the occurrence of new lesions follows a particular sinusoidal pattern over time: however, this has not been supported by a more recent study [Truyen *et al.* 1995a]. Although there is considerable variation in the amount of MRI activity over time, a regular or predictable pattern of change has not emerged. Little is known about the factors which lead to these variations in disease activity; one small study indicated that activity may be modified during pregnancy [van Walderveen *et al.* 1994].

Serial spinal cord imaging has also been carried out in this group [Thorpe *et al.* 1996a]. Ten patients with early relapsing-remitting multiple sclerosis had monthly gadolinium enhanced MRI scans of brain and cord for 12 months. Over this period there were 11 clinical relapses, 153 active brain lesions (94% enhancing) and 18 active cord lesions (60% enhancing). There was a strong association between the occurrence of active brain and cord lesions. Cord lesions were more likely to be symptomatic (six of the 18) than were brain lesions (only one of the 153 was associated with clinical symptoms). Progressive cord atrophy over the 12-month period was not seen in this group.

6.6.2   Benign multiple sclerosis

Serial studies of this population show that patients have fewer lesions over time than the early relapsing-remitting group (average five to six per patient per year). Furthermore, only one-third of new lesions show enhancement with Gd-DTPA [Thompson *et al.* 1992; Kidd *et al.* 1994]. This would seem to suggest that with increasing duration of disease a proportion of patients have fewer lesions, and those that do occur are less inflammatory. This would be in keeping with the clinical view that in some patients activity decreases with disease duration. A further factor is that patients in this group tend to be older than the relapsing-remitting patients. However, in the studies mentioned, age alone did not appear to explain the reduction in MRI activity.

6.6.3   Secondary progressive multiple sclerosis

Patients in this group move from the relapsing-remitting group because they develop slow progression, though many continue to have frequent relapses. It may be important to distinguish between those who relapse and those who do not. Early serial studies indicated that the majority of patients continued to have a high frequency of new lesions similar to that seen in the relapsing-remitting group. In Thompson's study [Thompson *et al.* 1991] 12 patients were followed over six months with fortnightly enhanced scans for the first three months and monthly scans for the remaining three months. The total number of new lesions was 109, corresponding with 18.2 lesions per patient per year and 87% enhanced (Figure 3.9). It has become clear, however, that there is a wide range of MRI activity in this group, and frequent new lesions tend to be seen in those who continue to have relapses. There is a subgroup who progress slowly but do not have any superimposed relapses and very little activity on MRI, behaving not dissimilarly to the primary progressive group [Kidd *et al.* 1996]. This again raises important issues with regard to the development of disability which will be discussed in more detail in a later section.

Spinal cord activity in this subgroup has recently been studied in nine patients over a 12-month period [Kidd *et al.* 1996]. This revealed very little new activity in the cord, with only two new lesions and one enlarging lesion seen compared with 112 new brain lesions. Change in cross-sectional area of the cord was also measured over time at C5, T2, T7 and T12 levels. The median reduction in cord area was -2.62 mm^2 but there was a very wide range of -17.1 to $+6.7$ mm^2. Progressive atrophy, particularly at the C5 level, was most marked in patients who developed increasing disability over this time, though this was not significant ($p = 0.08$). There was also an apparent increase in cord size in some patients, suggesting some methodological difficulties.

6.6.4   Primary progressive multiple sclerosis

There was particular interest in this small subgroup of patients given that cross-sectional studies suggest that they may have distinct MRI characteristics. The first serial study of this group [Thompson *et al.* 1991] followed 12 patients over a six-month period with fortnightly enhanced scans for the first three months and monthly scans for the remaining three months. This demonstrated for the first time that although these patients were deteriorating clinically, few new lesions were seen on MRI and those that did occur were small, 78% being less than 5 mm. Most surprisingly, little if any enhancement was seen. Twenty new lesions were seen in the 12 patients, giving a mean of 3.3 lesions per patient per year. Only one of the 20 lesions showed enhancement with Gd-DTPA. In a subsequent study of ten patients, scanned monthly for 12 months, 14 of 20 new brain lesions enhanced [Kidd *et al.* 1996]. Taking the two studies together, only 15/40 (38%) of new lesions enhanced. Similar findings have subsequently been seen in a number of other MR centres. The low frequency of enhancement with Gd-DTPA suggests that lesions in primary progressive multiple sclerosis are likely to be of a less inflammatory nature, though with some inflammation present, than those seen in relapsing-remitting and secondary progressive multiple sclerosis, a suggestion supported by a recent comparative post-mortem study of the two progressive forms of the disease [Révèsz *et al.* 1994]. Two recent studies of the potential for triple dose Gd-DPTA to demonstrate a higher proportion of enhancing lesions in primary progressive MS have given conflicting results [Filippi *et al.* 1995a; Silver *et al.* 1996].

There is also a group of patients who although predominantly primary progressive have a single episode of acute deterioration either at the onset or during the course of the disease. Such patients may best be described as transitional. A recent study has suggested that the MR characteristics of this group are identical to the primary progressive patients [Filippi *et al.* 1995f].

Serial MRI of the spinal cord in primary progressive MS demonstrated a similar finding to that seen in the secondary progressive group, with only three new lesions seen over a 12-month period in ten patients. A proportion of patients showed no new lesions on MRI of brain or spinal cord despite clear clinical deterioration. Progressive atrophy, however, was seen in the majority of patients, with a median change in cord area of -5.39mm^2 (range -20.45 to $+5.15$ mm^2). As with the secondary progressive group there was no significant relationship between the development of cord atrophy at the C5 level and disability ($p = 0.08$).

6.7   Cognitive/MRI correlates

Having been ignored and even denied for decades, cognitive dysfunction has now been well described in a number of recent studies. It occurs in 40% of patients in population based studies and 50–65% of patients who attend multiple sclerosis clinics [Rao *et al.* 1993]. The pattern of abnormalities includes deterioration in short-term memory, sustained attention, conceptual/abstract reasoning and speed of information processing with relative sparing of speech functions. This range of dysfunction is typical of pathology affecting the white matter, reflecting a subcortical rather than a cortical pattern. Cognitive impairment appears to relate to disease duration *per se* but there are conflicting results as to whether it relates to the development of disability [Heaton *et al.* 1985; Beatty & Goodkin 1990; Beatty *et al.* 1990; Rao *et al.* 1991a, b]. As with all manifestations of multiple sclerosis there is considerable individual variation.

Abnormalities of short-term memory and attention have been documented in patients who present with clinically isolated syndromes suggestive of multiple sclerosis [Callanan *et al.* 1989; Lyon-Caen *et al.* 1986] A five-year follow-up study of these patients has suggested that cognitive decline is linked to the disease course and, whilst deterioration in attention and memory functions has occurred in those who have entered the progressive phase, there is little evidence of deterioration in those who have not developed further neurological symptoms [Feinstein *et al.* 1992a, c]. This is in keeping with the finding that patients with secondary progressive MS have greater cognitive impairment that those with relapsing-remitting disease [Heaton *et al.* 1985; Rao *et al.* 1987]. A more recent study suggested that patients with primary progressive multiple sclerosis may have less cognitive impairment than age and disability matched secondary progressive patients [Comi *et al.* 1995].

What of the relationship between cranial MRI and cognitive impairment? It might be expected that this would be somewhat closer than the relationship between MRI and disability given the site of the abnormalities seen in multiple sclerosis. Overall the results have been disappointing, though a relationship between the overall severity of cognitive impairment and the extent of abnormalities on MRI has been documented [Franklin *et al.* 1988; Anzola *et al.* 1990; Ron *et al.* 1991; Pozzilli *et al.* 1991a, b]. However, with more accurate quantification techniques a more significant relationship has emerged, with Rao [Rao *et al.* 1989] reporting an association between total lesion area and 18 cognitive variables. One of the main components of frontal lobe activity, executive functioning, has also been studied and a number of aspects including conceptual reasoning, spatial working memory and strategic planning have been shown to correlate with lesion load in the frontal lobes [Arnett *et al.* 1994; Foong *et al.* in press]. A significant correlation between atrophy of the corpus callosum and various cognitive deficits, most notably a reduction in the speed of information processing, has been found [Huber *et al.* 1987; Rao *et al.* 1989]

Specific correlations between particular deficits and sites of pathology have proved more elusive. This may be in part due to limitations in quantitative assessment together with the difficulties of disentangling the effect of a given lesion in the context of more widespread pathology. A recent case study by Rozewicz *et al.* [1994] demonstrated non-dominant hemisphere abnormalities in a patient with a left parietal lesion during an acute relapse. Improvement was seen with resolution of the lesion. Other complicating factors which may influence the relationship include the pathological heterogeneity of lesions together with the inability of MRI to detect subtle pathological change. In this context it is interesting to note that a significant relationship between elevated T1 relaxation times in normal appearing frontal white matter and cognitive impairment has been found in patients with secondary progressive disease [Feinstein *et al.* 1992a].

Few serial studies have been carried out comparing change in cognitive function with serial MRI activity. One such study compared a small number of patients with early relapsing-remitting and benign multiple sclerosis with controls over a six-month period [Feinstein *et al.* 1993]. The results were influenced by continuing practice effect throughout the study, which was evident in both the multiple sclerosis population and the controls. There was marked variation in cognitive impairment between patients with identical lesion loads. However, those patients with high levels of MRI activity did show evidence of deteriorating cognitive function. This deterioration often occurred without any change in the EDSS. There were also a number of patients who deteriorated in the EDSS without any change in cranial MRI or cognitive function.

Taken together these studies suggest that there is a closer relationship between brain MRI and cognitive function than there is with sensorimotor function, a finding previously documented using positron emission tomography [Brooks *et al.* 1984]. With further improvement in quantification techniques and pathological specificity, a closer correlation between MRI abnormalities and cognitive dysfunction is likely to be seen [Langdon *et al.* 1996].

6.8 Mechanisms underlying acute relapse

Serial studies suggest that approximately 70–80% of clinical relapses are associated with new lesions. The corollary is however not true in that only 10–20% of new lesions are associated with clinically detectable activity. In serial studies there is a significantly higher number of active lesions per scan during relapse than during remission (3.9 vs 1.4, $p = 0.001$ [Thorpe *et al.* 1996a]). There is little evidence to differentiate the MRI activity of relapses which resolve completely from those with sequelae. However, it is likely that lesions with evidence of tissue destruction such as persisting low signal on T1-weighted images are more likely to be associated with poor recovery [Youl *et al.* 1991a; van Walderveen *et al.* 1995].

What has MRI taught us of the mechanisms underlying relapse and remission? Optic neuritis is a useful model to study the relationship between pathological change and symptom production, given that all nerve fibres subserve the same function. There is the added benefit of being able to assess function with neurophysiological techniques (visual evoked potential, VEP) as well as with MRI (see Section 2.4). Youl *et al.* studied ten patients within two weeks of the onset of symptoms [Youl *et al.* 1991b]. All affected nerves enhanced, and one month later all but two had ceased to do so. In other words the clinical features of the optic neuritis were associated with the enhancing (inflammatory) phase. Further information was acquired from the VEPs. In the acute stage there was a marked reduction in amplitude and an increase in latency, indicating both conduction block and demyelination. After enhancement ceased, the delay persisted but the amplitude had significantly increased. This observation suggests that inflammation plays a crucial role in the production of symptoms in acute relapse, possibly mediated by cytokines [McDonald 1994]. It may well be that the resolution of inflammation and oedema may be responsible for the re-establishment of conduction and clinical remission. Studies using the technique of magnetisation decay analysis have indicated that a component of the disappearing element of the acute lesion on PD/T2-weighted scans is likely to be oedema.

6.9   The development of disability

The main concern of any patient with multiple sclerosis is whether or not they will develop severe disability, become wheelchair bound and lose their independence. Disability may result from two mechanisms which may occur separately or in parallel: incomplete recovery from relapse and slow, insidious progression. In relapsing-remitting multiple sclerosis disability results entirely from the former while in primary progressive disease the latter is entirely responsible. In secondary progressive multiple sclerosis both mechanisms may occur, though it is apparent that some patients stop having relapses and simply show slow progression. Such clinical studies as exist suggest that the onset of the progressive phase of the disease is the main determining factor in the development of disability [Kurtzke *et al.* 1977; Confavreux *et al.* 1980; Weinshenker *et al.* 1989a, b] though incomplete remission has also been shown to make a contribution [Runmarker & Andersen 1993]. What insights does MRI give us into the development of disability? From the cross-sectional studies of the individual clinical subgroups it is clear that there is little correlation between the extent of MRI abnormality on a PD/T2-weighted scan and disability in the individual patient, with the extremes being a patient with benign disease who has extensive abnormality on brain MRI and on the other hand the patient with primary progressive multiple sclerosis who is wheelchair bound with a Kurtzke of 6.5, but has minimal abnormality on MRI. Many serial studies which have been carried out have not shown a relationship between the development of new lesions on MRI and the worsening of disability. However, these studies are limited by small numbers of patients and short duration of follow-up (usually six months). If the duration of follow-up is lengthened and patients are seen early in their disease course then a relationship between MRI abnormality and the development of disability may be established. This is well demonstrated by a study of 89 patients presenting with clinically isolated syndromes suggestive of MS such as optic neuritis [Morrissey *et al.* 1993a] which showed a significant relationship between the number of lesions on MRI on initial presentation and disability as measured by Kurtzke's EDSS at five years. Of the 18 patients with an EDSS of 3 or more at five year follow-up all but three had four or more lesions on their initial MRI. This finding was supported by a semi-quantitative study carried out on the same group of patients which showed a significantly larger median volume of abnormality on MRI at presentation in patients who were disabled at five years compared with those who were not ($p = 0.005$)[Filippi *et al.* 1994a].

The situation is less clear-cut in patients with established multiple sclerosis. Paty followed up 18 patients four years after a six-month study and showed that those who had more MRI lesions during the study were more disabled at follow-up [Paty *et al.* 1992a] (Table 5.4). Recently 22 primary and secondary progressive patients were followed up five years after a six-month serial MRI study [Losseff *et al.* 1995a]. There was no relationship between the extent of PD/T2-weighted MRI abnormality at the outset of the study and disability five years later. However, in the secondary progressive group there was a relationship between both the number of new enhancing lesions and the number of relapses which developed over the six-month study period and the resulting change in disability five years later ($p = 0.05$). Patients with primary progressive multiple sclerosis showed no relationship whatever between MRI activity and subsequent change in disability.

Studies involving larger numbers of patients have also been more encouraging. Filippi carried out a meta-analysis of 281 patients from four centres with clinically definite multiple sclerosis, all of whom had serial scans at an interval of between two and three years [Filippi *et al.* 1995d]. Despite the fact that there were significant differences between the centres in relation to the clinical characteristics of the patients, the use of immunosuppressive therapy and the MR protocols, a significant relationship between the development of disability and MRI activity (defined as new and enlarging lesions on PD/T2-weighted images – gadolinium was not used) over the study period was demonstrated ($p = 0.02$). This relationship was more evident in the relapsing-remitting patients than in those with secondary progressive disease, suggesting that there may be different mechanisms for disability at different stages of the disease. A study of 44 patients over a two-year period [Kidd *et al.* 1992] did not show any relationship between the development of disability and the accumulation of T2-weighted abnormality. This study demonstrated high MRI activity in patients with relapsing-remitting multiple sclerosis and low activity in those with primary progressive disease. However, in the secondary progressive group, while high activity was seen in those who continued to have relapses, patients who were deteriorating without relapse had very low activity, almost identical to the primary progressive group. These studies would suggest that disability which results from incomplete recovery from relapse may well relate to MRI activity, while disability which is progressive in nature and not associated with relapse does not. What then is the mechanism of disability underlying progressive deterioration?

Abnormalities seen on conventional PD/T2–weighted MRI give no indication as to the underlying pathology of the lesion and, as is well documented, there is a marked pathological heterogeneity of lesions in multiple sclerosis ranging from those with relative preservation of axons (gliotic lesions) to those in whom there is much expanded extracellular space and consequent severe axonal loss (Figure 6.4). It is reasonable to assume that in the latter there will be severe, irreversible disability. The role of axonal loss in the development of irreversible disability is supported by the detection of spinal cord atrophy (indicating axonal loss) in patients with progressive disease, and by the suggestion that increasing atrophy over time may be associated with worsening disability [Kidd *et al.* 1993; Kidd *et al.* 1996]. A closer relationship between MRI abnormalities and disability may therefore be expected when more pathologically specific imaging techniques are used.

6.9.1   T2 magnetisation decay analysis

This technique, which allows the differentiation between gliotic lesions (mono-exponential curve) and lesions associated with expanded extracellular space and axonal loss

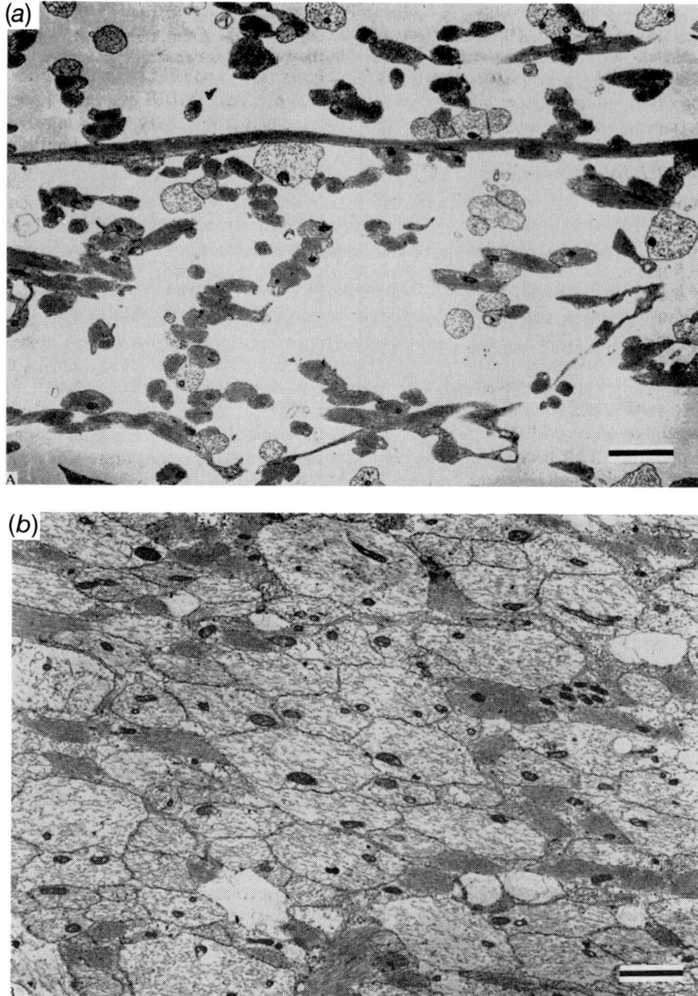

Figure 6.4 *Pathological specimens reveal two extreme types of multiple sclerosis lesion: (a) 'open' lesion with marked axonal loss and a grossly expanded extracellular space. (b) 'closed' lesion with complete demyelination, relative axonal preservation, intense gliosis and no expansion of the extracellular space. (From Barnes et al. 1991, by permission of Oxford University Press.)*

(bi-exponential curve), has been used in a study of chronic lesions known to be more than two years old. Half had mono-exponential T2 decay curves while in the remainder they were bi-exponential [Barnes *et al.* 1991]. The prediction that lesions associated with mono-exponential decay curves were gliotic while those with bi-exponential decay had a markedly expanded extracellular space (i.e. oedema) had been confirmed in earlier histopathological/MR correlative studies [Barnes *et al.* 1986, 1987, 1988], and in a post-mortem multiple sclerosis case, the association of expanded extracellular space and axonal loss was demonstrated [Barnes *et al.* 1991] (Figure 6.4). When this technique was used to study six disabled people with secondary progressive multiple sclerosis and five patients with benign disease, the majority (75%) of large lesions in the former group had a bi-exponential decay curve, while this was a relatively rare finding (12.5%) in the latter group [Filippi *et al.* 1994b].

6.9.2   Magnetisation transfer imaging

Images generated by this technique are derived from bound rather than free protons and therefore give an indication of tissue integrity. As the majority of bound protons are attached to myelin this technique may give a measure of myelin breakdown. Results are expressed as a magnetisation transfer (MT) ratio and the lower the ratio the greater the tissue destruction. This technique was used in a group of 43 patients which included all four clinical subgroups with a wide range of disability [Gass *et al.* 1994]. The average lesion MT ratio was significantly higher in the subgroup with benign disease when compared with the secondary progressive sub group ($p = 0.01$) and in mildly disabled (EDSS ≤ 3) compared with severely disabled patients (EDSS ≥ 5, $p = 0.001$) (Table 6.1). In the whole cohort there was a strong inverse correlation between disability, as measured on Kurtzke's EDSS, and the average lesion MT ratio (Spearman Rank Ccorrelation coefficient $= -0.44$, $p = 0.006$) (Figure 6.5). A recent follow-up after 18 months in eight benign and eight secondary progressive patients from the original cohort did not show any change in MT ratios in existing lesions; however, there was a significantly lower MT ratio in the new lesions that developed in the secondary progressive group during this follow-up period [HM Lai, unpublished observations].

6.9.3   Unenhanced T1-weighted spin echo imaging

Loss of tissue structure within a lesion may also result in markedly prolonged T1 relaxation time resulting in hypointensity on T1-weighted images (see Section 2.2.5 and Figure 2.1). This is supported by a recent study which showed that the MT ratio of hypointense lesions (27.3%) was significantly lower than that of isointense lesions (33.1%; $p = 0.0001$) [Hiehle *et al.* 1995]. In a recent study of 19 patients with multiple sclerosis who underwent two T1-weighted spin echo images separated by a two-year interval, a significant relationship was detected between increased disability (on the EDSS) and an increased volume of low signal lesions (Spearman Rank correlation coefficient $= 0.74$, $p = <0.002$) [van Walderveen *et al.* 1995]. After a further year of follow-up this relationship was seen in patients with secondary progressive multiple sclerosis but not in those with relapsing-remitting disease [Truyen *et al.* 1995b].

Table 6.1 *Magnetisation transfer ratios of multiple sclerosis lesions in different clinical subgroups*

	ERR	Be	SP	PP
Patient no.	11	11	11	10
Mean EDSS	2.9	2.7	6.1	4.8
(range)	(1.5–6.5)	(1.5–3.0)	(5.0–8.0)	(3.0–7.0)
Mean MTR	24.8%	25.4%	23.7%	24.2%
(range)	(21–28)	(23–27)	(21–26)	(20–27)

(MTR of normal control white matter = 31%)

Note:
ERR = early relapsing-remitting
Be = benign
SP = secondary progressive
PP = primary progressive
MTR = magnetisation transfer ratio
EDSS = Kurtzke expanded disability status scale
Source:
(From A. Gass *et al.* 1994, reprinted from *Annals of Neurology* V36, pp. 62–67, by permission of Little, Brown & Co. Inc.)

6.9.4 Proton MR spectroscopy

As mentioned earlier (Section 6.1) acute lesions show a marked though partially reversible reduction in the N-acetyl aspartate peak (NAA), suggesting axonal dysfunction [Davie *et al.* 1994a]. A recent study has looked at absolute NAA levels in relation to cerebellar function [Davie *et al.* 1995]. A comparison of 11 multiple sclerosis patients with longstanding cerebellar dysfunction and 11 without cerebellar signs demonstrated a highly significant decrease in the NAA levels from the cerebellum in the former group (Figure 3.25). There was a negative correlation between NAA concentration and both the EDSS ($r = -0.52$, $0.025 > p > 0.01$) and cerebellar function ($r = -0.49$, $0.05 > p > 0.02$). These reduced levels were similar to those found in patients with autosomal dominant cerebellar ataxia who were studied at the same time. A second important finding was a significant correlation between the degree of cerebellar atrophy and cerebellar dysfunction ($r = 0.54$, $0.02 > p > 0.01$), as had previously been seen in the spinal cord. Six of the ataxic multiple sclerosis patients were followed up after six months and in all the low NAA concentration persisted, suggesting that it is likely to reflect irreversible pathology (i.e. axonal loss).

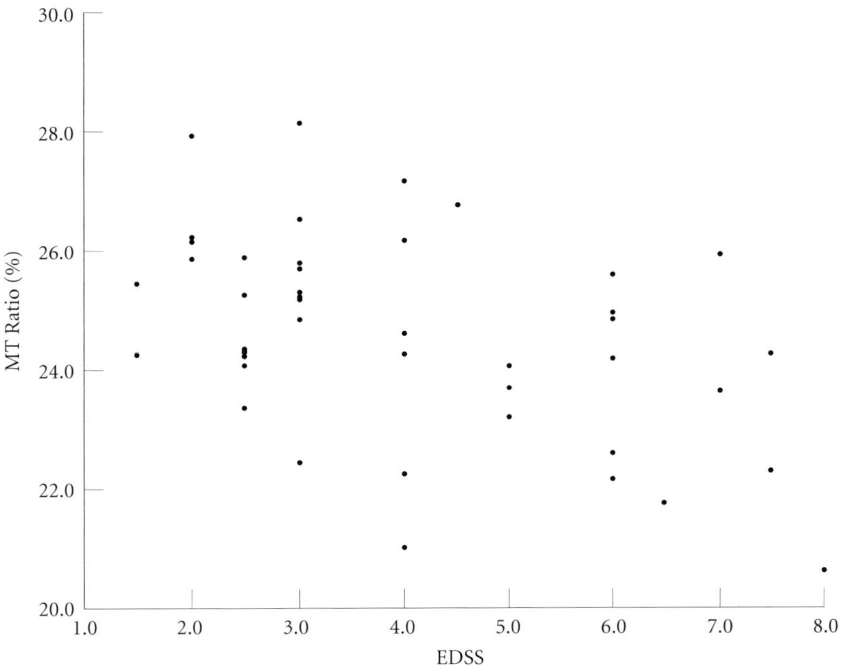

Figure 6.5 *Relationship between the mean magnetisation transfer ratio of multiple sclerosis lesions and EDSS. (From Gass et al. 1994, reprinted from* Annals of Neurology *V36, pp. 62–7, by permission of Little, Brown & Co. Inc.)*

6.9.5   Atrophy

There has been some encouraging recent work carried out addressing the methodological difficulties in measuring spinal cord atrophy [Losseff *et al.* 1995b, 1996a]. By concentrating on the upper cervical cord, which is relatively constant in size, and using a semi-automated outlining technique applied to axial reformats from a volume-acquired, inversion-prepared gradient echo sequence, intra-observer reproducibility error has been reduced to 0.6%. A cross-sectional study of 60 patients using this technique has shown a strong correlation between cord area and EDSS ($r = -0.7$) (Figure 6.6) [Losseff *et al.* 1996a]. As a logical sequence to his spinal cord work, Losseff has also developed a new technique to measure cerebral volume at the periventricular level. The method combines histogram-based automatic thresholding with sequences of morphological operations that distinguish the brain from surrounding tissues. When applied to 18 months of serial data from patients involved in a negative treatment trial, a significant relationship between the development of atrophy and increasing disability was demonstrated ($p < 0.05$) [Losseff *et al.* 1996b].

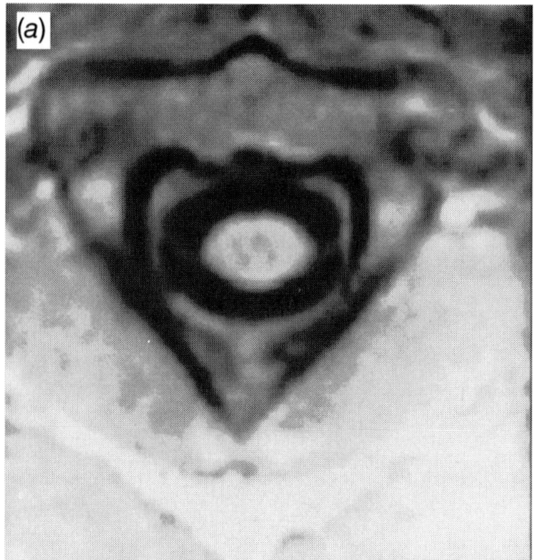

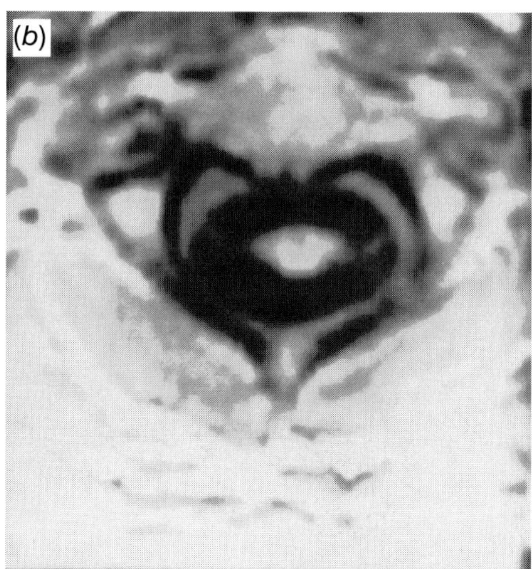

Figure 6.6 *3 mm thick axial image through C2, reconstructed from an inversion recovery prepared, volume acquired, gradient echo sequence. There is low signal in the subarachnoid space, which clearly delineates the spinal cord and allows for semi-automated outlining of the cord using a threshold technique. (a) Normal size cord in a patient with benign multiple sclerosis and EDSS=1. (b) Atrophic cord in a patient with secondary progressive multiple sclerosis and EDSS=8. (From Losseff et al. 1996, by permission of Oxford University Press.)*

6.9.6 Diffusion imaging

Despite the obvious potential of this technique there have been few clinically based studies carried out. A recent study of 12 patients with benign and 13 with secondary progressive disease did not detect any difference between the lesions in the two groups [Lai *et al.* 1995].

6.10 Conclusion

In summary, there are a number of lines of evidence to implicate axonal loss in the development of disability, and there is an increasing need to develop techniques which allow its detection and which can be easily incorporated into clinical practice. This is of importance in monitoring patients, particularly in the context of therapeutic trials [McDonald *et al.* 1994]. In this regard the potential ease of measuring hypointense lesions on T1-weighted images is particularly attractive.

7   Monitoring treatment trials

Donald W Paty, David H Miller

7.1   Introduction

Early in the experience with MRI in multiple sclerosis, intermittent scans showed that previously seen stable lesions could be seen to increase in size and new asymptomatic lesions could be seen to come and go [Johnson *et al.* 1984; Li *et al.* 1984]. It quickly became apparent that disease activity, as measured by MRI, could be quite dramatic and was often subclinical. The implications of such findings for therapeutic monitoring were obvious. The present chapter concentrates on this aspect of the use of MRI in multiple sclerosis, in four sections: (i) a review of natural history serial studies which provide the basis for defining trial protocols; (ii) a consideration of the implications of the clinical–MRI relationships summarised in the previous two chapters for the interpretation of MRI findings in trials; (iii) a summary of MRI results from clinical trials performed to date; (iv) recommendations for the use of MRI in clinical trials.

7.2   Natural history serial studies

7.2.1   Serial MRI studies for natural history of activity of disease

Systematic serial studies combining frequent neurological and MRI examinations have been carried out in a number of centres (see Table 7.1).
MRI lesions can be defined as follows:

(i) *Enhancing lesions seen on T1-weighted scans*
Enhancement (i.e. hyperintensity) occurs in some lesions after injecting gadolinium chelates; the remaining non-enhancing lesions are isointense or hypointense compared with normal white matter. There are three types of enhancing lesion:

(1) *New lesion*: first ever enhancement in a lesion.

Table 7.1 *Systematic serial MRI natural history studies*

Senior author	GD	Year	Patient	Type of findings
1) Isaac	o	1988	RR	MRI activity 5 times the clinical activity rate
2) Willoughby	o	1989	RR	MRI activity 5 times the clinical activity rate
3) Koopmans	o	1989a	RP	MRI activity was high in RP patients
4) Miller	+	1988a	RR	MRI activity higher than clinical. All new MRI lesions enhanced
5) Kermode	+	1990a	RR	Gd enhancement can precede standard MRI lesion
6) Bastianello	+	1990	Mixed	All new lesions enhanced
7) Wiebe	+	1990	Mixed	Spinal MRI of limited value since it increased the yield of activity by only 20%
8) Harris	+	1991	RR	MRI activity greater than clinical
9) Thompson	+	1991	PP	Pattern differs from RR and RP. These primary CP patients have a low number of small non-enhancing new lesions
10) Thompson	+	1992	RR	Early RR and benign MS are different
11) Barkhof	+	1992b	Mixed	MRI activity 10 times clinical
12) Capra	+	1992	RR	MRI activity much greater than clinical
13) McFarland	+	1992	RR	Marked fluctuation month to month in MRI activity
14) Smith	+	1993	RR	Continuation of Harris study. Lesion activity comes in 'bursts'
15) Smith	+	1993	RR	Proposed pre- and post-treatment analysis
16) Miller	+	1993c	RR & RP	Gadolinium increased MRI activity by 60% when compared to T2 analysis alone
17) Kidd	+	1994	RR	Benign patients had less activity than early RR
18) Khoury	+	1994	Mixed	Clinical and MRI activity correlated
19) van Walderveen	o	1994	RR-preg	↓ in MRI activity correlated in 3rd trimester of pregnancy
20) van Walderveen	+	1995	Mixed	T1 lesions correlated better than T2 with clinical severity.

Note:

GD =   Gadolinium was used

RR =   Relapsing and remitting

RP =   Relapsing progressive (chronic progressive after a relapsing start)

PP =   Primary chronic progressive (progressive from outset without relapses)

(2) *Recurrent lesion*: new enhancement in a lesion in which there had been an earlier episode of enhancenent that had resolved.

(3) *Persistent lesion*: the same lesion was enhancing on the previous scan.

Enhancement can occur alone or with any of the lesion changes listed below on PD/T2-weighted scans:

(ii) *Lesions seen on the PD/T2-weighted scan*

(1) *New lesion*: new lesions can be seen on the PD/T2 and on the T1 unenhanced scan. Most enhance for the first two to six weeks. Many of these lesions enlarge over time and then become smaller over time (within two months).

(2) *Stable lesion*: these lesions do not change from one scan to the next.

(3) *Reappearing lesion:* lesions that reappear at the same site from which an earlier lesion had disappeared (disappearance and hence reappearance on PD- or T2-weighted scans is unusual with high field strength machines $\geq$ 0.5T)

(4) *Enlarging lesion*: lesions having a significant increase in size from a previously seen stable appearance. Most of these enlarging lesions also enhance for a few weeks.

Any new, enhancing or enlarging lesions can be considered to be signs of advancing pathology, indicating an increase in disease activity. However, a distinction should be made between persistent activity and new or recurrent activity. Persistent MRI activity suggests prolonged pathological activity that probably should be weighted more than short duration activity, e.g. lesions that enhance on two consecutive monthly scans can be given more weighting than those that enhance on a single scan. However, *it is the new enhancing or new PD/T2 or T1 lesion that is probably the most important one,* because, if a putative therapy can significantly slow or stop new lesion formation it may be able to prevent progression of the disease. In addition however, once new lesions have formed there may be inevitable pathological changes that occur within those lesions, such as demyelination, gliosis or axonal loss, that would require a different therapeutic strategy from the one that would prevent new lesions (mostly inflammatory) from forming in the first place. *Recurrent* activity may also be important in producing irreversible damage, and it can reasonably be considered a subset of new lesion activity.

The first systematic study of asymptomatic unenhanced MRI activity was in seven relapsing patients [Isaac *et al.* 1988]. Some of the patients were disabled, but most functioned completely independently. The patients were examined by monthly carefully repositioned and reproducible unenhanced MRI scans over six months. Five clinical relapses occurred in three patients. In contrast there were 17 new, enlarging or recurrent MRI lesions (MRI activity events) seen during the study. All activity was new or recurrent; persisting activity was not counted (i.e. an active lesion was counted just once, at its first appearance). Seventeen out of the 36 (48%) follow-up examinations had MRI activity events. The mean clinical relapse rate was 1.4 relapses per patient per year. The rate for the appearance of new MRI lesions was 4.9 new lesions per patient per year. The total MRI lesion activity rate was 8.0 activity events per patient per year. The total MRI activity rate was 3.4 times the clinical activity rate.

Another study included nine patients with minimally disabling but actively relapsing disease [Willoughby *et al.* 1989]. Each patient had a careful interim history along with neurological and unenhanced MRI examinations done once every two weeks for an average of five months. Clinically detected activity was minimal, with three instances in which asymptomatic changes in neurological findings were detected. One patient had two minor spinal cord sensory relapses. Six of the patients had MRI activity. There were ten new lesions and two enlarging lesions. All of the MRI activity (12 events) was asymptomatic. The clinical relapse rate was 0.53 relapses per patient per year. The MRI activity rate was 3.2 activity events per patient per year. The frequency of MRI activity was 2.6 positive MRI examinations per patient per year. There were 83 follow-up MRI examinations and ten of those examinations (12%) showed evidence of active lesions. The total MRI activity rate in this study was also six times the clinical relapse rate.

A third study included eight severely disabled patients in the progressive phase of multiple sclerosis [Koopmans *et al.* 1989b]. Patients were selected because of documented chronic deterioration over the previous year. Seven of the eight patients had begun with relapsing disease and could be considered secondary progressive (SP). All patients had histories, physical examinations and MRI examinations once every two weeks over a period of six months. There were 98 follow-up unenhanced MRI examinations during which time no clinical relapses were seen. However, 25 new MRI lesions developed. There were also 61 instances in which previously seen stable MRI lesions increased in size. There were thus 86 MRI activity events during the study (note that a continuous increase in size (persistent activity) over several scans was counted as only a single activity event). Fifty of the 98 follow-up scans (50%) showed evidence for increasing disease activity by this method.

The average MRI activity rate in the three studies was 30% active scans. This rate was almost exactly the same as that seen in the placebo arm of the interferon β-1b clinical trial [Paty *et al.* 1993].

A number of gadolinium enhanced MRI serial studies have also been reported (see Table 7.1). In these studies up to 90% of new MRI lesions enhanced with gadolinium. Occasionally an enhancing area was seen before the standard MRI lesion was seen [Kermode *et al.* 1990a]. In one study, spinal cord imaging added about 20% to the MRI activity rate based on the standard head MRI scans [Wiebe *et al.* 1990]. Miller *et al.* [1993c] compared Gd enhancement with ordinary PD/T2 lesion evaluation for sensitivity in detecting MRI activity. They studied 19 relapsing-remitting and seven secondary progressive (total 26 patients) who had monthly MRI evaluations over four months each. One (#26) patient was an outlier with 144 active lesions, most (88%) detected by enhancement occurring within T2 lesions that did not change in size. Eighty-three per cent (83%) of the active lesions in patient #26 were newly active and 17% persistently active. In the other 25 cases there were 106 active lesions: 68 (64%) were detected only by enhancement, 16 (15%) were detected only by T2 changes, and 22 (21%) were detected by both techniques. Of the 106 active lesions detected in the 25 patients noted above, 82 (77%) were newly active and 24 (23%) were persistently active.

The Queen Square group [Thompson *et al.* 1990b] have also reported profound MRI activity differences among several clinical categories of patient. Primary progressive patients had the lowest rate of activity (very few lesions were enhancing) at 3.3 active lesions per patient per year. The next highest rate was for benign patients (DSS < 3 at > 10 years) who had 8.8 *new* lesions per patient per year. Typical relapsing-remitting and secondary progressive patients had 17.2 and 18.2 *new* lesions per patient per year respectively.

The data from most serial studies have shown that the rate of lesion activity varies widely among patients with some extreme outliers as noted above. Unfortunately, the rate of development of new and/or otherwise active lesions also varies considerably over time in individual patients. Some patients can be active over several months and then be totally inactive for the next several months. Harris *et al.* [1991] and Smith *et al.* [1993] have called these activity periods 'bursts' of activity. It is also clear that much more activity is seen on high field scanners using thinner (3–5 mm thick) slices. Figure 3.9 shows an example of serial MRI activity obtained in a secondary progressive patient using monthly T2-weighted and gadolinium enhanced scanning on a 0.5 T system.

The optimum scanning frequency for activity measurements is a compromise between the information obtained versus cost and compliance. It also depends heavily on the scanner and sequences used. The following experience is based on using the low field (0.15 T) system with low resolution, 10 mm slice thickness and PD/T2-weighted scans alone in Vancouver. It was found that the scanning frequency most likely to give good, detailed information is once every two weeks. Assuming that no lesion activity lasts less than two weeks, 100% of new and active lesions are detectable at two weeks' scanning frequency. In an examination of the impact of scanning frequency, Koopmans *et al.* [unpublished observations] found (in unenhanced scans) that 67% of lesion activity was seen with scans performed every four weeks and 40% of lesion activity was seen with scans performed every six weeks. Longer scanning intervals reduced the detection of active lesions even more. There was less impact on new lesion activity than on other forms of unenhanced activity. Conversely, 36% of active lesions had a duration of activity of less than four weeks, another 28% between four and six weeks, and another 7% between six and eight weeks. Scanning at yearly intervals allowed at least 33% of the new lesions to be seen, [Koopmans *et al.* unpublished observations] (relatively more of the enlarging activity was lost) and if the number of patients evaluated is large, highly significant therapeutic results can be detected, as in the interferon β-1b clinical trial.

At Queen Square, three patients have undergone weekly PD/T2-weighted and gadolinium enhanced scans for three months on a 1.5 T system with 5 mm thick slices [Lai *et al.* 1996]. On weekly scans 38 new enhancing lesions were seen, but only 16 new PD/T2 lesions, confirming the greater sensitivity of enhancement for lesion activity reported earlier [Miller *et al.* 1993c]. Although two lesions enhanced on only a single scan (proving that enhancement can occur for less than two weeks), monthly scans revealed 33 new enhancing lesions. Thus, assuming that weekly scanning is 100% sensitive for activity, 87% of new enhancing lesions were seen on monthly scans. The monthly interval is a practical one for patients and is now widely used in treatment trials using scanners within the usual range of available field strengths (0.5 –1.5 tesla).

The NIH Neuroimmunology Group [McFarland *et al.* 1992; Smith *et al.* 1993] have proposed a unique method of activity assessment. They suggest determining the number of enhancing lesions by monthly scanning on untreated patients for six months. They then do a post-treatment activity analysis (Boot Strap) for comparison. This single crossover design is more powerful than a parallel groups, placebo-controlled design because there is less intra-patient variation in MRI activity over time than there is inter-patient variation. A limitation of the single crossover design is the tendency for regression towards the mean if (as often happens) patients are selected because they have recently active disease either clinically or on MRI; simultaneous, placebo-controlled, parallel groups will thus provide more certain proof of treatment effect. Nevertheless, the results of a study from the same group [Stone *et al.* 1995a] showed that open label interferon β-1b dramatically reduced the enhancement rate in a group of relapsing patients that they had been studying for MRI natural history prior to starting on therapy. Since that result is consistent with published studies [Paty *et al.* 1993] the methodology may indeed be sound, especially where, as in the NIH patients, there has been a long run-in period of observation prior to treatment.

7.2.2   MRI quantitative lesion load studies

Several studies have compared the severity (extent) of disease on the MRI scan of the head with the degree of clinical severity [Huber *et al.* 1987; Franklin *et al.* 1988; Kiel *et al.* 1988]. The correlation between clinical impairment and the MRI quantitative study measures has not been precise. Several computer assisted methods for measuring the abnormal areas seen on the MRI scan have been developed in order to follow the evolution of the extent of pathology over time [Paty 1987, 1988 a, b]. An operator controlled computer assisted method of analysis has been shown to be reproducible, to show an expected increase in lesion load over time and to be sensitive to treatment effects [Paty *et al.* 1993]. In the analysis of the scans a radiologist experienced in serial MRI evaluation indicates the number, size, and distribution of lesions for each subject. After all lesions are identified, localised and named, they are marked on the MRI hard copy film for subsequent quantitation.

For quantitation purposes, a technician with a known reproducibility record traces the margins of the lesions using a track ball tracing system. The PD- and T2-weighted scans are used to identify the lesions; however, the tracing of lesions is done only on the PD-weighted (long TR, short TE) scan. The reason for that restriction is that, on the PD-weighted scan, the CSF is dark or neutral with white matter, allowing contrast with the

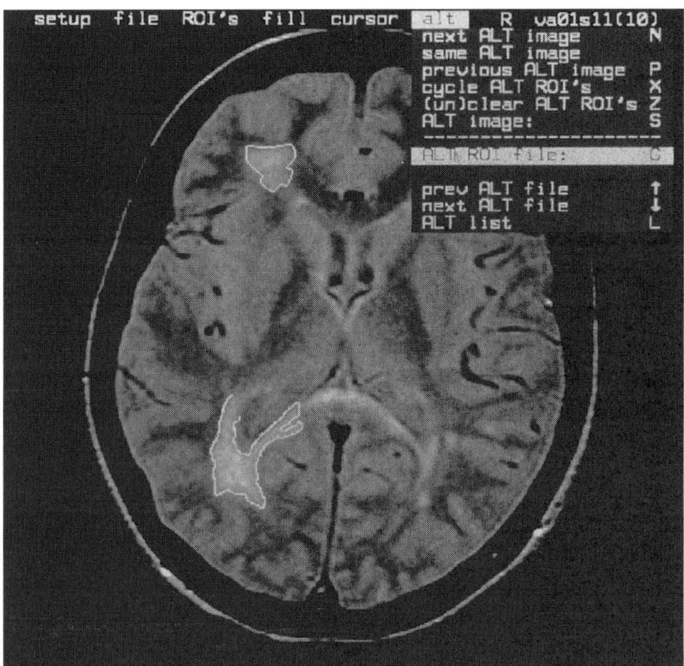

Figure 7.1 *MR image shows two multiple sclerosis lesions which have been out-lined manually on a computer screen at the University of British Columbia Multiple Sclerosis/MRI Study Group.*

higher signal of the lesions – thus the periventricular lesion load can be more easily identified and traced. The area of each lesion (Region of Interest [ROI]), is displayed on a computer monitor, using the radiologist's markings on the film as a guide. Repeated tracings on the same image, spaced over days or weeks, by an experienced and skilled technician can measure the MRI lesions with a reproducibility error of less than 6%. The inter-observer error is much greater (17–30%). Therefore a single observer is used for each study in order to keep variability to a minimum.

By using this method a computer based description of the area of the lesions slice by slice in square millimetres can be obtained. The computer is programmed to calculate individual lesion (ROI) area, total lesion area per slice and total lesion area from all head slices in each patient. At the end of the process all of the abnormal areas traced (ROIs) are added up, slice by slice, in order to obtain an overall index of the extent of the disease in mm^2. Figure 7.1 shows how the quantitation process is done. Figure 7.2 shows what an entire slice quantitation looks like.

Van Walderveen *et al.* [1995] have recently suggested that changes in the extent of hypointense, non-enhancing lesions seen on gadolinium enhanced T1-weighted scans correlates better with change in clinical impairment than does the extent of the change in lesions seen on the PD/T2-weighted scans. This difference is probably because many

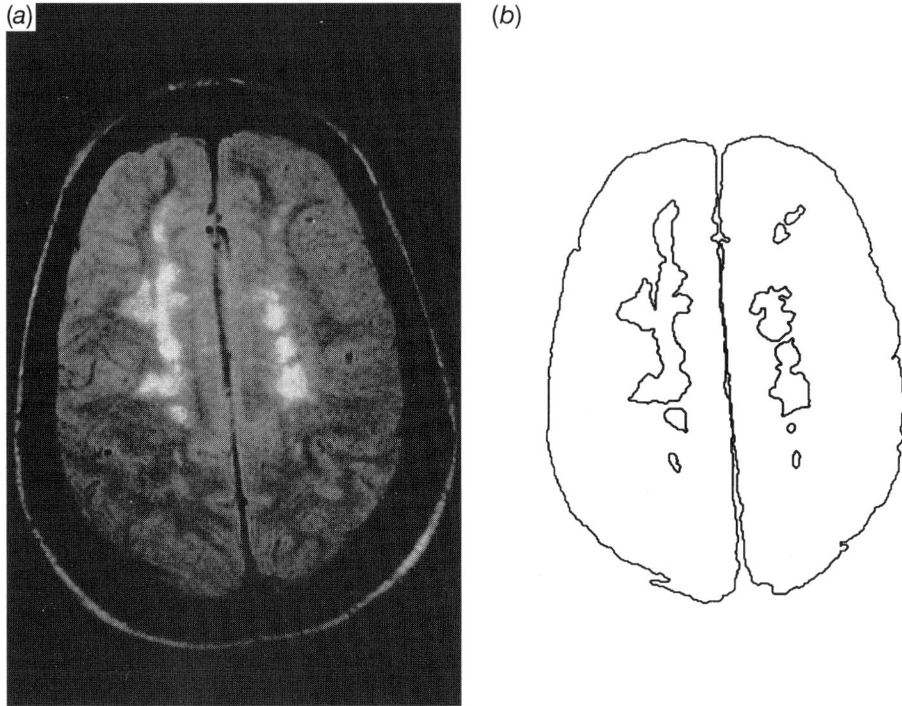

Figure 7.2 *(a) A single slice shows multiple sclerosis lesions; (b) the result of lesion segmentation by manual outlining is displayed.*

of the hypointense lesions seen on the T1 scan tend to be more chronic and pathologically more severe than those lesions seen only on the PD/T2 scan. All lesions seen on unenhanced T1-weighted scans are also seen on PD/T2; however, there are a significant number of lesions seen on PD/T2 that are not seen on T1. The portion of lesions seen on PD/T2 but not on T1 are probably less destructive pathologically. Some may only be inflammatory, and therefore, one can speculate that anti-inflammatory therapies would be less likely to exert an effect on the non-enhancing hypointense T1 lesions than on the PD/T2-weighted scans (*enhancing* lesions on T1-weighted scans are however inflammatory and anti-inflammatory therapy should exert an effect on these).

There are many automated and semi-automated methods proposed for measuring lesion size, and some of these are listed in Table 7.2. The manual method described above has been validated as showing the expected increase in lesion load over time and being sensitive to a treatment effect. The automated methods use a variety of strategies and have many virtues, e.g. improved precision and being less time consuming. However, it is possible that some automatic methods, though reproducible, may miss a treatment effect, e.g. the margin of the lesion might be where the treatment effect is located and the eye (as employed using manual tracing) may be more sensitive than the computer for detecting subtle changes. The various methods need to be compared and contrasted in a

Table 7.2 *Several methods of measuring the lesion load on MRI*

Date	Author	Description of quantative method	Units reported
1985	Paty	Manual tracing of each lesion slice by slice summed	mm^2
1987	Paty	Manual tracing of each lesion slice by slice summed	mm^2
1989b	Koopmans	Manual tracing of each lesion slice by slice	mm^2
1989	Kapouleas	Low level segmentation, 3×3 gradient operator edge detection with editing	Voxels
1990	Baumhefner	Manual tracing	mm^2
1992	Pannizzo	Segmentation algorithms with fat suppression with editing	Pixels
1992	Haughton	4 sequence intensities plotted vs echo time squares	T1 and T2 intensities
1992	Wicks	Threshold on T2 images	mm^3
1992	Swirsky-Sacchetti	Total lesion area (TLA) manual	mm^2
1992	Kamber	Brain tissue probability model with lesion segmentation	Proportions
1993	Jackson (Narayana)	T2 and MTR images with contrast segmentation	cm^3
1994	Gass	MTR/threshold with editing	mm^2
1994	Arnold	Summed NAA for whole brain (shows progressive decrease over time)	NAA/Cr ratios
1994	Zuk/Atkins	Registration to match surfaces	Proportions
1994	Guttmann	4D segmentation algorithm	mm^3
1994	Mitchell	2D histogram using proton density and T2-weighted intensities	3D
1995	Cohen	3D connectivity: 'fuzzy logic'	mm^3
1996	Johnston/Atkins	Model based on volume segmentation	
1996	Grimaud	Comparison of manual with thresholding and contouring	mm^3

Table 7.3 *Selected correlations from the final report of the IFN 1ß study (1995; Table 8)*

Measure 1 (1)	Comparisons with	Measure 2 (2)	Spearman rank correlation coefficient (Table 8)	*p* value
Baseline EDSS		Baseline MRI area	0.218	<0.001
End point EDSS		End point MRI area	0.257	<0.001
Change in EDSS		Change in MRI area	0.229	<0.001
Baseline Scripps (NRS)*		Baseline MRI area	−0.249	<0.001
End point Scripps		End point MRI area	−0.277	<0.001
Change in Scripps		Change in MRI area	−0.213	<0.001
Exacerbation Rate		Change in MRI area	0.203	<0.001

Note:

Reference: IFNB Study Group, 1995, *Neurology*, 45, 1277–85

*NRS = Neurological Rating Scale (Scripps scale)

cooperative project with the goal of identifying the ability of each to be both sensitive to changes over time and sensitive to treatment effects.

7.3   Clinical MRI correlations: implications for treatment trials

A detailed review of the correlations between clinical and MRI findings has been presented in Chapters 5 and 6. In addition, some correlations have been noted in two clinical trials in which quantitative studies showed clear-cut increases in lesion load of at least 10% per year [Koopmans *et al.* 1992; The IFNB 1b Study Group 1995].

In the cyclosporin trial, the mean MRI lesion load increase was 25% per year; in addition, even though there was no MRI treatment effect [Koopmans *et al.* 1992], the change in MRI lesion load and the change in EDSS were weakly correlated ($r = 0.186, p = 0.018$).

In the interferon β-1b trial, there were numerous correlations between a number of MRI and clinical parameters. These associations were modest but statistically significant (Table 7.3). The patients with the highest relapse rate (> 1.5 per patient per year) had the greatest change in EDSS and the greatest change in MRI lesion load. The most important of those correlations was that the change in EDSS correlated significantly, albeit weakly, with the change in MRI lesion load. It is not understood why the MRI activity rates were affected much more profoundly by the treatment than was the clinical attack rate;

perhaps future experience with variable doses of drug, and with additional drugs that approach different aspects of the immune response, may help in understanding this dilemma, as may the implementation of MR techniques that are more specific for the disabling pathology in multiple sclerosis, namely demyelination and axonal loss.

The above studies plus those summarised in Chapters 5 and 6 confirm that conventional PD/T2-weighted and gadolinium enhanced MRI findings have only modest correlations with the clinical status and course in established multiple sclerosis (although there are more impressive correlations in patients with clinically isolated syndromes). In spite of the limited correlations, the sensitive and objective way in which MRI detects pathological activity has made it a useful tool to monitor therapy. A recent Task Force of the US National Multiple Sclerosis Society has prepared guidelines for the use of MRI in therapeutic trials (see also Section 7.5.3), and included the following four position statements which adequately summarise the current viewpoint of the authors of this book:

(1) MRI is a highly sensitive marker of pathological activity in relapsing-remitting and secondary progressive multiple sclerosis.

(2) There are significant correlations emerging between a number of MR and clinical parameters, although in established multiple sclerosis the relationship between short-term MRI activity and long-term disability is still uncertain.

(3) A high sensitivity makes MRI an excellent tool for rapid screening of therapies aimed at suppressing new pathological activity in relapsing-remitting and secondary progressive multiple sclerosis. Because the long-term relationship between MRI and disability is still uncertain, MRI data should not be the definitive determinant of therapeutic efficacy. A clinically significant endpoint must be shown. MRI should be used to select appropriate patients with clinically isolated syndromes for trials of therapy aimed at delaying the evolution to definite multiple sclerosis.

(4) There are still evolving major improvements in the resolution and sensitivity of MR imaging, and in new techniques to monitor demyelination and neuronal damage and to quantify lesion load. Further studies are needed in ongoing treatment trials to determine whether these new techniques will prove to be more strongly predictive of clinical outcome.

7.4   Recent use of MRI in clinical trials (Tables 7.3, 7.4 and 7.5)

An important application of serial MRI quantitative measurements is in clinical trials. Clinical trials in multiple sclerosis have long been hampered by the lack of an objective measurement of lesion load. As noted above, neurological findings (impairment) and functional deficits (disability) at best indicate the anatomical localisation of some of the multiple sclerosis lesions and give some approximation of the extent of their severity. However, the bulk of lesions are silent to the neurological examination. Therefore, in order to have a more objective approach to clinical trials, quantitative MRI methods have been used several times. The first clinical treatment trials to be monitored by MRI were performed from 1985 to 1990 [Kappos *et al.* 1988; Paty 1987, 1988, etc.; Kastrukoff *et al.* 1990; Koopmans *et al.* 1992].

There are analogous methods in clinical and MRI outcome measures for clinical trials. Clinical acute phase measures are counting and otherwise measuring relapses, while chronic phase measures utilise neurological impairment measures such as the EDSS. In order to be certified as chronic, the measure must be confirmed after an interval of three to six months.

MRI acute phase measures are activity measures counting active lesions over time.

Table 7.4 *MRI activity measures used in the IFNß 1b (1993 & 1995) clinical trial in RRMS*

MRI measure	N	Duration	Placebo vs low dose vs high dose			*p* value
			PLAC	LD	HD	(Plac vs HD)
Vancouver cohort (6-weekly scans)						
% active scans/patient						
(median)	52	2 yrs	29.4	11.8	5.9	0.0170
% active scans/group						
(mean)	52	2 yrs	30.0	15.0	15.0	0.001
Annual rate new lesions						
(median)	52	2 yrs	2.0	0.5	0.5	0.0085
Annual rate all active lesions						
(median)	52	2 yrs	3.0	1.0	0.5	0.0234
*All patients** (annual scans)						
Activity rate all active lesions						
(mean)	217	4 yrs	6.44	3.92	3.08	0.001
Activity rate new lesions*						
(mean)	217	4 yrs	3.57	2.01	1.80	0.001
Lesion load measure	217	2 yrs	11.9	12.4	−5.6	0.0015
% from baseline (median)		3 yrs	21.0	6.1	−3.8	0.0002
		4 yrs	18.7	11.7	0.8	0.005

Note:

* Data from R Koopmans, G Zhao, D Li & D Paty, in preparation (1996) 'Interferon beta-1b decreases MS lesion activity in relapsing-remitting patients as detected by yearly MRI.'

RRMS=relapsing remitting MS.

Table 7.5 *Serial MRI studies in the evaluation of clinical trials*

	Senior Author	Year	Agent used	GD used	Type of PT	Findings
1)	Paty	1993	IFNB 1b	o	RR	MRIs every 6 weeks over 2 years revealed a significant treatment effect
2)	Durelli	1994	IFNA(r)	o	RR	MRIs at 6 months revealed a significant treatment effect
3)	Bastianello	1994	Mitoxantrone	+	RR	5 MRIs over 1 year revealed a trend but not a significant treatment effect
4)	Stone	1995a	IFNB 1b	+	RR	Pre- and post-treatment (open label) enhanced studies revealed a marked treatment effect
5)	Sipe	1994	Cladribine	+	SP	Less enhancement in treated subjects
6)	Moreau	1994	Campath-1H	+	SP	Pre- and post-treatment (open label) enhanced studies revealed a marked treatment effect
7)	Wiles	1994	TLI irradiation	o	SP/PP	Marginal effect
8)	Milligan	1994	Isoprinosine	o	RR/SP	No effect
9)	Edan	1995	Mitoxantrone	+	SP/RR	Marked (80–90%) reduction in number of enhancing lesions over 6 months in mitoxantrone treated group

Note

RR = relapsing-remitting

SP = secondary progressive

PP = primary progressive

GD = gadolinium enhancement

MRI chronic phase measures have applied lesion load (burden of disease) quantitation. However, the confirmation rule applied to chronic clinical measures has not been applied as yet to MRI.

7.4.1   Alpha lymphoblastoid interferon

In a prospective evaluation of 100 patients during a placebo-controlled therapeutic trial of alpha lymphoblastoid interferon [Kastrukoff *et al.* 1990; Koopmans *et al.* 1993b] 63 of the subjects had quantitative MRI evaluations at entry, at six months, and at two years. The MRI quantitation technique was used to analyse the MRI changes that occurred over that time. The changes in the lesion load ranged from -50% to $+62\%$ over two years. The mean change in extent was $+10\%$ over baseline ($p = 0.02$). The results were disappointing in that no significant treatment effect was seen at two years in either the clinical or MRI measurements. However, at six months there was a trend toward a treatment effect on the MRI detected lesion load ($p = 0.0628$). In addition, the activity analysis showed that the number of active lesions on MRI was highest in the placebo group at both six months and 24 months ($p = > 0.05$) but that the differences were not overall statistically significant at two years ($p = > 0.75$). The possible treatment effect was most pronounced in the subgroup who had large MRI lesion load at baseline ($p = 0.019$). This clinical trial experience showed that both the quantitative measure of disease burden and the analysis of individual lesion changes contributed important information to the assessment of outcome. Most important, there was a statistically significant increase in MRI detected lesion load, as expected, in both groups (treatment and placebo) over the two years.

7.4.2   Cyclosporin A

Similar quantitative methods were applied in this collaborative therapeutic trial. In order to do the MRI analysis in multicentre studies, computer software was developed to read the MRI tape formats from the various manufacturers including GE, Siemens, Fonar, Diasonics, Picker, and Phillips [Paty 1988a]. The cyclosporin trial did not show a robust clinical therapeutic effect [The Multiple Sclerosis Study Group 1990], but did show an increase in MRI lesion load with time and a significant correlation between change in MR and change in EDSS [Koopmans *et al.* 1992].

MRI measurements expressed as per cent change from baseline showed their greatest variability in patients with the smallest lesion load at baseline. That finding was not a surprise since the addition of a few small lesions in such a case would cause a small absolute change but a large percentage change. However, a separate analysis done for patients with large 'disease burden' at baseline and those with minimal 'disease burden' at baseline did not change the outcome of the study.

7.4.3   Interferon β-1b (Tables 7.3 and 7.4)

The manual computer assisted MRI quantitation method was used in the IFNB-1b placebo-controlled clinical trial in relapsing patients [Paty *et al.* 1993; The IFNB Study Group 1993]. Interferon β-1b was submitted to a multicentre, randomised double-blind, placebo-controlled trial in 372 ambulatory patients with relapsing and remitting multiple sclerosis. Mildly or moderately disabled patients with at least two exacerbations in the previous two years were accepted. One third of the patients received placebo, one third received 1.6 million international units (MIU) and one third received 8 MIU self-administered by sub-cutaneous injections every other day. The primary endpoints were the difference in exacerbation rates between treated and placebo groups and the proportion of patients remaining exacerbation free. The secondary endpoints included quantitative yearly PD/T2-weighted MRI scans in all patients, and frequent (once every six weeks) MRI scans for analysis of disease activity in a sub-cohort of 52 patients at The University of British Columbia (UBC). The numbers of new and enlarging lesions were determined in all scans (every six weeks) over two years in the Vancouver cohort and yearly in all patients. Gadolinium enhancement was not available at the start of the study so was not used as an activity measure. Table 7.4 shows some of the MRI outcome measures used in the study.

The annual exacerbation rate for patients receiving placebo was 1.27 exacerbations per patient per year during the first two years of the study. Patients receiving 1.6 MIU had 1.17 exacerbations per patient per year. Those patients receiving the high dose (8 MIU) of interferon β-1b had an exacerbation rate of 0.84 exacerbations per patient per year. The exacerbation rates were significantly lower in both treatment groups when compared with the placebo group ($p = 0.0086$). There was a two-fold reduction in the frequency of moderate and severe attacks in the high dose treatment group. The high dose treatment group had 36 patients who were exacerbation free at two years compared with only 18 patients in the placebo group. The overall neurological impairment (EDSS score) changed very little from baseline in both the placebo and treatment arms. A statistically significant change in disability as a treatment effect could not be discerned in this trial.

MRI analyses were carried out in 327 of the 372 patients. Baseline MRI characteristics were the same in all treatment groups. The MRI results support the clinical results showing a significant reduction in disease activity as measured by the number of active scans (median 80% reduction, $p = 0.0082$) and the appearance of new lesions. In addition, there was an equally significant reduction in MRI lesion load (using computer assisted quantitative methods) in the treatment group as compared with the placebo group (mean group difference was 23% from baseline, $p = 0.0001$).

In a further double-blind controlled follow-up for four years the study continued to show a 30% reduction in relapse rate in the high dose treatment group. However, the reduced patient numbers due to drop out reduced the statistical significance especially since the patients who dropped out had the highest rates of activity on MRI [The IFNB Study Group 1995]. The yearly MRI quantitation and the MRI activity rates after four years continued to show a significant reduction in both measures in the high dose treatment group in spite of the lower numbers of patients remaining in the trial [The IFNB Study Group 1995].

The measure that was most sensitive to treatment effect was the MRI activity rate (see Table 7.4). The Vancouver cohort of 52 patients showed a significant treatment effect at the end of one year in both lesion activity and lesion load measures [Paty *et al.* 1994]. The earliest indication of treatment effect was the percentage of active scans in each treatment group at each scanning interval. At six weeks into the study the placebo group had 30% active scans, compared to 15% in both treatment groups. This difference was not statistically significant at six weeks (the first scanning interval) but the trend continued throughout the study and the cumulative differences became significant at the one year mark. The delay in statistical significance can be attributed to the small sample size. The difference remained significant throughout the second year of the study. The overall activity rate, the active scan rate, and the new lesion rate were all statistically significantly depressed by the treatment.

An activity analysis (new and enlarging lesions) also done on the yearly scans from all sites showed a significant treatment effect at both doses [Koopmans *et al.* 1994]. However, the yearly scans do not identify the time of onset of the treatment effect or the consistency of treatment effect throughout the study.

For some reason the MRI activity measurements in the Vancouver cohort of the trial did not distinguish between the two drug doses. The lesion load measure, however, did show a dose effect.

Quantitative lesion loads were also calculated on the subgroup of patients who completed four or more years (at least five yearly scans). In this cohort the placebo group showed a statistically significant increase in lesion load from baseline to year one, year one to year two, and year two to year three. The difference from year three to year four was not statistically significant while the comparison between placebo and high dose treated groups remained significantly different throughout the study. An analysis of those patients who dropped out prior to year four showed that their increase on the lesion load measure and their clinical measures were much higher than the mean. Those findings suggested that the patients who dropped out were, on the whole, those that were doing the worst. The clinical and MRI correlations from the four-year trial data are summarised in Table 7.3.

In summary, a combination of clinical and MRI results showed that interferon β-1b has a partial beneficial effect on the course of relapsing-remitting multiple sclerosis. However the effect was much greater on MRI than clinical measurements. For example, the mean relapse rate was decreased by 34% in the high dose treatment group while the mean percentage active scan rate was reduced by 55%, the median active scan rate by 80%, the median new lesion rate by 70% and the mean new lesion rate by 62%. It is a sobering contrast to note that there was no statistically significant effect of treatment on the progression of neurological impairment. The necessary further studies are underway in order to discern the long-term effect of this therapy on progression in impairment in patients with secondary progressive disease.

7.4.4   Interferon α-2a

Recently Durelli and his colleagues [1994] have reported a pilot trial with interferon α-2a monitored by MRI showing a significant treatment effect over six months. They treated 20 patients with relapsing-remitting MS with 9 million IU intra-muscularly every other day for six months. There were 27 MRI events in the placebo group and one in the treated group ($p = < 0.01$). Eight per cent of the treated group and 75% of the placebo group had active scans. Production of gamma interferon was also reduced in the treatment group. These findings should be further examined and confirmed in a large clinical trial using both frequent scanning for activity and quantitative lesion load measures for chronic changes.

7.4.5   Interferon β-1a

Jacobs *et al.* [1994, 1996] have reported a trial in relapsing MS with once per week intra-muscular injection of interferon β-1a that showed a slowing in progression of disability, a 30% reduction in relapse rate and a decrease in enhancing lesions on yearly scans as a therapeutic effect [Simon *et al.* 1995]. The analysis over two years did not show the expected increase in PD/T2 lesion load over time or a therapeutic effect on T2 lesion load. Those findings may reflect differences in methodology for measuring PD/T2 lesion load, or it may be that the MRI effect was less pronounced than the interferon β-1b trial.

   In another small study, intramuscular interferon β-1a was given weekly for three months to six patients while six other patients received placebo [Rudge *et al.* 1995]; in all patients monthly gadolinium enhanced scans were performed for nine months, starting three months before treatment began and stopping three months after treatment had ceased. There was a non-significant increase in MRI activity during the treatment phase in the six patients treated with interferon β-1a.

7.4.6   Corticosteroids

In small, uncontrolled studies of patients in acute relapse, high dose intravenous methylprednisolone has been found to rapidly and markedly suppress gadolinium enhancement in lesions that were enhancing prior to starting treatment. This effect was generally accompanied by clinical improvement [Miller *et al.* 1992c; Barkhof *et al.* 1991, 1992c; Burnham *et al.* 1991]. The effect on enhancement appears to be transient (one week or so after three days of intravenous methylprednisolone [Miller *et al.* 1992c]). In these uncontrolled studies, no obvious effect was noted on pre-existing PD/T2 lesions (although their size was not measured quantitatively), or on the development of new disease activity.

7.4.7   Campath-1H

Using a run-in period of scanning pre-treatment as control data, a dramatic reduction in lesion activity was seen in seven patients treated with Campath-1H, an anti-lymphocyte antibody [Moreau *et al.* 1994]. During a three-month run-in period, there was a total of 27 new enhancing or PD/T2 lesions; in the first three months post treatment there were 13 lesions, and in the next three months only two new lesions appeared. While this study illustrates the power of MRI to observe treatment effects in small cohorts, its significance is limited by the well-known hazards of using patients as their own control. Patients were required to display MRI activity in order to be treated; thus the cohort is biased towards being 'active' at entry, and it is possible that the result is partly due to regression towards the mean and not solely a treatment effect.

7.4.8   Cladribine

A larger study, which did include a control group, reported stabilisation of T2 lesion load in patients treated with cladribine, whereas lesion load increased in the control group [Sipe *et al.* 1994]. However, the groups were not matched for lesion load at entry, and the mean lesion load was substantially higher in the cladribine group. Furthermore, the reproducibility of the lesion load measurements was not reported. A more favourable outcome for the treated group in terms of ongoing enhancement during the study is difficult to interpret as the proportions in each group who displayed enhancement on the entry scan were not stated.

7.4.9   Mitoxantrone

A placebo-controlled trial of mitoxantrone in relapsing-remitting multiple sclerosis over one year revealed that the mean numbers of new and enhancing lesions in the treated group were respectively 40% and 60% less than in the placebo group [Bastianello *et al.* 1994]. However, this difference was not statistically significant, perhaps because of the small sample size (13 treated with mitoxantrone and 12 placebo). A more recent multicentre French study used gadolinium enhanced monthly scans for two months prior to the start of treatment and for six months during treatment; 20 patients received monthly intravenous methylprednisolone alone while 20 received monthly methylprednisolone and mitoxantrone. There was a dramatic reduction in the number of enhancing lesions (by 80–90%) in the mitoxantrone group [Edan *et al.* 1995].

7.4.10   Linomide

In a double-blind, placebo-controlled study of the immunomodulating agent linomide, 30 secondary progressive patients were followed with clinical assessments and monthly T2-weighted and gadolinium enhanced MRI for six months. The percentage of patients with new enhancing lesions was 75% in the placebo and 33% in the linomide group ($p <$ 0.021) [Karussis *et al.* 1996]. Some clinical benefits were also noted. A reduction in MRI activity of a similar magnitude was also reported in a group of relapsing-remitting patients [Andersen *et al.* 1996].

7.4.11   Results from other recent trials

The lack of or at best minor effects on MRI activity of isoprinosine [Milligan *et al.* 1994] and total lymphoid irradiation [Wiles *et al.* 1994] supported the clinical assessment that these therapies are not useful in multiple sclerosis. Serial quantitative MRI analysis was performed in a small subgroup of patients participating in the North American, placebo-controlled trial of Copolymer-1 in relapsing-remitting multiple sclerosis; there was a non-significant trend suggesting reduced MRI activity in the Copolymer-1 treated patients, but the sample size was too small to draw definite conclusions [Cohen *et al.* 1995]. Finally, serial monthly MRI studies showed no reduction in MRI activity in recent placebo-controlled trials of deoxyspergualin [Kappos *et al.* 1995] and chimeric anti-CD4 antibodies [Barkhof *et al.* 1995].

7.4.12   Trials in progress

Statistical calculations have suggested that substantial sample sizes (e.g. 2 $\times$ 30–50) are needed to demonstrate a moderate (50–70%) reduction in active lesions in a parallel design placebo-controlled study [McFarland *et al.* 1992; Nauta *et al.* 1994]. Such studies are now being frequently undertaken to evaluate new therapies. The positive MRI results seen recently with a number of agents in such studies (e.g. linomide and mitoxantrone) does provide a rationale for examining them further in a large-scale trial which has a definitive clinical endpoint. Herein lies a key role of MRI in treatment monitoring – to provide a preliminary measure of therapeutic efficacy at the pathological level, long before it is possible to evaluate confidently the clinical effect. Nevertheless, given the modest long-term relationship between MRI and disability in established multiple sclerosis, it is prudent for the present that disability remains the definitive measure of therapeutic efficacy.

7.5   A guide to the application of MR techniques in therapeutic trials

Experience with trials in the past few years has clearly shown that clinical monitoring, though concentrating on the aspect most relevant to the patient, is not sensitive or precise enough to give rapid and accurate indications of the therapeutic effect. Today, combined clinical and MRI monitoring is providing a wealth of new insights into the monitoring paradigm.

Several years ago a European committee on the use of MRI to monitor clinical trials in multiple sclerosis [Miller *et al.* 1991b] made the following suggestions:

(1) That MRI monitoring of treatment trials is appropriate.

(2) That such monitoring studies can be done in periods as short as six months where MRI parameters are the primary outcome.

(3) That gadolinium enhancement adds 10% or more to the activity determined by unenhanced PD/T2 scanning and should be done routinely (subsequent work suggests that the additional yield with gadolinium is nearer 100% [Miller *et al.* 1993c]).

(4) That scanning every four weeks should be the standard interval for preliminary studies of the efficacy of treatment on pathological activity.

(5) That preliminary MRI outcome studies should be confined to early relapsing-remitting or secondary progressive multiple sclerosis, as MRI activity is greatest in these cohorts.

The European group subsequently proposed a database for recording lesion activity in the context of clinical trials [Barkhof *et al.* 1993]. In addition, Nauta *et al.* [1994] have made sample size calculations based on previously published natural history studies at Queen Square and Amsterdam, utilising 23 relapsing–remitting or secondary progressive patients having monthly scans for six months. Individual patients had 0% to 100% active scans (on average 40% of the scans were active); three of the 23 (13%) had no MRI activity. They calculated that for treatment efficacy of 80% in a parallel groups, placebo-controlled study, the required sample size was 2×20 if followed for four months (200 scans), 2×30 if followed for three months (180 scans) or 2×50 if followed for one month (200 scans). For a treatment efficacy of 60%, 2×40 patients for six months (560 scans), 2×50 for four months (500 scans), or 2×75 for two months (450 scans) would be needed.

It may not be absolutely necessary to do routine enhanced studies in all clinical trials [Paty 1988a, b; Paty *et al.* 1992b; Miller *et al.* 1992d] as evidenced by the success of the interferon β-1b relapsing and remitting trial in which gadolinium was not used. Routine axial PD/T2-weighted scans alone can identify many active lesions in serial studies, and enhanced scans add to the cost and complexity in both time and invasiveness. It is likely, however, that gadolinium enhancement improves reliability (as well as sensitivity): it is not uncommon to confirm that a lesion is active when unambiguous enhancement is seen but the corresponding PD/T2-weighted change was only equivocal. It is often especially difficult to decide whether or not a PD/T2 lesion is enlarging, since repositioning errors can readily change its appearance [Goodkin *et al.* 1992]. If one is doing a study in which knowledge of the frequency and degree of disruption of the blood–brain barrier is critical, then enhancement is essential. In addition, enhancement, spectroscopy, T2 relaxation, and other MR techniques may help to provide evidence for the mechanism of action of drugs found to be effective by conventional PD/T2-weighted scanning. If there is a differential effect between these various MR measurements, that difference may give an indication as to where the drug exerts its effect, e.g. at the bloood–brain barrier, to reduce inflammation, to reduce demyelination, or in the final analysis, to reduce axonal loss.

The sections that follow are a guide to the analysis of MR images in systematic studies for both MRI activity and lesion load. These comments are placed in the context of the clinical outcomes also being measured and their associated problems.

7.5.1 Acute dynamic activity

7.5.1.1 *Clinical monitoring for acute dynamic activity*

Clinical relapses can be identified as new symptoms accompanied by appropriate neurological signs usually evolving to a maximum state over a few days [Schumacher *et al.* 1965]. There is a 70% likelihood for acute relapses to recover, at least partially [Rose *et al.* 1970]. The Schumacher Committee defined relapses very carefully and the original articles should be read for details. Symptoms should appear in the absence of fever or other metabolic upset. Symptoms that appear and resolve coincident with fever are usually categorised as a *pseudo relapse.* Pseudo relapses are due to reversible failure of conduction in demyelinated areas due to changes in the microenvironment. For example, increased temperature or increased rate of firing of an axon can result in temporary conduction block (Waxman 1988).

Relapses must be over 24 hours in duration and are usually defined as lasting up to a month. Some relapses last longer than a month. However, a new relapse can only be diagnosed after one month has passed from the onset of the previous relapse. This one-month rule is arbitrary but is generally acknowledged. New data from MRI monitoring has shown that new lesions can occur at a very rapid rate, and some day we may be forced to drop the one-month rule. Perhaps two weeks is more appropriate.

Various methods have been used to quantitate relapses. Perhaps the best method is that devised by Millar [1973], who used a formula that considered the severity of individual symptoms and signs plus duration to derive a relapse severity score. Recent clinical studies have used changes in the Scripps impairment score to measure the severity of relapses [The IFNB Study Group 1993]. The degree of change in the Scripps impairment score was used to categorise the severity of relapses as mild, moderate, or severe. This method seemed to work well in the interferon β-1b trial in relapsing and remitting disease. Clinical dynamic activity can be measured as relapses per month, quarter, or year and expressed as activity per patient, per group, or as per cent activity overall. Since relapse rates vary widely among patients in a skewed fashion, results should be expressed as both the mean and the median ($\pm$ SD).

7.5.1.2   *MR monitoring for acute dynamic activity*

7.5.1.2.1   *Types of active lesion.*   A distinction should be made between new and persistent lesion activity: the former term is used when the activity first appears, the latter term when the same lesion continues to be active on follow-up scans. When a lesion has been active, then becomes inactive, and then becomes active again, the term recurrent activity may be used. When both PD/T2-weighted and gadolinium enhanced scans are obtained, new, recurrent and persistent active lesions are defined as follows:

(1) *New active lesions*: either new enhancement on gadolinium enhanced T1-weighted scans (regardless of whether there is a corresponding change on the PD/T2-weighted scans) or new non-enhancing lesions on the PD/T2-weighted scans or newly enlarging non-enhancing lesions on the PD/T2-weighted scans. Of these three types of new active lesion, new enhancing lesions are by far the most common (over 90% of total) when scanning at monthly intervals.

(2) *Recurrent active lesions*: either new enhancement where there had been a previous episode of enhancement or a new PD/T2 lesion where there had been a previous lesion that had disappeared. Neither category is common, and the latter is extremely rare on high field scanners.

(3) *Persistent active lesions*: either continued enhancement of a new enhancing lesion at follow-up or continued enlargement on follow-up of a non-enhancing new or enlarging lesion on PD/T2-weighted MRI. At monthly intervals about one-third of new enhancing lesions continue to enhance at follow-up, but persistent non-enhancing activity on PD/T2-weighted scans is extremely rare.

7.5.1.2.2   *Types of Activity to monitor.*   One can look at total number of active lesions, or the number of new, recurrent or persistently active lesions. Also the number of active scans (i.e. it contains at least one active lesion) can be studied, as can the number of active patients (i.e. having at least one active lesion during the study). The results can then be expressed as absolute numbers, or percentages per patient, scan, group, or over time.

7.5.2 Chronic dynamic activity

7.5.2.1 *Clinical monitoring for chronic changes:*

This method of evaluation is the most problematic [Willoughby & Paty 1988]. Chronic clinical impairment is the feature that is of most concern to the physician and to the patient since it is the feature that causes disability. However, it is clear that the type and degree of impairment is dependent on the severity of only a few specific lesions located in specific tracts. There are many lesions in silent areas of the nervous system that are biologically important but not so clinically important. Therefore, even though the impairment scales measure clinically relevant neurological deficits, they do not give a very good indication as to the total involvement in the nervous system by the multiple sclerosis pathological process.

It is probably not possible to devise a clinical scale that reflects the total extent of involvement by the pathological process. In addition, the most frequently used clinical impairment scale (the EDSS) [Kurtzke 1983] is notoriously insensitive to change.

Also, the addition of measures of cognitive, emotional and quality of life factors to the standard neurological scoring systems will help in providing some sort of assessment of the global involvement. How one can make these clinical measures more sensitive to pathological change is not apparent at this time. Combining all measures into a single global index of severity such as the EDSS may not be the answer. In order to increase sensitivity, one must be able to measure changes due to fluctuation in individual lesions, because it is at the individual lesion level that the fundamental pathological changes occur.

7.5.2.2 *MRI monitoring for chronic changes*

The methods available today to measure chronic MRI changes are usually limited to determining the extent of the lesions on the T_1– or PD/T_2-weighted scan by defining the border of the lesion (lesions) by visual or semi-automated algorithms. The lesions seen on PD/T_2-weighted scans have heterogeneous pathology. As noted in Section 7.2.2, van Walderveen and colleagues [1995] have tried to limit the heterogeneity by measuring only the hypointense lesions seen on the T_1-weighted scan. The lesions seen on the T_1 scan are much less extensive than those seen on the PD/T_2 scans and probably reflect a subgroup of the most severe lesions. The T_1 measures may exclude some of the less destructive or purely inflammatory lesions which are present on the PD/T_2-weighted scan. However, acute lesions may show transient hypointensity on T_1-weighted scans which reverses with follow-up – thus T_1 hypointensity does not mean there is always irreversible tissue damage.

It must be remembered that the exact pathology that is being measured by T_1– and PD/T_2-weighted scans is still unknown. In future, as technical problems are overcome, it will be important to use other MR techniques which are probably more specific to severe tissue damage and in particular irreversible demyelination and axonal loss, the pathological substrates of permanent disability. The putative techniques are listed in Table 5.5, and discussed in Chapters 5 and 6.

7.4.3   Guidelines of The United States Multiple Sclerosis Society
MRI Task Force 1996

Already, it can be said that a quantitative approach to MRI activity by measuring active lesions in frequent scans and by measuring the lesion load will be complementary and additive to the clinical evaluation and is now considered an important outcome measure in all clinical studies (Whitaker *et al.* 1995). Under the auspices of the Medical Advisory Board of The United States National Multiple Sclerosis Society, a Task Force has recently developed detailed guidelines for using MRI to monitor the treatment of multiple sclerosis [Miller *et al.* 1996]. Summary position statements from the Task Force have already been presented (Section 7.3). The Task Force has developed MRI protocols for three types of trial (see Appendices 1–3):

(1) *Exploratory trials in established multiple sclerosis (Appendix 1).* It is recommended that MRI measurements be the primary outcome in such trials.

(2) *Definitive trials in established multiple sclerosis (Appendix 2).* MRI measurements are proposed as a secondary outcome, the primary outcomes being clinical, most often progression in disability or the relapse rate.

(3) *Trials in patients presenting with clinically isolated syndromes (Appendix 3).* The primary outcome of this study is the proportion of patients developing clinically definite multiple sclerosis over the next two to three years. MRI has a crucial role in identifying and selecting those patients with a high risk of developing multiple sclerosis over this period. Follow-up scans are proposed as a secondary outcome measure.

Figure 7.3 provides a flow diagram for the use of MRI in assessing new therapies, from initial screening to definitive trials, in patients with established multiple sclerosis. The interested reader is referred to the paper for full details concerning these protocols [Miller *et al.* 1996].

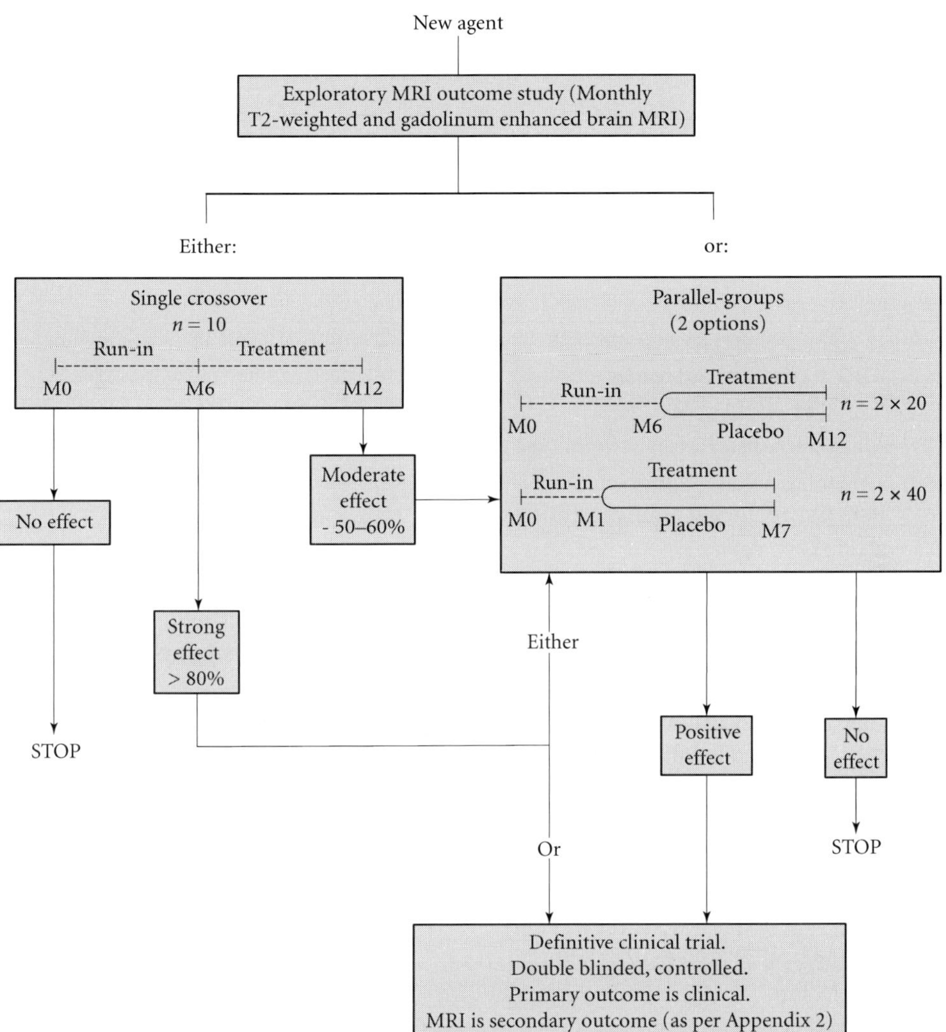

Figure 7.3 *Suggested procedures for MRI evaluation of new experimental therapies in relapsing-remitting and secondary progressive multiple sclerosis (prepared by the MRI Task Force of the United States Multiple Sclerosis Society). (From Miller et al. 1996, reprinted from* Annals of Neurology *V39, pp. 6–16, by permission of Little, Brown & Co. Inc.)*

Appendix 1
Preliminary trials in established multiple sclerosis

(a) MRI is primary outcome.

(b) Main outcome: lesion activity (see text for definitions).

(c) Patients: relapsing-remitting and secondary progressive multiple sclerosis aged 18–50 years.

(d) Design (see Figure 7.3).

EITHER	single crossover with ten patients*, using six months of run-in and six months of treatment;
OR	parallel groups, 2 × 20 patients*, with six months of run-in followed by six months treatment;
OR	parallel groups, 2 × 40 patients[†], with one month of run-in followed by six months of treatment.

(e) Core protocol: monthly PD/T2-weighted fast SE and gadolinium enhanced brain MRI.

(f) Duration 7–12 months (see above).

(g) Optional: T1 and PD lesion load six-monthly.

NB. The sample sizes in (d) were estimated to provide a greater than 80% chance of demonstrating a 50–60% reduction in the number of active lesions by therapy. They are based on the MRI findings, without selection according to MRI activity, in two small untreated groups of patients with relapsing-remitting or secondary progressive multiple sclerosis [McFarland *et al.* 1992*; Nauta *et al.* 1994[†]]. Because of the marked variations in MRI activity between and within patients over time, differences in the definition of active lesions*[†], and differences in statistical methodology, they should be regarded as approximate estimates only. Further analysis of larger untreated cohorts is needed to obtain more reliable sample size estimates for the various designs and clinical subgroups.

* Active lesions defined as new and persistently enhancing lesions; using this definition, 85% of scans contained active lesions. Slightly higher sample sizes were calculated when using new enhancing lesions only as the outcome.

[†] Active lesions defined as new enhancing and new or enlarging non-enhancing lesions; 42% of scans contained active lesions.

(Appendices 1–3 reprinted from Miller *et al.* 1996, *Annals of Neurology* V39, pp. 6–16, by permission of Little, Brown & Co. Inc.)

Appendix 2
Definitive trials in established multiple sclerosis.

(a) MRI is secondary outcome.

(b) Main MR outcome: change in T1 and PD lesion load using either manual outlining or semi-automated techniques which have been validated for their accuracy and reproducibility.

(c) Patients:

      EITHER   relapsing-remitting and secondary progressive;

      OR   primary progressive.

(d) Design: parallel groups.

(e) Core protocol: unenhanced PD/T2- and T1-weighted conventional SE brain MRI for six to twelve-month intervals in all patients.[*]

(f) Duration 2–3 years.

(g) Optional: yearly gadolinium enhanced brain MRI.

(h) Optional: monthly PD/T2-weighted and gadolinium enhanced brain MRI for six months at beginning and end in a subset of patients.

(i) Optional: putative markers of demyelination and neuronal damage (Table 5.5) six- to 12-monthly in a subset of patients.

---

[*] The sample size (typically several hundred patients) will be determined by the primary clinical outcomes being sought. In general, large numbers of patients will also be needed to demonstrate significant treatment effects on changes in total MRI lesion load, and it therefore seems prudent that the core MRI protocol be applied to all patients.

Appendix 3
Trials in clinically isolated syndromes

(a)   MRI is secondary outcome measure (the suggested primary outcome is the proportion of patients who develop clinicallly definite multiple sclerosis during the study).

(b)   Main MR outcomes:
(i) change in T1 and PD lesion load using either manual outlining or validated semi-automated techniques;
(ii)new or enlarging lesions seen on PD/T2-weighted scans.

(c)   Age 18 to 45 (the upper age limit chosen to reduce the likelihood of age-related vascular abnormalities on MRI).

(d)   Entry MRI criteria:

EITHER   four or more non-enhancing cerebral white matter lesions on PD/T2-weighted brain MRI at presentation;

OR   three cerebral white matter lesions, at least one of which enhances;

OR   two non-enhancing cerebral white matter lesions and one or more infratentorial lesions.

(e)   Design: parallel groups, placebo-controlled.

(f)   Core protocol: six- or 12-monthly unenhanced PD/T2- and T1-weighted conventional SE brain MRI in all patients*.

(g)   Duration: three years.

(h)   Optional: monthly PD/T2-weighted and gadolinium enhanced brain MRI for six months at beginning and end in a subset of patients.

* The sample size will be determined by the primary clinical outcomes being sought. Substantial numbers of patients will probably be needed to demonstrate significant treatment effects on changes in total MRI lesion load, and it therefore seems prudent that the core MRI protocol be applied to all patients.

References

Adams CWM, Poston RN & Buk SJ (1989). Pathology, histochemistry and immunocytochemistry of lesions in acute multiple sclerosis. *Journal of the Neurological Sciences*, 92, 291–306.

Adams C (1989). In: *A Colour Atlas of Multiple Sclerosis and Other Demyelinating Disorders.* Ipswich, Wolfe.

Adams RD & Kubik CS (1952). The morbid anatomy of the demyelinative diseases. *American Journal of Medicine* 12, 510–46.

Ahn SS, Mantello MT, Jones KM, *et al.* (1992). Rapid MR imaging of the pediatric brain using the fast-spin echo technique. *American Journal of Neuroradiology*, 13, 1169–77.

Aisen AM, Gabrielsen TO and McCune WJ (1985a). MR imaging of systemic lupus erythematosus involving the brain. *American Journal of Radiology*, 144, 1027–31.

Aisen AM, Martel W, Gabrielsen TO, *et al.* (1985b). Wilson disease of the brain: MR imaging. *Radiology*, 157, 137–41.

Alcock NS & Hoffman HL (1962). Recurrent encephalomyelitis in childhood. *Archives of Diseases in Childhood*, 37, 40–4.

Alexander EL, Craft C, Dorsch C, *et al.* (1982). Necrotizing arteritis and spinal subarachnoid hemorrhage in Sjogren syndrome. *Annals of Neurology*, 11, 632–5.

Alexander EL, Beall SS, Gordon B, *et al.* (1988). Magnetic resonance imaging of cerebral lesions in patients with Sjogren syndrome. *Medicine (Baltimore)*, 108, 815–23.

Allen IV, Glover G & Anderson R (1981). Abnormalities in the macroscopically normal white matter in cases of mild or spinal multiple sclerosis. *Acta Neuropathologica*, suppl VII, 176–8.

Allen IV (1991). Pathology and its implications. In: *McAlpine's Multiple Sclerosis*, 2nd edn, ed. WB Matthews, pp 341–90. London, Churchill Livingstone.

Alperovich A, Hors J, Lyon-Caen O, *et al.* (1992). Multiple sclerosis in 54 twinships: concordance rate is independent of zygosity. *Annals of Neurology*, 32, 724–7.

Aminoff MJ & Logue V (1974). The prognosis of patients with spinal vascular malformations. *Brain*, 97, 211–18.

Anzola GP, Bevilacquia L, Cappa SF, *et al.* (1990). Neuropsychological assessment in patients with relapsing-remitting multiple sclerosis and mild functional impairment: correlation with magnetic resonance imaging. *Journal of Neurology, Neurosurgery and Psychiatry*, 53, 142–5.

Andersen O, Lycke J, Tolleson PO, *et al.* (1996). Linomide reduces the rate of active lesions in relapsing-remitting multiple sclerosis. *Neurology*, 47, 895–900.

April RS and Vansonnenberg E (1976). A case of neuromyelitis optica (Devic's syndrome) in systemic lupus erythematosus. *Neurology*, 26, 1066–70.

Arnett PA, Rao SM, Bernardin L, *et al.* (1994). Relationship between frontal lobe lesions and Wisconsin Card Sorting Test performance in patients with multiple sclerosis. *Neurology*, 44, 420–5.

Arnold DL, Matthews PM, Francis G and Antel J (1990). Proton magnetic resonance spectroscopy of human brain *in vivo* in the evaluation of multiple sclerosis: assessment of the load of the disease. *Magnetic Resonance in Medicine*, 14, 154–9.

Arnold DL, Matthews PM, Francis G, *et al.* (1992). Proton magnetic resonance spectroscopic imaging for metabolic characterisation of plaques in multiple sclerosis. *Annals of Neurology*, 31, 235–41.

Arnold DL, Riess GT, Matthews PM, *et al.* (1994). Use of proton magnetic resonance spectroscopy for monitoring disease progression in multiple sclerosis. *Annals of Neurology*, 36, 76–82.

Atlas SW, Grossman RI, Goldberg HJ, Hackney DB, Bilaniuk LT and Zimmerman RA (1986). MR diagnosis of acute disseminated encephalomyelitis. *Journal of Computer Assisted Tomography*, 8, 381–4.

Awad IA, Spetzler RF, Hodak JA, Awad CA, Carey R (1986). Incidental subcortical lesions identified on magnetic resonance imaging in the elderly. I. Correlation with age and cerebrovascular risk factors. *Stroke*, 17, 1084–9.

Balaban RS & Ceckler TL (1992). Magnetization transfer

contrast in magnetic resonance imaging. *Magnetic Resonance Quarterly*, 8, 116–17.

Banna M & El-Ramahi K (1991). Neurologic involvement in Behçet disease: imaging findings in 16 patients. *American Journal of Neuroradiology*, 12, 791–6.

Baratti C, Barkhof F, Hoogenraad F and Valk J (1994). Fluid attenuated inversion recovery (FLAIR) sequence in multiple sclerosis: contrast parameters in a steady state and comparison with spin echo sequences. *Proceedings of The Society of Magnetic Resonance*, 1, 544.

Barbosa S, Blumhardt LD, Roberts N, *et al.* (1994). Magnetic resonance relaxation time mapping in multiple sclerosis: normal appearing white matter and the 'invisible' lesion load. *Magnetic Resonance Imaging*, 12, 33–42.

Barkhof F, Hommes OR, Scheltens P and Valk J (1991). Quantitative MRI changes in gadolinium-DTPA enhancement after high-dose intravenous methylprednisolone treatment in multiple sclerosis. *Neurology*, 41, 1219–22.

Barkhof F, Valk J, Hommes O, *et al.* (1992a). Gadopentate dimeglumine enhancement of multiple sclerosis lesions on long TR spin-echo images at 0.6 T. *American Journal of Neuroradiology*, 13, 1257–9.

Barkhof F, Scheltens P, Frequin ST, *et al.* (1992b). Relapsing-remitting multiple sclerosis: sequential enhanced MR imaging vs clinical findings in determining disease activity. *American Journal of Radiology*, 159, 1041–7.

Barkhof F, Frequin STFM, Hommes OR, *et al.* (1992c). A correlative triad of gadolinium-DTPA MRI, EDSS, and CSF-MBP in relapsing/remitting multiple sclerosis patients treated with high-dose intravenous methylprednisolone. *Neurology*, 42, 63–7.

Barkhof F, Thompson AJ, Kappos L, *et al.* (1993). Database for serial magnetic resonance imaging in multiple sclerosis. *Neuroradiology*, 35, 362–6.

Barkhof F, Filippi M, Tas MW, *et al.* (1994). Towards specific MR imaging criteria for early MS. In: *Proceedings of European Committee for Treatment and Research in Multiple Sclerosis*, 10th Congress, p. 9. Athens, University Studio Press.

Barkhof F, Thompson AJ, Hodgkinson S, *et al.* (1995). Double-blind, placebo-controlled, MR monitored exploratory trial of chimeric anti-CD4 antibodies in MS. *Journal of Neuroimmunology*, suppl 1, 15.

Barnard RO and Trigg M (1974). Corpus callosum in multiple sclerosis. *Journal of Neurology, Neurosurgery and Psychiatry*, 37, 1259–64.

Barnes D, McDonald WI, Johnson G, *et al.* (1986). NMR imaging of experimental cerebral oedema. *Journal of Neurology, Neurosurgery and Psychiatry*, 49, 1341–7.

Barnes D, McDonald WI, Johnson G, *et al.* (1987). Quantitative nuclear magnetic resonance imaging: characterisation of experimental cerebral oedema. *Journal of Neurology, Neurosurgery and Psychiatry*, 50, 125–33.

Barnes D, McDonald WI, Landon DN and Johnson G (1988). The characterization of experimental gliosis by quantitative nuclear magnetic resonance imaging. *Brain*, 111, 83–94.

Barnes D, Munro PMG, Youl BD, *et al.* (1991). The longstanding MS lesion. A quantitative MRI and electron microscopic study. *Brain*, 114, 1271–80.

Barratt HJ, Miller DH and Rudge P (1988). The site of the lesion causing deafness in multiple sclerosis. *Scandinavian Audiology* 17, 67–71.

Bastianello S, Pozzilli C, Bernardi S, *et al.* (1990). Serial study of gadolinium-DTPA MRI enhancement in multiple sclerosis. *Neurology*, 40, 591–5.

Bastianello S, Pozzilli C, D'Andrea F, *et al.* (1994). A controlled trial of mitoxantrone in multiple sclerosis: serial MRI evaluation at one year. *Canadian Journal of Neurological Science*, 21, 266–70.

Bateman DE, White JE, Elrington G, *et al.* (1987). Three further cases of Lyme disease. *British Medical Journal*, 294, 548–9.

Bauer HJ & Hanefeld FA (1993). *Multiple Sclerosis: its Impact from Childhood to Old Age*. London, WB Saunders.

Baumhefner RW, Tourtellotte WW, Syndulcho K, *et al.* (1990). Quantitative MS plaque assessment with MRI. Its correlation with clinical parameters, EPs, and intra blood–brain barrier. *Archives of Neurology*, 47, 19–26.

Beatty WW & Goodkin DE (1990). Screening for cognitive impairment in multiple sclerosis: an evaluation of the Mini-Mental State Examination. *Archives of Neurology*, 47, 297–301.

Beatty WW, Goodkin DE, Hertsgaard D & Monson N (1990). Clinical and demographic predictors of cognitive performance in multiple sclerosis: Do diagnostic type, disease duration and disability matter? *Archives of Neurology*, 47, 305–8.

Beaulieu C & Allen PS (1994). Determinants of anisotropic water diffusion in nerves. *Magnetic Resonance in Medicine*, 31, 394–400.

Beck RW, Cleary PA, Anderson MM jr, *et al.* (1992). A randomised, controlled trial of corticosteroids in the treatment of acute optic neuritis. *New England Journal of Medicine*, 326, 581–8.

Beck RA & Cleary PA (1993). Optic neuritis treatment trial: one-year follow-up results. *Archives of Ophthalmology*, 111, 773–5.

Beck RW, Cleary PA, Trobe JD, *et al.* (1993). The effect of corticosteroids for acute optic neuritis on the subsequent development of multiple sclerosis. *New England Journal of Medicine*, 329, 1764–9.

Beck RW (1995). The Optic Neuritis Treatment Trial: three year follow-up results. *Archives of Ophthalmology*, 113, 136.

Bergin JD (1957). Rapidly progressing dementia in

disseminated sclerosis. *Journal of Neurology, Neurosurgery and Psychiatry*, 20, 285–92.

Bick U, Ullrich K, Stober U, *et al.* (1991). Disturbed myelination in patients with treated hyperphenylalaninaemia: disturbed myelination or toxic oedema? *European Journal of Pediatrics*, 150, 185–9.

Bielschowsky M (1903). Zur histologie der multiplen sklerose. *Neurologisches Zentralblatt*, 770.

Bird GLA, Meadows J, Goka J, *et al.* (1990). Cyclosporin-associated akinetic mutism and extrapyramidal syndrome after liver transplantation. *Journal of Neurology, Neurosurgery and Psychiatry*, 53, 1068–71.

Birken DL & Oldendorf WH (1989). N-acetyl-L-aspartate: a literature review of a compound prominent in ¹H-NMR spectroscopic studies of brain. *Neuroscience and Biobehavioural Reviews*, 13, 23–31.

Black JA, Felts P, Smith KJ, *et al.* (1991). Distribution of sodium channels in chronically demyelinated spinal cord axons: Immuno-ultrastructral localization and electrophysiological observations. *Brain Research*, 544, 59–70.

Bloch F, Hansen WW and Packard ME (1946). Nuclear induction. *Physics Reviews*, 69, 127.

Boggild MD, Williams R, Haq N & Hawkins CP (1995). Cortical plaques visualised by fluid-attenuated inversion recovery imaging in relapsing multiple sclerosis. *Journal of Neurology*, 242 (suppl 2), S6.

Bogousslavsky J, Fox AJ, Carey LS, *et al.* (1986). Correlates of brain-stem oculomotor disorders in multiple sclerosis (magnetic resonance imaging). *Archives of Neurology*, 43, 460–3.

Bostock H & Sears TA (1978). The internodal axon membrane: electrical excitability and continuous conduction in segmental demyelination. *Journal of Physiology*, 280, 273–301.

Bostock H & McDonald WI (1982). Recovery and function after demyelination. In: Sears TA (ed.) *Neuronal-Glial Cell Inter-relationships*. Berlin, Springer Verlag, pp. 287–302.

Bradley WG & Whitty CW (1968). Acute optic neuritis: prognosis for the development of multiple sclerosis. *Journal of Neurology, Neurosurgery and Psychiatry*, 31, 10–18.

Brant-Zawadski M, Fein G, van Dyke C, *et al.* (1985). MR imaging of the ageing brain: patchy white-matter lesions and dementia. *American Journal of Neuroradiology*, 6, 675–82.

Brinkmeier H, Kaspar A, Wiethölter H, Rüdel R (1992). Interleukin-II inhibits sodium currents in human muscle cells. *Pflügers Archiv European Journal of Physiology*, 420, 621–3.

Bronstein AM, Morris J, du Boulay GH, *et al.* (1990a). Abnormalities of horizontal gaze. Clinical, oculographic and magnetic resonance imaging findings. I. Abducens palsy. *Journal of Neurology, Neurosurgery and Psychiatry*, 53, 194–9.

Bronstein AM, Rudge P, Gresty MA, *et al.* (1990b). Abnormalities of horizontal gaze. Clinical, oculographic and magnetic resonance imaging findings. II. Gaze palsy and internuclear ophthalmoplegia. *Journal of Neurology, Neurosurgery and Psychiatry*, 53, 200–7.

Brooks DL, Leenders KL, Head G, *et al.* (1984). Studies on regional cerebral oxygen utilisation and cognitive function in multiple sclerosis. *Journal of Neurology, Neurosurgery and Psychiatry* 47, 1182–91.

Brosnan CF, Litwak MS, Schroeder CE, *et al.* (1989). Preliminary studies of cytokine-induced functional effects on the visual pathways in the rabbit. *Journal of Neuroimmunology*, 25, 227–39.

Brownell B & Hughes JT (1962). The distribution of plaques in the cerebrum in multiple sclerosis. *Journal of Neurology, Neurosurgery and Psychiatry*, 25, 315–20.

Burnham JA, Wright RR, Dreisbach J and Murray RS (1991). The effect of high dose steroids on MRI gadolinium enhancement in acute demyelinating lesions. *Neurology*, 41, 1349–54.

Butler EG and Gilligan BS (1989). Obstructive hydrocephalus caused by multiple sclerosis. *Clinical and Experimental Neurology*, 26, 219–23.

Bye AME, Kendall BE & Wilson J (1985). Multiple sclerosis in childhood. *Developmental Medicine and Child Neurology*, 27, 215–22.

Cadoux-Hudson TAD, Kermode A, Rajagopalan B, *et al.* (1991). Biochemical changes within a multiple sclerosis plaque in vivo. *Journal of Neurology, Neurosurgery and Psychiatry*, 54, 1004–6.

Callanan MM, Logsdail SJ, Ron MA and Warrington EK (1989). Cognitive impairment in patients with clinically isolated lesions of the type seen in MS: A psychometric and MRI study. *Brain*, 112, 361–74.

Campi A, Filippi M, Comi G, *et al.* (1995). Acute transverse myelopathy: spinal and cranial MR study with clinical follow-up. *American Journal of Neuroradiology*, 16, 115–23.

Capra R, Marciano N, Vignolo LA, *et al.* (1992). Gadolinium-pentacetic acid magnetic resonance imaging in patients with relapsing-remitting multiple sclerosis. *Archives of Neurology*, 49, 687–9.

Carswell,R. (1838). *Pathological Anatomy: Illustrations of the Elementary Forms of the Disease*. London, Longman, Orme, Brown, Green and Longman.

Charcot M. (1868). Histologie de la sclérose en plaques. *Gazette des Hôpitaux*, Paris, 141, 554–5, 557–8.

Christiansen P, Frederiksen JL, Henriksen O and Larsson HBW (1992). Gd-DTPA enhanced lesions in the brain of patients with acute optic neuritis. *Acta Neurologica Scandinavica*, 85, 141–6.

Chusid MJ, Williamson SJ, Murphy JV & Ramey LS (1979). Neuromyelitis optica (Devic disease) following varicella infection. *Journal of Pediatrics*, 95, 737–8.

Cleary MA, Walter JH, Wraith JE, *et al.* (1994). Magnetic

resonance imaging of the brain in phenylketonuria. *Lancet*, 344, 87–90.

Cline HE, Lorensen WE, Kikinis R, *et al.* (1990). Three-dimensional segmentation of MR images of the head using probability and connectivity. *Journal of Computer Assisted Tomography*, 14, 1037–45.

Cohen JA, Grossman RI, Udupa JK, *et al.* (1995). Assessment of the efficacy of copolymer-1 in the treatment of MS by quantitative MRI. *Journal of Neuroimmunology*, suppl 1, 31.

Cohen MM, Lessell S & Wolf PA (1979). A prospective study of the risk of developing multiple sclerosis in uncomplicated optic neuritis. *Neurology*, 29, 208–13.

Collins DL, Neelin P, Peters TM and Evans AC (1994). Automatic 3D intersubject registration of MR volumetric data in standardized Talairach space. *Journal of Computer Assisted Tomography*, 18, 192–205.

Comi G, Filippi M, Martinelli V, *et al.* (1995). Brain MRI correlates of cognitive impairment in primary and secondary progressive multiple sclerosis. *Journal of Neurological Science*, 132, 222–7.

Compston DAS, Batchelor JR, Earl CJ and McDonald WI (1978). Factors influencing the risk of multiple sclerosis developing in patients with optic neuritis. *Brain*, 101, 495–511.

Confavreux C, Aimard G & Devic M (1980). Course and prognosis of multiple sclerosis assessed by computerised data processing of 349 patients. *Brain*, 103, 281–300.

Constable RT & Gore JC (1992). The loss of small objects in variable TE imaging: implications for FSE, RARE and EPI. *Magnetic Resonance in Medicine*, 28, 9–24.

Constantino A, Black SE, Carr T, *et al.* (1986). Dorsal midbrain syndrome in multiple sclerosis with magnetic resonance imaging correlation. *Canadian Journal of Neurological Science*, 13, 62–5.

Cowan J, Ormerod IEC & Rudge P (1990). Hemiparetic multiple sclerosis. *Journal of Neurology, Neurosurgery and Psychiatry*, 53, 675–80.

Cruickshank JK, Rudge P, Dalgleish AG, *et al.* (1989). Tropical spastic paraparesis and human T cell lymphotropic virus type I in the United Kingdom. *Brain*, 112, 1057–90.

Curé JK, Cromwell LD & Case JL (1990). Auditory dysfunction caused by multiple sclerosis: detection with MR imaging. *American Journal of Neuroradiology*, 11, 817–20.

Curnes JT, Laster DW, Ball MR, *et al.* (1986). MRI of radiation injury to the brain. *American Journal of Radiology*, 147, 119–24.

Davie CA, Hawkins CP, Barker GJ, *et al.* (1994a). Serial proton magnetic spectroscopy in acute multiple sclerosis lesions. *Brain*, 117, 49–58.

Davie CA, Barker GJ, Brenton D, *et al.* (1994b). Proton

magnetic resonance spectroscopy in adult cases of phenylketonuria. *Journal of Neurology, Neurosurgery and Psychiatry*, 57, 1292.

Davie CA, Barker GJ, Webb S, *et al.* (1995). Persistent functional deficit in multiple sclerosis and autosomal dominant cerebellar ataxia is associated with axonal loss. *Brain*, 118, 1583–92.

Davies SEC, Newcombe J, Williams SR, *et al.* (1995). High resolution proton NMR spectroscopy of multiple sclerosis lesions. *Journal of Neurochemistry*, 64, 742–8.

Dawson JW (1916). The histology of disseminated sclerosis. *Transactions of the Royal Society Edinburgh* 50, 417–740.

Dawson DM (1992). Antineoplastic drugs. In: *Diseases of the Nervous System. Clinical Neurobiology*, 2nd edn, vol 2, eds AK Asbury, GM McKhann & WI McDonald, pp. 1121–9. Philadelphia: WB Saunders.

Dietrich RB & Bradley WG jr (1988). Iron accumulation in the basal ganglia following severe ischaemic-anoxic insults in children. *Radiology*, 168, 203–6.

Doran M & Bydder GM (1990). Magnetic resonance: perfusion and diffusion imaging. *Neuroradiology*, 32, 392–8.

Dorwat RH, Frank JA, Dwyer AJ, *et al.* (1986). CNS imaging with short TI inversion recovery pulse sequence: sensitivity compared to T-2 weighted spin echo images. *Proceedings of The Society of Magnetic Resonance in Medicine*, 1, 9–10.

Dousset V, Grosman R, Ramer KN, *et al.* (1992). Experimental allergic encephalomyelitis and multiple sclerosis: lesion characterization with magnetization transfer imaging. *Radiology*, 182, 483–91.

Dousset V, Brochet B, Vital F, *et al.* (1994). Imaging including diffusion and magnetization transfer of chronic relapsing experimental encephalomyelitis – correlation with immunological and pathological datas. *Proceedings of the Society of Magnetic Resonance*, 2, 1401.

Dousset V, Brochet B, Vital A, *et al.* (1995). Lysolecithin-induced demyelination in primates: preliminary in vivo study with MR and magnetization transfer. *American Journal of Neuroradiology*, 16, 225–31.

Drayer BP, Burger P, Hurwitz B, *et al.* (1987). Reduced signal intensity on MR images of thalamus and putamen in multiple sclerosis: increased iron content? *American Journal of Neuroradiology*, 8, 413–19.

Drayer BP (1988). Imaging of the aging brain: part I. Normal findings. *Radiology*, 166, 785–96.

Duda EE, Huttenlocher PR & Patronas NJ (1980). CT of subacute sclerosing panencephalitis. *American Journal of Neuroradiology*, 1, 35–8.

Dunn V, Bale JF, Zimmerman RD, *et al.* (1986). MRI in children with post infectious disseminated encephalomyelitis. *Magnetic Resonance Imaging*, 4, 25–32.

Durelli L, Bongioanni MR, Cavallo R, *et al.* (1994). Chronic systemic high-dose recombinant interferon alpha-2a reduces exacerbation rate, MRI signs of disease activity, and lymphocyte interferon gamma production in relapsing-remitting multiple sclerosis. *Neurology*, 44, 406–13.

Ebers GC, Bulman DE, Sadovnick AD, *et al.* (1986). A population based study of multiple sclerosis in twins. *New England Journal of Medicine*, 315, 1638–42.

Edan G & French and British Multiple Sclerosis Mitoxantrone Trial Group (1995). Demonstration of the efficacy of mitoxantrone (MTX) using MRI in MS patients with very active disease. *Journal of Neuroimmunology*, suppl 1, 16.

Edelstein WA, Hutchison JMS, Johnson G, Redpath T (1980). Spin warp NMR imaging and applications to human whole-body imaging. *Physical Medicine and Biology*, 25, 751–6.

Edzes HT & Samulski ET (1977). Cross relaxation and spin diffusion in the proton NMR of hydrated collagen. *Nature*, 265, 521–3.

Ellis SG & Verity MA (1979). Central nervous system involvement in systemic lupus erythematosus: a review of neuropathological findings in 57 cases. *Seminars in Arthritis and Rheumatism*, 8, 212–21.

Eng J, Ceckler TL & Balaban RS (1991). Quantitative H magnetisation transfer imaging in vivo. *Magnetic Resonance in Medicine*, 17, 304–14.

England JD, Gamboni F, Levinson SR and Finger TE (1990). Changed distribution of sodium channels along demyelinated axons. *Proceedings of the National Academy of Science, USA*, 87, 6777–80.

Enzmann DR & Rubin JB (1988). Cervical spine: MR imaging with a partial flip angle, gradient-refocused pulse sequence. Part II. Spinal cord disease. *Radiology*, 166, 473–8.

Erdem E, Carlier R, Idir ABC, *et al.* (1993a) Gadolinium-enhanced MRI in central nervous system Behçet's disease. *Neuroradiology*, 35, 142–4.

Erdem E, Carlier R, Delvalle A, *et al.* (1993b). Gadolinium-enhanced MRI in Whipple's disease. *Neuroradiology*, 35, 581–3.

Fazekas F, Offenbacher H, Fuchs S, *et al.* (1988). Criteria for an increased specificity of MRI interpretation in elderly subjects with suspected multiple sclerosis. *Neurology*, 38, 1822–5.

Fazekas F (1989). Magnetic resonance signal abnormalities in asymptomatic individuals: their incidence and functional correlate. *European Neurology*, 29, 164–8.

Feinstein A, Kartsounis LD, Miller DH, *et al.* (1992a). Clinically isolated lesions of the type seen in multiple sclerosis: a cognitive, psychiatric, and MRI follow-up study. *Journal of Neurology, Neurosurgery and Psychiatry*, 55, 869–76.

Feinstein A, du Boulay GH & Ron MA (1992b). Psychotic illness in multiple sclerosis: a clinical and magnetic resonance imaging study. *British Journal of Psychiatry*, 161, 680–5.

Feinstein A, Youl BD, Ron MA. (1992c). Acute optic neuritis. A cognitive and magnetic resonance imaging study. *Brain*, 115, 1403–15.

Feinstein A, Ron M & Thompson AJ (1993). A serial study of psychometric and magnetic resonance imaging changes in multiple sclerosis. *Brain*, 116, 569–602.

Ferbert A, Busse D & Thron A (1991). Microinfarction in classic migraine? A study with magnetic resonance imaging findings. *Stroke*, 22, 1010–14.

Filippi M, Horsfield MA, Morrissey SP, *et al.* (1994a). Quantitative brain MRI lesion load predicts the course of clinically isolated syndromes suggestive of multiple sclerosis. *Neurology*, 44, 635–41.

Filippi M, Barker GJ, Horsfield MA, *et al.* (1994b). Benign and secondary progressive multiple sclerosis; a preliminary quantitative MRI study. *Journal of Neurology*, 241, 246–51.

Filippi M, Campi A, Martinelli V, *et al.* (1995a). Comparison of triple dose versus standard dose gadolinium-DTPA for detection of MRI enhancing lesions in patients with primary progressive multiple sclerosis. *Journal of Neurology, Neurosurgery and Psychiatry*, 59, 540–4.

Filippi M, Horsfield MA, Bressi S, *et al.* (1995b). Intra- and inter-observer agreement of brain MRI lesion volume measurements in multiple sclerosis. A comparison of techniques. *Brain*, 118, 1593–1600.

Filippi M, Horsfield MA, Campi A, *et al.* (1995c). Resolution-dependent estimates of lesion volumes in magnetic resonance imaging studies of the brain in multiple sclerosis. *Annals of Neurology*, 38, 749–754.

Filippi M, Paty DW, Kappos L, *et al.* (1995d). Correlations between changes in disability and T2-weighted brain MRI activity in multiple sclerosis: a follow-up study. *Neurology*, 45, 255–60.

Filippi M, Campi A, Mammi S, *et al.* (1995e). Brain magnetic resonance imaging and multimodal evoked potentials in benign and secondary progressive multiple sclerosis. *Journal of Neurology, Neurosurgery and Psychiatry*, 58, 31–7.

Filippi M, Campi A, Martinelli V, *et al.* (1995f). A brain MRI study of different types of chronic-progressive multiple sclerosis. *Acta Neurologia Scandinavica*, 91, 231–3.

Filippi M. Yousry T, Baratti C, *et al.* (1996a). Quantitative assessment of MRI lesion load in multiple sclerosis. A comparison of conventional spin echo with fast fluid attenuated inversion recovery. *Brain*, 119, 1349–1355.

Filippi M, Yousry T, Campi A, *et al.* (1996b). Comparison of triple dose versus standard dose gadolinium-DTPA for detection of MRI enhancing lesions in multiple sclerosis. *Neurology*, 46, 379–384.

Finelli DA, Hurst GC, Gullapali RP and Bellon EM (1994a). Improved contrast of enhancing brain lesions on postgadolinium, T1-weighted spin-echo images with use of magnetization transfer. *Radiology*, 190, 553–9.

Finelli DA, Hurst GC, Karsman BA, *et al.* (1994b). Use of magnetization transfer for improved contrast on gradient-echo images of the cervical spine. *Radiology*, 193, 165–71.

Fog T (1965). The topography of plaques in multiple sclerosis with special reference to cerebral plaques. *Acta Neurologica Scandinavica*, 41 (suppl 15), 1–161.

Foong J, Rozewicz L, Quaghebeur G, *et al.* (1997). Executive function in multiple sclerosis: the role of frontal lobe pathology. *Brain*, in press.

Ford B, Tampieri D & Francis G (1992). Long term follow-up of acute partial transverse myelopathy. *Neurology*, 42, 250–2.

Francis DA, Compston DAS, Batchelor JR, McDonald WI (1987). A reassessment of the risk of multiple sclerosis developing in patients with optic neuritis after extended follow-up. *Journal of Neurology, Neurosurgery and Psychiatry*, 50, 758–65.

Frank JA, Stone LA, Smith ME, *et al.* (1994). Serial contrast-enhanced magnetic resonance imaging in patients with early relapsing-remitting multiple sclerosis: implications for treatment trials. *Annals of Neurology*, 36, S86–S90.

Franklin GM, Heaton RK, Nelson LM, *et al.* (1988). Correlation of neuropsychological and MRI findings in chronic/progressive multiple sclerosis. *Neurology*, 38, 1826–9.

Frederiksen JL, Larsson HBW, Olesen J, Stigsby B (1991). MRI, VEP, SEP and biothesiometry suggest monosymptomatic acute optic neuritis to be a first manifestation of multiple sclerosis. *Acta Neurologica Scandinavica*, 83, 343–50.

Friedman DP & Taraglino LS (1993). Amyotrophic lateral sclerosis: hyperintensity of the corticospinal tracts on MR images of the spinal cord. *American Journal of Radiology*, 160, 604–6.

Gass A, Barker GJ, Kidd D, *et al.* (1994). Correlation of magnetisation transfer ratio with clinical disability in multiple sclerosis. *Annals of Neurology*, 36, 62–7.

Gass A, Barker GJ, MacManus DG, *et al.* (1995). High resolution magnetic resonance imaging of the anterior visual pathway in patients with optic neuropathies using fast spin echo and phased array local coils. *Journal of Neurology, Neurosurgery and Psychiatry*, 58, 562–9.

Gawne-Cain ML, O'Riordan JL, Thompson AJ, Moseley IF, & Miller DH (1997). Multiple sclerosis lesion detection in the brain: a comparison of fast fluid attenuated inversion recovery and conventional T2 weighted dual spin echo. *Neurology*, in press.

Gean-Marton AD, Venzia LG, Marton KL, *et al.* (1991). Abnormal corpus callosum: a sensitive and specific indicator of multiple sclerosis. *Radiology*, 180, 215–21.

Gerard G & Weisberg LA (1986). MRI periventricular lesions in adults. *Neurology*, 36, 998–1001.

Gilbert JJ & Sadler M (1983). Unsuspected multiple sclerosis. *Archives of Neurology*, 40, 533–6.

Goodin DS, Rowley HA & Olney RK (1988). Magnetic resonance imaging in amyotrophic lateral sclerosis. *Annals of Neurology*, 23, 418–20.

Goodkin DE, Hertsgaard D, Rudick RA (1990). Exacerbation rates and adherence to disease type in a prospectively followed up population with multiple sclerosis. *Archives of Neurology*, 46, 1107–12.

Goodkin DE, Ross JS, VanderBrug Medendorp S, *et al.* (1992). MRI lesion enlargement in multiple sclerosis: disease-related activity, chance occurrence, or measurement artifact. *Archives of Neurology*, 49, 261–4.

Greenan TJ, Grossman IR & Goldberg HI (1992). Cerebral vasculitis: MR imaging and angiographic correlation. *Radiology*, 182, 65–72.

Greenfield JG & King LS (1936). Observations on the histopathology of the cerebral lesions in disseminated sclerosis. *Brain*, 59, 445–58.

Griffin JW, Cornblath DR, Alexander E, *et al.* (1990). Ataxic sensory neuropathy and dorsal root ganglionitis associated with Sjogren's disease. *Annals of Neurology*, 27, 304–15.

Grimaud J, Millar J, Thorpe JW, *et al.* (1995). Signal intensity on MRI of basal ganglia in multiple sclerosis. *Journal of Neurology, Neurosurgery and Psychiatry*, 59, 306–8.

Grimaud J, Lai M, Thorpe JW, *et al.* (1996). Evaluation of a computer assisted quantification of MS lesions in cranial MRI. *Magnetic Resonance Imaging*, 14, 495–505.

Grossman RI, Gonzales-Scarano F, Atlas SW, *et al.* (1986). Multiple sclerosis: gadolinium enhancement in MR imaging. *Radiology*, 161, 721–5.

Grossman, RI, Lisak RP, Macchi PJ and Joseph PM (1987). MR of acute experimental allergic encephalomyelitis. *American Journal of Neuroradiology*, 8, 1045–8.

Grossman RI, Lenkinski RE, Ramer KN, *et al.* (1992). MR proton spectroscopy in multiple sclerosis. *American Journal of Neuroradiology*, 13, 1535–43.

Guttmann CRG, Kikinis R, Metcalf D & Jolesz FA (1994). Automated volumetric and morphologic analysis of the evolution of focal multiple sclerosis. *Journal of Magnetic Resonance Imaging* 4(P), 88.

Guttmann CRG, Ahn SS, Hsu L, *et al.* (1995). The evolution of multiple sclerosis lesions on serial MR. *American Journal of Neuroradiology*, 16, 1481–91.

Hajnal JV, Bryant DJ, Kasuboski L, *et al.* (1992). Use of fluid attenuated inversion recovery (FLAIR) pulse sequences in MRI of the brain. *Journal of Computer Assisted Tomography*, 16, 841–4.

Hallgren B & Sourander P (1958). The effects of age on the

non-haemin iron in the human brain. *Journal of Neurochemistry*, 3, 41–51.

Halliday AM (1993). *Evoked Potentials in Clinical Testing*. Second edition. Edinburgh, Churchill Livingstone.

Handler MS, Johnson LM, Dick AR and Batnitzky S (1993). Neurosarcoidosis with unusual MRI findings. *Neuroradiology*, 35, 146–8.

Hansen K & Lebech AM (1992). The clinical and epidemiological profile of Lyme Neuroborreliosis in Denmark 1985–1990: a prospective study of 187 patients with *Borrelia burgdorferei* specific intrathecal antibody production. *Brain*, 115, 399–423.

Harding AE (1984). *The Hereditary Ataxias and Related Disorders*. Edinburgh, Churchill Livingstone.

Harding AE, Sweeney MG, Miller DH, *et al.* (1992). Occurrence of a multiple sclerosis-like illness in women who have Leber's hereditary optic neuropathy mitochondrial DNA mutation. *Brain*, 115, 979–89.

Harris JO, Frank JA, Patronas N, *et al.* (1991). Serial gadolinium-enhanced magnetic resonance imaging scans in patients with early, relapsing-remitting multiple sclerosis: implications for clinical trials and natural history. *Annals of Neurology*, 29, 548–55.

Haughton VM, Yetkin FZ, Rao SM, *et al.* (1992). Quantitative MR in the diagnosis of multiple sclerosis. *Magnetic Resonance in Medicine*, 26, 71–8.

Hawke SHB, Hallinan JM & McLeod JG (1990). Cranial magnetic resonance imaging in chronic demyelinating polyneuropathy. *Journal of Neurology, Neurosurgery and Psychiatry*, 53, 794–6.

Hawkins CP, Munro PMG, Mackenzie F, *et al.* (1990a). Duration and selectivity of blood–brain barrier breakdown in chronic relapsing experimental allergic encephalomyelitis studied by gadolinium-DTPA and protein markers. *Brain*, 113, 365–78.

Hawkins CP, McDonald WI, Revesz T, *et al.* (1990b). Myelin breakdown products detected by magnetic resonance imaging in man. *Journal of Physiology*, 426, 43P.

Hawkins CP, Mackenzie F, Tofts PS, *et al.* (1991). Patterns of blood–brain barrier breakdown in inflammatory demyelination. *Brain*, 114, 801–10.

Hawkins CP, Munro PMG, Landon DN, McDonald WI (1992). Metabolically dependent blood–brain barrier breakdown in chronic relapsing experimental allergic encephalomyelitis. *Acta Neuropathologica*, 83, 630–5.

Hawkins CP, McLaughlin L, Kendall BE & McDonald WI (1993). Pathological findings correlated with MRI in HIV infection. *Neuroradiology*, 35, 264–8.

Heaton RK, Nelson LM, Thompson DS, *et al.* (1985). Neuropsychological findings in relapsing/remitting and chronic/progressive multiple sclerosis. *Journal of Consulting and Clinical Psychology*, 53, 103–10.

Hendrix LE, Kneeland JB, Haughton VM, *et al.* (1990). MR imaging of optic nerve lesions: value of gadopentate dimeglumine and fat-suppression technique. *American Journal of Neuroradiology*, 11, 749–54.

Hennig J, Naureth A & Freidberg H (1986). RARE imaging: a fast imaging method for clinical MR. *Magnetic Resonance in Medicine*, 3, 823–33.

Hiehle JF, Grossman RI, Ramer KN, *et al.* (1995). Magnetization transfer effect in MR-detected multiple sclerosis lesions: comparison with gadolinium-enhanced spin-echo images and nonenhanced T1-weighted images. *American Journal of Neuroradiology*, 16, 69–77.

Hill JM & Switzer RC III (1984). The regional distribution and cellular localization of iron in the rat brain. *Neuroscience*, 11, 595–603.

Hoeck A, Demmel U, Schicha H, *et al.* (1975). Trace element concentration in the human brain. *Brain*, 98, 49–64.

Hornabrook RSL, Miller DH, Newton MR, *et al.* (1992). Frequent involvement of the optic radiation in patients with acute isolated optic neuritis. *Neurology*, 42, 77–9.

Horowitz AL, Kaplan RD, Grewe G, *et al.* (1989). The ovoid lesion: a new MR observation in patients with MS. *American Journal of Neuroradiology*, 10, 303–5.

Horsfield MA, Davie C, Tofts PS and Miller DH (1994). The role of diffusion in NMR imaging of the CNS. *Argomenti di Neurologia*, 4, 84–9.

Howard RS, Wiles CM, Hirsch NP, *et al.* (1992). Respiratory involvement in multiple sclerosis. *Brain*, 115, 479–94.

Huber SJ, Paulson GW, Shuttleworth EC, *et al.* (1987). Magnetic resonance imaging correlates of dementia in multiple sclerosis. *Archives of Neurology*, 44, 732–6.

Husted CA, Matson GB, Adams DA, *et al.* (1994a). In vivo detection of myelin phospholipids in multiple sclerosis with phosphorous magnetic resonance spectroscopic imaging. *Annals of Neurology*, 36, 239–41.

Husted CA, Goodin DS, Hugg JW, *et al.* (1994b). Biochemical alterations in multiple sclerosis lesions and normal appearing white matter detected by in vivo ^{31}P and ^{1}H spectroscopic imaging. *Annals of Neurology*, 36, 157–65.

Imakita S, Nishimura T, Naito H, *et al.* (1987). Magnetic resonance imaging of human cerebral infarction: enhancement with Gd-DTPA. *Neuroradiology*, 29, 422–9.

Isaac C, Li DK, Genton M, *et al.* (1988). Multiple sclerosis: a serial study using MRI in relapsing patients. *Neurology*, 38, 1511–15.

Jackson JA, Leake DR & Schneiders NJ (1985). Magnetic resonance imaging in multiple sclerosis: results in 32 cases. *American Journal of Neuroradiology*, 6, 171–6.

Jackson EF, Narayana PA, Wolinsky JS & Doyle TJ (1993). Accuracy and reproducibility in volumetric analysis of multiple sclerosis lesions. *Journal of Computer Assisted Tomography*, 17, 200–5.

Jacobs L, Kinkel PR & Kinkel WR (1986). Silent brain lesions in patients with isolated optic neuritis. A clinical and nuclear magnetic resonance imaging study. *Archives of Neurology*, 43, 452–5.

Jacobs L, Munschauer FE & Kaba SE (1991). Clinical and magnetic resonance imaging in optic neuritis. *Neurology*, 41, 15–19.

Jacobs L, Cookfair D, Rudick RA, *et al.* (1994). Results of a phase III trial of intramuscular recombinant beta interferon as treatment for multiple sclerosis. *Annals of Neurology*, 36, 259.

Jacobs LD, Cockfair DL, Rudick RA, *et al.* (1996). Intramuscular interferon beta-1a for disease progression in relapsing multiple sclerosis. *Annals of Neurology*, 39, 285–94.

Johnson G, Miller DH, MacManus D, *et al.* (1987). STIR sequence in NMR imaging of the optic nerve. *Neuroradiology*, 29, 238–45.

Johnson MA, Li DKB, Bryant DJ & Payne JA (1984). Magnetic resonance imaging: serial observations in multiple sclerosis. *American Journal of Neuroradiology*, 5, 495–9.

Johnson M, Maciunas R, Dutt P, *et al.* (1989). Granulomatous angiitis masquerading as a mass lesion: magnetic resonance imaging and stereotactic findings in a patient with occult Hodgkin's disease. *Surgical Neurology*, 31, 49–53.

Johnson RT and Richardson EP (1968). The neurological manifestations of systemic lupus erythematosus. *Medicine (Baltimore)*, 47, 337–69.

Johnston B, Atkins MS, Mackiewich B and Anderson M (1996). Segmentation of multiple sclerosis lesions in intensity-corrected multispectral MRI. *Institute of Electric and Electronic Engineering Transactions on Medical Imaging*, 15, 154–169.

Jones KM, Mulkern RV, Mantello MV, *et al.* (1992). Evaluation of brain haemorrhage: comparison of fast spin echo and conventional dual spin-echo images. *Radiology*, 182, 53–8.

Kaltreider HB & Talal N (1969). The neuropathy of Sjogren's syndrome. *Annals of Internal Medicine*, 70, 751–62.

Kamber M, Collins DL, Shinghal R, *et al.* (1992). Model-based 3D segmentation of multiple sclerosis lesions in dual-echo MRI data. *Proceedings of the International Society for Optical Engineering. Visualization in Biomedical Computing*, 1808, 590.

Kapouleas I (1989). Automatic detection of multiple sclerosis lesions in MRI brain images. In: Kingsland LC (ed.) *Proceedings of the 1990 Symposium on Computer Applications in Medical Care. Institute of Electric and Electronic Engineering.* Washington DC, Computer Society Press, pp. 739–45.

Kapouleas I, Grossman RI, Kessler D, *et al.* (1993). Techniques for quantitation and comparison of multiple sclerosis lesions in serial MRI studies. *Neurology*, 43(suppl), A246.

Kappos L, Stadt D, Ratzka M, *et al.* (1988). Magnetic resonance imaging in the evaluation of treatment in multiple sclerosis. *Neuroradiology*, 30, 299–302.

Kappos L, Radu EW, Haas J, *et al.* (1995). Deoxyspergualin (DSG) in MS: second interim analysis of the European multicentre study. *Journal of Neurology*, 242(suppl 2), S23.

Karussis D, Meiner Z, Lehmann D, *et al.* (1996). Treatment of secondary progressive multiple sclerosis with the immunomodulator linomide. A double-blind placebo-controlled study with monthly magnetic resonance imaging evaluation. *Neurology*, 47, 341–6.

Kastrukoff LF, Oger JJF, Hashimoto SA, *et al.* (1990). Systemic lymphoblastoid interferon therapy in chronic progressive multiple sclerosis. I. Clinical and MRI evaluation. *Neurology*, 40, 479–86.

Katz D, Taubenberger JK, Canella B, *et al.* (1993). Correlation between magnetic resonance imaging findings and lesion development in chronic, active multiple sclerosis. *Annals of Neurology*, 34, 661–9.

Kermode AG, Plant GT, MacManus DG, *et al.* (1989a). Behçet's disease with slowly enlarging midbrain mass on MRI: resolution following steroid therapy. *Neurology*, 39, 1251–2.

Kermode AG, Moseley IF, Kendall BE, *et al.* (1989b). Magnetic resonance imaging in Leber's optic neuropathy. *Journal of Neurology, Neurosurgery and Psychiatry*, 52, 671–4.

Kermode AG, Thompson AJ, Tofts P, *et al.* (1990a). Breakdown of the blood–brain barrier precedes symptoms and other MRI signs of new lesions in multiple sclerosis: pathogenetic and clinical implications. *Brain*, 113, 1477–89.

Kermode AG, Tofts P, Thompson AJ, *et al.* (1990b). Heterogeneity of blood–brain barrier changes in multiple sclerosis: an MRI study with gadolinium-DTPA enhancement. *Neurology*, 40, 229–35.

Kermode AG, Rudge P, Thompson AJ, *et al.* (1990c). MRI of the thoracic cord in tropical spastic paraparesis. *Journal of Neurology, Neurosurgery and Psychiatry*, 53, 710.

Kesselring J, Ormerod IEC, Miller DH, du Boulay EPGH and McDonald WI (1989a). *Magnetic resonance imaging in multiple sclerosis. An atlas of diagnosis and differential diagnosis.* Stuttgart: Thieme.

Kesselring J, Miller DH, MacManus DG, *et al.* (1989b). Quantitative magnetic resonance imaging in multiple sclerosis: the effect of high dose intravenous methylprednisolone. *Journal of Neurology, Neurosurgery and Psychiatry*, 52, 14–17.

Kesselring J, Miller DH, Robb SA, *et al.* (1990). Acute disseminated encephalomyelitis: MRI findings and the distinction from multiple sclerosis. *Brain*, 113, 291–320.

Khaw KT, Manji H, Britton J & Schon F (1991).

Neurosarcoidosis: Demonstration of meningeal disease by gadolinium enhanced magnetic resonance imaging. *Journal of Neurology, Neurosurgery and Psychiatry*, 54, 499–502.

Khoury SJ, Guttmann CRG, Oray EJ, *et al.* (1994). Longitudinal MRI in multiple sclerosis: correlation between disability and lesion burden. *Neurology*, 44, 2120–4.

Kidd, D., Thompson, A.J., Miller, D.H., *et al.* [1992]. MRI activity in multiple sclerosis: a two year study. *Journal of Neurology, Neurosurgery, and Psychiatry* 55: 1213.

Kidd D, Thorpe JW, Thompson AJ, *et al.* (1993). Spinal cord MRI using multi-array coils and fast spin echo. II: findings in multiple sclerosis. *Neurology*, 43, 2632–7.

Kidd D, Thompson AJ, Kendall BE, *et al.* (1994). Benign form of multiple sclerosis: MRI evidence for less frequent and less inflammatory disease activity. *Journal of Neurology, Neurosurgery and Psychiatry*, 57, 1070–2.

Kidd, D., Thorpe, J.W., Kendall, B.E., *et al.* (1996). MRI dynamics of brain and spinal cord in progressive multiple sclerosis. *Journal of Neurology, Neurosurgery and Psychiatry*, 60, 15–19.

Kiel MK, Greenspun B & Grossman RI (1988). Magnetic resonance imaging and degree of disability in multiple sclerosis. *Archives of Physical Medicine and Rehabilitation*, 69, 11–3.

King PH and Bragdon AC (1991). MRI reveals multiple reversible lesions in an attack of acute intermittent porphyria. *Neurology*, 41, 1300–2.

Kirkpatrick JB & Hayman LA (1987). White matter lesions in MR imaging of clinically healthy brains of elderly subjects: possible pathological basis. *Radiology*, 162, 509–11.

Klockgether T, Schroth G, Diener H-C & Dichgans J (1990). Idiopathic cerebellar ataxia of late onset: natural history and MRI morphology. *Journal of Neurology, Neurosurgery and Psychiatry*, 53, 297–305.

Koo EH & Massey EW (1988). Granulomatous angiitis of the central nervous system: protean manifestations and response to treatment. *Journal of Neurology, Neurosurgery and Psychiatry*, 51, 1126–33.

Koopmans RA, Li DKB, Oger JJF, *et al.* (1989a). Chronic progressive multiple sclerosis: serial magnetic resonance brain imaging over six months. *Annals of Neurology*, 26, 248–56.

Koopmans RA, Li DKB, Grochowski EW, *et al.* (1989b). Benign versus chronic progressive multiple sclerosis: magnetic resonance imaging features. *Annals of Neurology*, 25, 74–81.

Koopmans RA, Li DKB, Zhao GJ, *et al.* (1992). MRI assessment of cyclosporine therapy of MS in a multicenter trial. *Neurology*, 42(suppl 3), 210.

Koopmans RA, Li DKB, Zhu G, *et al.* (1993a). Magnetic resonance spectroscopy of multiple sclerosis: in-vivo detection of myelin breakdown products. *Lancet*, 341, 631–2.

Koopmans RA, Li DKB, Redekop WK, *et al.* (1993b). The use of magnetic resonance imaging in monitoring interferon therapy of multiple sclerosis. *Journal of Neuroimaging*, 3, 163–8.

Koopmans RA, Zhao GJ, Paty DW & Li DKB (1994). Lesion activity assessment by yearly serial MRI in monitoring a therapeutic trial of interferon beta in the treatment of relapsing and remitting MS. *Neurology*, 44(Suppl 2), A392.

Kruse B, Barker PB, van Zijl PCM, *et al.* (1994). Multislice proton magnetic resonance spectroscopic imaging in X-linked adrenoleucodystrophy. *Annals of Neurology*, 36, 595–608.

Kurtzke JF, Beebe GW, Nagler B, *et al.* (1977). Studies on the natural history of multiple sclerosis – 8. Early prognostic features of the later course of the illness. *Journal of Chronic Disease*, 30, 819–30.

Kurtzke JF (1983). Rating neurologic impairment in multiple sclerosis: an expanded disability status scale (EDSS). *Neurology*, 33, 1444–52.

Lai HM, Horsfield M, Barker GJ, *et al.* (1995). Diffusion coefficient measurements in lesions and normal appearing white matter of patients with benign and secondary progressive multiple sclerosis and in normal controls. *Journal of Neurology*, 242, S120.

Lai HM, Hodgson T, Gawne-Cain M, *et al.* (1996). A preliminary study into the sensitivity of disease activity detection by serial weekly magnetic resonance imaging in multiple sclerosis. *Journal of Neurology, Neurosurgery and Psychiatry*, 60, 339–41.

Landy PJ (1983). A prospective study of the risk of developing multiple sclerosis in optic neuritis in a tropical and subtropical area. *Journal of Neurology, Neurosurgery and Psychiatry*, 46, 659–61.

Lane RJM, Roche SW, Leung AAW, *et al.* (1988). Cyclosporin neurotoxicity in cardiac transplant recipients. *Journal of Neurology, Neurosurgery and Psychiatry*, 51, 1434–7.

Langdon DW, Grimaud J, Barker GJ *et al.* (1996). Correlation of multiparameter measures with cognitive dysfunction in multiple sclerosis: a preliminary study. *Journal of Neurology*, 243 (2), S82.

Larsson HBW, Frederiksen J, Kjaer L, *et al.* (1988). In vivo determination of T1 and T2 in the brain of patients with severe but stable multiple sclerosis. *Magnetic Resonance in Medicine*, 7, 43–55.

Larsson HBW, Christiansen P, Jensen M, *et al.* (1991). Localized in vivo proton spectroscopy in the brain of patients with multiple sclerosis. *Magnetic Resonance in Medicine*, 22, 23–31.

Larsson HBW, Thomsen C, Frederiksen J, *et al.* (1992). In vivo magnetic resonance diffusion measurement in the brain of patients with multiple sclerosis. *Magnetic Resonance Imaging*, 10, 7–12.

Lassman H (1983). *Comparative Neuropathology of Chronic Experimental Allergic Encephalomyelitis and MS*. Berlin, Springer.

Lassman H, Suchanek G & Ozawa K (1994). Histopathology and the blood–cerebrospinal fluid barrier in multiple sclerosis. *Annals of Neurology*, 36, S42–S46.

Lauterbur PC (1973). Image formation by induced local interactions: examples employing nuclear magnetic resonance. *Nature*, 242, 190–1.

Lee DH, Simon JH, Szumowski J, *et al.* (1991). Optic neuritis and orbital lesions: lipid-suppressed and chemical shift MR imaging. *Radiology*, 179, 543–6.

Lee KH, Hashimoto SA, Hooge JP, *et al.* (1991). Magnetic resonance imaging of the head in the diagnosis of multiple sclerosis: a prospective 2-year follow-up with comparison of clinical evaluation, evoked potentials, oligoclonal banding, and CT. *Neurology*, 41, 657–60.

Leifer D, Buonanno FS & Richardson EP (1990). Clinicopathologic correlations of cranial magnetic resonance imaging of periventricular white matter. *Neurology*, 40, 911–8.

Lexa FJ, Grossman RI & Rosenquist AC (1993). Detection of early axonal degeneration in mammalian central nervous system by magnetization transfer techniques in magnetic resonance imaging. *Annals of the New York Academy of Sciences*, 679, 336–40.

Li DKB, Mayo J, Fache S, *et al.* (1984). Early experience in nuclear magnetic resonance imaging of multiple sclerosis. *Annals of the New York Academy of Science*, 436, 483–6.

Lim L, Ron MA, Ormerod IEC, *et al.* (1988). Psychiatric and neurological manifestations of systemic lupus erythematosus. *Quarterly Journal of Medicine*, 66, 27–38.

Lipton HL & Teasdall RD (1973). Acute transverse myelopathy in adults. *Archives of Neurology*, 28, 252–7.

Loevner LA, Grossman RI, McGowan JC, *et al.* (1995). Characterization of multiple sclerosis plaques with T1-weighted MR and quantitative magnetization transfer. *American Journal of Neuroradiology*, 16, 1473–9.

Logsdail SJ, Callanan MM & Ron MA (1988). Psychiatric morbidity in patients with clinically isolated lesions of a type seen in multiple sclerosis: a clinical and MRI study. *Psychological Medicine*, 18, 355–64.

Losseff NA, Kingsley DPE, Kendall BE, *et al.* (1995a). Serial magnetic resonance imaging (MRI) in multiple sclerosis (MS): a five year follow-up study. *Journal of Neurology*, 242, S7.

Losseff NA, Lai M, Miller DH, *et al.* (1995b). The prognostic value of serial axial cord area measurement by magnetic resonance imaging (MRI) in multiple sclerosis. *Journal of Neurology*, 242(suppl 2), S110.

Losseff NA, Webb SL, O'Riordan JI, *et al.* (1996a). Spinal cord atrophy and disability in multiple sclerosis: a new reproducible and sensitive MRI method with potential to monitor disease progression. *Brain*, 119, 701–708.

Losseff NA, Wang L, Lai HM, *et al.* (1996b) Progressive cerebral atrophy in MS: a serial MRI study. *Brain*, 119, 2009–2019.

Lublin, F.D. & Reingold, S.C. (1996). Defining the clinical cause of multiple sclerosis: results of an international survey. *Neurology*, 46, 907–910.

Lukes SA, Crooks LE, Aminoff MJ, *et al.* (1983). Nuclear magnetic resonance imaging in multiple sclerosis. *Annals of Neurology*, 13, 592–601.

Lumsden CE (1970). The neuropathology of multiple sclerosis. In: *The Handbook of Clinical Neurology*, vol. 9, eds. PJ Vinken & GW Bruyn, pp. 217–309. Amsterdam, North Holland.

Lynch SG, Rose JW, Smoker W, Petajan JH (1990). MRI in familial multiple sclerosis. *Neurology*, 40, 900–3.

Lyon-Caen O, Jouvent R, Hauser S, *et al.* (1986). Cognitive dysfunction in recent onset demyelinating disease. *Archives of Neurology* 43, 1138–41.

McAlpine D (1964). The benign form of multiple sclerosis. *British Medical Journal*, 2, 1029–32.

McDonald WI & Sears TA (1970). The effects of experimental demyelination on conduction in the central nervous system. *Brain*, 93, 583–98.

McDonald WI, Miller DH and Barnes D (1992). The pathological evolution of multiple sclerosis. *Neuropathology and Applied Neurobiology*, 18, 319–34.

McDonald WI (1993). The dynamics of multiple sclerosis. The Charcot lecture. *Journal of Neurology*, 240, 28–36.

McDonald WI (1994). The pathological and clinical dynamics of multiple sclerosis. *Journal of Neuropathology and Experimental Neurology*, 53, 338–43.

McDonald WI, Miller DH and Thompson AJ (1994). Are magnetic resonance findings predictive of clinical outcome in therapeutic trials in multiple sclerosis? The dilemma of interferon-beta. *Annals of Neurology*, 36, 14–18.

McFarland HF, Frank JA, Albert PS, *et al.* (1992). Using gadolinium-enhanced magnetic resonance imaging lesions to monitor disease activity in multiple sclerosis. *Annals of Neurology*, 32, 758–66.

MacKay A, Whittal K, Adler J, *et al.* (1994). In vivo visualization of myelin water in brain by magnetic resonance. *Magnetic Resonance in Medicine*, 31, 673–7.

McLean BN, Miller D, Thompson EJ (1995). Oligoclonal banding of IgG in the cerebrospinal fluid, bloood–brain barrier function and MRI findings in patients with sarcoidosis, systemic lupus erythematosus and Behçet's disease involving the nervous system. *Journal of Neurology, Neurosurgery and Psychiatry*, 58, 548–54.

Magalhaes ACA, Caramelli P, Menezes JR, *et al.* (1994).

Wilson's disease: MRI with clinical correlation. *Neuroradiology*, 36, 97–100.

Mandler RN, Davis LE, Jeffery DR & Kornfield MK (1993). Devic's neuromyelitis optica: a clinicopathological study of 8 patients. *Annals of Neurology*, 34, 162–8.

Marti-Fabregas J & Pujol J (1990). Selective involvement of the pyramidal tract on magnetic resonance imaging in primary lateral sclerosis. *Neurology*, 40, 1799–800.

Martinelli V, Comi G, Filippi M, *et al.* (1991). Paraclinical tests in acute-onset optic neuritis: basdal data and results of short term follow-up. *Acta Neurologica Scandinavica*, 84, 231–6.

Mathews VP, King JC, Elster AD and Hamilton CA (1994). Cerebral infarction: effects of dose and magnetization transfer saturation at gadolinium-enhanced MR imaging. *Radiology*, 190, 547–52.

Matthews PM, Tampieri D, Berkovic SF, *et al.* (1991). MRI shows specific abnormalities in the MELAS syndrome. *Neurology*, 41, 1043–6.

Matthews WB (1991). Clinical aspects. In: *McAlpine's Multiple Sclerosis*, 2nd edn, ed. WB Matthews, pp. 43–300. London, Churchill Livingstone.

Melki PS, Mulkern RV, Panych LP, & Jolesz FA (1991). Comparison of the FAISE method with conventional dual spin-echo images. *Journal of Magnetic Resonance Imaging*, 1, 319–26.

Melki PS, Jolesz FA & Mulkern RV (1992). Partial RF echo-planar imaging with the FAISE method. II. Contrast equivalence with spin-echo sequences. *Magnetic Resonance in Medicine*, 26, 342–54.

Metha RC, Pike BG and Enzmann DR (1995). Improved detection of enhancing and nonenhancing lesions of multiple sclerosis with magnetization transfer. *American Journal of Neuroradiology*, 16, 1771–8.

Millar JH, Zilkha KJ, Langman MJ, *et al.* (1973). Double-blind trial of linoleate supplementation of the diet in multiple sclerosis. *British Medical Journal*, 1, 765–8.

Miller DH, McDonald WI, Blumhardt LD, *et al.* (1987a). MRI of brain and spinal cord in isolated noncompressive spinal cord syndromes. *Annals of Neurology*, 22, 714–23.

Miller DH, Ormerod IEC, Gibson A, *et al.* (1987b). MR brain scanning in patients with vasculitis: differentiation from multiple sclerosis. *Neuroradiology*, 29, 226–31.

Miller DH, McDonald WI, Johnson G, *et al.* (1987c). Gadolinium-DTPA enhanced MRI of the brain and orbits in patients with clinically isolated optic neuritis. *Proceedings of The Society of Magnetic Resonance in Medicine*, 1, 143.

Miller DH (1988). MRI: sensitive and safe in diagnosing MS. *MRI Decisions*, 2, 17–24.

Miller DH, Rudge P, Johnson G, *et al.* (1988a). Serial gadolinium enhanced magnetic resonance imaging in multiple sclerosis. *Brain*, 111, 927–39.

Miller DH, Newton MR, van der Poel JC, *et al.* (1988b). Magnetic resonance imaging of the optic nerve in optic neuritis. *Neurology*, 38, 175–9.

Miller DH, Kendall BE, Barter S, *et al.* (1988c). Magnetic resonance imaging in central nervous system sarcoidosis. *Neurology*, 38, 378–83.

Miller DH, Ormerod IEC, McDonald WI, *et al.* (1988d). The early risk of multiple sclerosis after optic neuritis. *Journal of Neurology, Neurosurgery and Psychiatry*, 51, 1569–71.

Miller DH, Johnson G, Tofts PS, *et al.* (1989a). Precise relaxation times measurements of normal appearing white matter in inflammatory central nervous system disease. *Magnetic Resonance in Medicine*, 11, 331 6.

Miller DH, Ormerod IEC, Rudge P, *et al.* (1989b). The early risk of multiple sclerosis following isolated acute syndromes of the brainstem and spinal cord. *Annals of Neurology*, 26, 635–9.

Miller DH, Robb SA, Ormerod IEC, *et al.* (1990). Magnetic resonance imaging in inflammatory and demyelinating white matter diseases of childhood. *Developmental Medicine and Child Neurology*, 32, 97–107.

Miller DH, Austin SJ, Connelly A, *et al.* (1991a). Proton magnetic resonance spectroscopy of an acute and chronic lesion in multiple sclerosis. *Lancet*, 337, 58–9.

Miller DH, Barkhof F, Berry I, *et al.* (1991b). Magnetic resonance imaging in monitoring the treatment of multiple sclerosis: concerted action guidelines. *Journal of Neurology, Neurosurgery and Psychiatry*, 54, 683–8.

Miller DH, Buchanan N, Barker G, *et al.* (1992a). Gadolinium-enhanced magnetic resonance imaging of the central nervous system in systemic lupus erythematosus. *Journal of Neurology*, 239, 460–4.

Miller DH, Hornabrook RW & Purdie G (1992b). The natural history of multiple sclerosis: a regional study with some longitudinal data. *Journal of Neurology, Neurosurgery and Psychiatry*, 55, 341–6.

Miller DH, Thompson AJ, Morrissey SP, *et al.* (1992c). High dose steroids in acute relapses of multiple sclerosis: MRI evidence for a possible mechanism of therapeutic effect. *Journal of Neurology, Neurosurgery and Psychiatry*, 55, 450–3.

Miller DH, Barkhof F, Berry I, *et al.* (1992d). MRI in monitoring the treatment of multiple sclerosis: concerted action guidelines (Matters Arising). *Journal of Neurology, Neurosurgery and Psychiatry*, 55, 978.

Miller DH, MacManus DG, Bartlett PA, *et al.* (1993a). Detection of optic nerve lesions in optic neuritis using frequency-selective fat-saturation sequences. *Neuroradiology*, 35, 156–8.

Miller DH, Scaravilli F, Thomas DCT, *et al.* (1993b). Acute disseminated encephalomyelitis presenting as a solitary brainstem mass. *Journal of Neurology, Neurosurgery and Psychiatry*, 56, 920–2.

Miller DH, Barkhof F & Nauta JJP (1993c). Gadolinium enhancement increases the sensitivity of MRI in detecting disease activity in multiple sclerosis. *Brain*, 116, 1077–94.

Miller DH, Albert PS, Barkhof F, *et al.* (1996). Guidelines for using magnetic resonance techniques in monitoring the treatment of multiple sclerosis. *Annals of Neurology*, 39, 6–16.

Miller HG & Evans MJ (1953). Prognosis in acute disseminated encephalomyelitis: with a note on neuromyelitis optica. *Quarterly Journal of Medicine*, 22, 347–479.

Milligan NM, Miller DH and Compston DAS (1994). A placebo-controlled trial of isoprinosine in patients with multiple sclerosis. *Journal of Neurology, Neurosurgery and Psychiatry* 57, 164–8.

Milton WJ, Atlas SW, Lexas FJ, *et al.* (1991). Deep gray matter hypointensity patterns with aging in healthy adults: MR imaging at 1.5 T. *Radiology*, 181, 715–9.

Minderhoud JM, Mooyaart EL, Kamman RL, *et al.* (1992). In vivo phosphorous magnetic resonance spectroscopy in multiple sclerosis. *Archives of Neurology*, 49, 161–5.

Miro J, Pena-Sagredo JL, Berciano J, *et al.* (1990). Prevalence of Sjogren's syndrome in patients with multiple sclerosis. *Annals of Neurology*, 27, 582–4.

Mitchell JR, Karlick SJ, Lee DH & Fenster A (1994). Computer-assisted identification and quantification of multiple sclerosis lesions in MR imaging volumes in the brain. *Journal of Magnetic Resonance Imaging*, 4, 197–208.

Mochizuki A, Hamanouchi H, Murata M, *et al.* (1988). Medullary lesion revealed by MRI in a case of MS with respiratory arrest. *Neuroradiology*, 30, 574–6.

Moll C, Mourre C, Lazdunsky M & Ulrich J (1991). Increase of sodium channels in demyelinated lesions of multiple sclerosis. *Brain Research*, 556, 311–16.

Moreau T, Thorpe J, Miller D, *et al.* (1994). Preliminary evidence from magnetic resonance imaging for reduction in disease activity after lymphocyte depletion in multiple sclerosis. *Lancet*, 344, 298–301.

Morrissey SP, Miller DH, Kendall BE, *et al.* (1993a). The significance of brain magnetic resonance imaging abnormalities at presentation with clinically isolated syndromes suggestive of multiple sclerosis. A 5-year follow-up study. *Brain*, 116, 135–46.

Morrissey SP, Miller DH, Hermaszewski R, *et al.* (1993b). Magnetic resonance imaging of the central nervous system in Behçet's disease. *European Neurology*, 33, 287–93.

Motomura S, Tabira T & Kuriowa Y (1980). A clinical comparative study of multiple sclerosis and neuro-Behçet's syndrome. *Journal of Neurology, Neurosurgery and Psychiatry*, 43, 210–13.

Moulin D, Paty D & Ebers GC (1983). The predictive value of cerebrospinal fluid electrophoresis in 'possible' multiple sclerosis. *Brain*, 106, 809–16.

Mumford CJ, Wood NW, Kellar-Wood H, *et al.* (1994). The British Isles survey of multiple sclerosis in twins. *Neurology*, 44, 11–15.

Nabatame H, Fukuyama H, Akiguchi I, *et al.* (1988). Spinocerebellar degeneration: qualitative and quantitative MR analysis of atrophy. *Journal of Computer Assisted Tomography*, 1, 298–303.

Nauta JJP, Barkhof F, Thompson AJ & Miller DH (1994). Magnetic resonance imaging in monitoring the treatment of multiple sclerosis patients: statistical power of parallel-groups and crossover designs. *Journal of the Neurological Sciences*, 122, 6–14.

Nesbit GM, Forbes GS, Scheithauer BW, *et al.* (1991). Multiple sclerosis: Histopathologic and MR and/or CT correlation in 37 cases at biopsy and three cases at autopsy. *Radiology*, 180, 467–74.

Newcombe J, Hawkins CP, Henderson CL, *et al.* (1991). Histopathology of multiple sclerosis lesions detected by magnetic resonance imaging in unfixed postmortem central nervous system tissue. *Brain*, 114, 1013–23.

Newman NJ, Lott MT & Wallace DC (1991). The clinical characteristics of pedigrees of Leber's hereditary optic neuropathy with the 11778 mutation. *American Journal of Ophthalmology*, 111, 750–62.

Newton M, Cruickshank K, Miller DH, *et al.* (1987). Antibody to human T-lymphotropic virus type 1 in West-Indian-born UK residents with spastic paraparesis. *Lancet*, 329, 415–16.

Niendorf HP, Haustein J, Cornelius I, *et al.* (1991). Safety of gadolinium-DTPA: extended clinical experience. *Magnetic Resonance in Medicine*, 22, 222–8.

Nikolskelainen E, Frey H & Salmi A (1981). Prognosis of optic neuritis with special reference to cerebrospinal fluid immunoglobulins and measles virus antibodies. *Annals of Neurology*, 9, 545–50.

Noseworthy JH, Bass BH, Vandervoort MK, *et al.* (1989). The prevalence of primary Sjogren's syndrome in a multiple sclerosis population. *Annals of Neurology*, 25, 95–8.

Offenbacher H, Fazekas F, Schmidt R, *et al.* (1993). Assessment of MRI criteria for a diagnosis of MS. *Neurology*, 43, 905–9.

Olsen WL, Longo FM, Mills CM & Norman D (1988). White matter disease in AIDS: findings at MR imaging. *Radiology*, 169, 445–8.

Oppenheimer DR (1978). The cervical cord in multiple sclerosis. *Neuropathology and Applied Neurobiology* 4, 151–62.

O'Riordan JI, McDonald WI & Miller DH (1996a). The prognostic significance of brain MRI in clinically isolated syndromes suggestive of demyelination – a 10 year follow-up. *Journal of Neurology, Neurosurgery and Psychiatry* (abstract), 61, 214.

O'Riordan JI, Gallagher HL, Kingsley DPE, *et al.* (1996b).

Clinical, CSF and MRI findings in Devic's neuromyelitis optica. *Journal of Neurology, Neurosurgery and Psychiatry*, 60, 382–7.

Ormerod IEC, Roberts RC, du Boulay GH, *et al.* (1984). NMR in multiple sclerosis and cerebrovascular disease. *Lancet*, 324, 1134–5.

Ormerod IEC, McDonald WI, du Boulay GH, *et al.* (1986a). Disseminated lesions at presentation in patients with optic neuritis. *Journal of Neurology, Neurosurgery and Psychiatry*, 49, 124–7.

Ormerod IEC, Bronstein A, Rudge P, *et al.* (1986b). Magnetic resonance imaging in clinically isolated lesions of the brain stem. *Journal of Neurology, Neurosurgery and Psychiatry*, 49, 737–43.

Ormerod IEC, Miller DH, McDonald WI, *et al.* (1987). The role of NMR imaging in the assessement of multiple sclerosis and isolated neurological lesions: a quantitative study. *Brain*, 110, 1579–616.

Ormerod IEC, Waddy HM, Kermode AG, *et al.* (1990). Involvement of the central nervous system in chronic inflammatory demyelinating polyneuropathy: a clinical, electrophysiological and magnetic resonance imaging study. *Journal of Neurology, Neurosurgery and Psychiatry*, 53, 789–93

Ormerod IEC, Harding AE, Miller DH, *et al.* (1994). Magnetic resonance imaging in degenerative ataxic disorders. *Journal of Neurology, Neurosurgery and Psychiatry*, 57, 51–7.

Pannizzo F, Stallmeyer MJB, Friedman J, *et al.* (1992). Quantitative MRI studies for assessment of multiple sclerosis. *Magnetic Resonance in Medicine*, 24, 90–9.

Pastakia B, Polinsky R, DiChiro G, *et al.* (1986). Multiple system atrophy (Shy-Drager syndrome): MR imaging. *Radiology*, 159, 499–502.

Paty DW, Bergstrom J, Palmer M, *et al.* (1985). A quantitative magnetic resonance image of the multiple sclerosis brain. *Neurology*, 35(suppl 1), 137.

Paty DW (1987). Multiple sclerosis: Assessment of disease progression and effects of treatment. *Canadian Journal of Neurological Science*, 14, 518–20.

Paty DW (1988a). Trial measures in multiple sclerosis: The use of magnetic resonance imaging in the evaluation of clinical trials. *Neurology*, 38, 82–3.

Paty DW (1988b). Magnetic resonance imaging in the assessment of disease activity in multiple sclerosis. *Canadian Journal of Neurological Sciences*, 15, 266–72.

Paty DW, Oger JJF, Kastrukoff LF, *et al.* (1988). MRI in the diagnosis of MS: a prospective study of comparison with clinical evaluation, evoked potentials, oligoclonal banding, and CT. *Neurology*, 38, 180–5.

Paty DW, Koopmans RA, Redekop WK, *et al.* (1992a). Does the MRI activity rate predict the clinical course of MS? *Neurology*, 42 (suppl 3), 427.

Paty DW, Li DKB & Koopmans R (1992b). MRI in monitoring the treatment of multiple sclerosis: concerted action guidelines (Matters Arising). *Journal of Neurology, Neurosurgery and Psychiatry*, 55, 978.

Paty DW, Li DKB, The UBC MS/MRI Study Group & The IFNB Multiple Sclerosis Study Group (1993). Interferon beta-1b is effective in relapsing-remitting multiple sclerosis. II. MRI analysis result of a multicentre, randomized, double-blind, placebo-controlled trial. *Neurology*, 43, 662–7.

Paty DW, Li DK, Oger JJ, *et al.* (1994). Magnetic resonance imaging in the evaluation of clinical trials in multiple sclerosis. *Annals of Neurology*, 36 (Suppl), S95–6.

Perkin GD & Rose FC (1979). *Optic Neuritis and its Differential Diagnosis*. Oxford, Oxford University Press.

Phadke JG & Best PV (1983). Atypical and clinically silent multiple sclerosis: a report of 12 cases discovered unexpectedly at necropsy. *Journal of Neurology, Neurosurgery and Psychiatry*, 46, 414–20.

Phadke JG (1987). Survival pattern and cause of death in patients with multiple sclerosis: results from an epidemiological study in north east Scotland. *Journal of Neurology, Neurosurgery and Psychiatry*, 50, 523–31.

Pierot L, Sauve C, Leger J-M, *et al.* (1993). Asymptomatic cerebral involvement in Sjogren's syndrome: MRI findings of 15 cases. *Neuroradiology*, 35, 378–80.

Plant GT, Kermode AG, du Boulay EPGH & McDonald WI (1989). Spasmodic torticollis due to a midbrain lesion in a case of multiple sclerosis. *Movement Disorders*, 4, 359–62.

Plant GT, Kermode AG, Turano G, *et al.* (1992). Symptomatic retrochiasmal lesions in multiple sclerosis: clinical features, visual evoked potentials, and magnetic resonance imaging. *Neurology*, 42, 68–72.

Poser CM, Paty DW, Scheinberg L, *et al.* (1983). New diagnostic criteria for multiple sclerosis: guidelines for research protocols. *Annals of Neurology*, 13, 227–31.

Poser, CM (1983). *The Diagnosis of Multiple Sclerosis*. New York, Stratton–Verlag.

Poser S, Raun NE, Poser W (1982). Age at onset, initial symptomatology, and the course of multiple sclerosis. *Acta Neurologica Scandinavica*, 66, 355–62.

Powell T, Sussman JG & Davies Jones GA (1992). MR imaging in acute multiple sclerosis: ringlike appearance in plaques suggesting the presence of paramagnetic free radicals. *American Journal of Neuroradiology*, 13, 1544–6.

Pozzilli C, Bastianello S, Padovani A, *et al.* (1991a). Anterior corpus callosum atrophy and verbal fluency in multiple sclerosis. *Cortex*, 27, 441–5.

Pozzilli C, Passafiume D, Bernardi S, *et al.* (1991b). SPECT, MRI and cognitive functions in multiple sclerosis. *Journal of Neurology, Neurosurgery and Psychiatry*, 54, 110–15.

Prineas JW, Barnard RO, Kwon EE, *et al.* (1993a). Multiple

sclerosis: remyelination of nascent lesions. *Annals of Neurology*, 33, 137–51.

Prineas JW, Barnard RO, Revesz T, *et al.* (1993b). Multiple sclerosis. Pathology of recurrent lesions. *Brain*, 116, 681–93.

Pringle CE, Hudson AJ, Munoz DG, *et al.* (1992). Primary lateral sclerosis. Clinical features, neuropathology and diagnostic criteria. *Brain*, 115, 495–520.

Purcell EM, Torrey HC and Pound RV (1946). Resonance absorption by nuclear magnetic moments in a solid. *Physics Reviews*, 69, 37–8.

Rao SM, Hammeke TA and Speech TJ, (1987). Wisconsin speech test performance in relapsing/remitting and chronic/progressive multiple sclerosis. *Consulting and Clinical Psychology*, 55, 263–265.

Rao SM, Leo GJ, Haughton VM, *et al.* (1989). Correlation of magnetic resonance imaging with neuropsychological testing in multiple sclerosis. *Neurology*, 39, 161–6.

Rao SM, Leo GJ, Bernardin L and Unverzagt F (1991a). Cognitive dysfunction in multiple sclerosis.I. Frequency, patterns, and prediction. *Neurology*, 41, 685–91.

Rao SM, Leo GJ, Ellington L *et al.* (1991b). Cognitive dysfunction in multiple sclerosis. II. Impact on employment and social functioning. *Neurology*, 41, 692–96.

Rao SM, Reingold SC, Ron MA, *et al.* (1993). Workshop on neurobehavioural disorders in multiple sclerosis. Diagnosis, underlying disease, natural history, and therapeutic intervention. Bergamo, Italy, June 25–27, 1992. *Archives of Neurology*, 50, 658–62.

Redpath T, Smith FW and Adach J (1993). A double inversion recovery sequence for simultaneous suppression of lipid and fluid signals. *Proceedings of Society of Magnetic Resonance in Medicine*, 12th Annual Meeting, 3, 1194.

Révèsz T, Hawkins CP, du Boulay EPGH, *et al.* (1989). Pathological findings correlated with magnetic resonance imaging in subcortical arteriosclerotic encephalopathy (Binswanger's disease). *Journal of Neurology, Neurosurgery and Psychiatry*, 52, 1337–44.

Révèsz T, Kidd D, Thompson AJ, *et al.* (1994). A comparison of the pathology of primary and secondary progressive multiple sclerosis. *Brain*, 117, 759–65.

Rindfleisch E (1863). Histologisches Detail zu der grauen Degeneration von Gehirn und Rückenmark. (Zugleich ein Beitrag zu der Lehre von der Entstehung und Verwandlung der Zelle.) *Archiv für Pathologische Anatomie und Physiologie und für Klinische Medicin*, 26, 474–83.

Rizzo JF & Lessell S (1988). Risk of developing multiple sclerosis after uncomplicated optic neuritis: a long-term prospective study. *Neurology*, 38, 185–90.

Rodriguez M, Scheithauer BW, Forbes G & Kelly PJ (1993). Oligodendrocyte injury is an early event in lesions of multiple sclerosis. *Mayo Clinic Proceedings*, 68, 627–36.

Roemer PB, Edelstein WA, Hayes CE, *et al.* (1990). The NMR phased array. *Magnetic Resonance in Medicine*, 16, 192–225.

Ron MA & Logsdail SJ (1989). Psychiatric morbidity in multiple sclerosis: a clinical and MRI study. *Psychological Medicine*, 19, 887–95.

Ron MA, Callanan MM & Warrington EK (1991). Cognitive abnormalities in multiple sclerosis: a psychometric and MRI study. *Psychological Medicine*, 21, 59–68.

Ron MA & Feinstein A (1992). Multiple sclerosis and the mind. *Journal of Neurology, Neurosurgery and Psychiatry*, 55, 1–3.

Rose AS, Kuzma JW, Kurtzke JF, *et al.* (1970). Cooperative study in the evaluation of therapy in multiple sclerosis: ACTH vs. placebo. *Neurology*, 5, 1–59.

Rose MR, Ball JA & Thompson PD (1993). Magnetic resonance imaging in tonic spasms of multiple sclerosis. *Journal of Neurology*, 241, 115–17.

Rozewicz L, Langdon D, Davie CA, *et al.* (1994). Reversible cognitive impairment in multiple sclerosis. *Journal of Neurology*, 241(suppl 1), S59.

Rudge P, Miller D, Crimlisk H & Thorpe J (1995). Does interferon beta cause initial exacerbation of multiple sclerosis? *Lancet*, 345, 580.

Runge VM, Price AC, Kirshner HS, *et al.* (1984). Magnetic resonance imaging of multiple sclerosis: a study of pulse-technique efficiency. *American Journal of Radiology*, 143, 1015–26.

Runmarker B and Andersen O (1993). Prognostic factors in a multiple sclerosis incidence cohort with twenty-five years of follow-up. *Brain* 116, 117–134.

Rydberg RN, Hammond CA, Grimm RC, *et al.* (1994). Initial experience in MR imaging of the brain with a fast fluid-attenuated inversion-recovery pulse sequence. *Radiology*, 193, 173–80.

Rydberg JN, Reiderer SJ, Rydberg CH & Jack CR (1995). Contrast optimisation of fluid-attenuated inversion recovery (FLAIR) imaging. *Magnetic Resonance in Medicine*, 34, 868–77.

Sadovnick AD, Baird PA & Ward RH (1988). Multiple sclerosis: updated risks for relatives. *American Journal of Medical Genetics*, 29, 533–41.

Sadovnick AD, Armstrong H, Rice GPA, *et al.* (1993). A population-based study of multiple sclerosis in twins: update. *Annals of Neurology*, 33, 281–5.

Sale-Luis ML, Hormigo A, Mauricio C, *et al.* (1990). Magnetic resonance imaging in motor neurone disease. *Journal of Neurology*, 237, 471–4.

Sandberg-Wollheim M, Bynke H, Cronqvist S, *et al.* (1990). A long-term prospective study of optic neuritis: evaluation of risk factors. *Annals of Neurology*, 27, 386–93.

Sandhu FS & Dillon WP (1991). MR demonstration of leucoencephalopathy associated with mitochondrial encephalomyopathy: case report. *American Journal of Neuroradiology*, 12, 375–9.

Savoiardo M, Strada L, Girotti F, *et al.* (1990). Olivopontocerebellar atrophy: MR diagnosis and relationship to multisystem atrophy. *Radiology*, 174, 693–6.

Scheltens PH, Barkhof F, Valk J, *et al.* (1992). White matter lesions on magnetic resonance imaging in clinically diagnosed Alzheimer's disease. Evidence for heterogeneity. *Brain*, 115, 735–48.

Schumacher GA, Beebe G, Kibler RF, *et al.* (1965). Problems of experimental trials of therapy in multiple sclerosis: Report by the panel on the evaluation of experimental trials of therapy in multiple sclerosis. *Annals of the New York Academy of Medicine*, 122, 552–68.

Seltzer S, Mark AS and Atlas SW (1991). CNS sarcoidosis: evaluation with contrast-enhanced MR imaging. *American Journal of Neuroradiology*, 12, 1227–33.

Sharief MK & Thompson EJ (1991). The predictive value of intrathecal immunoglobulin synthesis and magnetic resonance imaging in acute isolated syndromes for subsequent development of multiple sclerosis. *Annals of Neurology*, 29, 147–51.

Shibasaki H & Kuroiwa Y (1969). Statistical analysis multiple sclerosis and neuromyelitis optica based on autopsied cases in Japan. *Folia Psychiatrica et Neurologica Japonica*, 23, 1–10.

Shoemaker EI, Lin Z-S, Rae-Grant AD & Little B (1994). Primary angiitis of the central nervous system: unusual MR appearance. *American Journal of Neuroradiology*, 15, 331–4.

Silver NC, Good CD, Barker GJ *et al.* (1996). Enhancing lesion detection in multiple sclerosis: effects of gadolinium dose, magnetization transfer and delayed scanning. *Journal of Neurology*, 243 (2), S69.

Simmonds A, Arridge SR, Barker GJ, *et al.* (1993). A multi-stage pipeline for segmentation of neurological MRI data. In: *Proceedings of The Society of Magnetic Resonance in Medicine*, 12th Annual Meeting, vol 2, p. 696. Berkeley, Society of Magnetic Resonance in Medicine.

Simon JH, Holtas SL, Schiffer RB, *et al.* (1986). Corpus callosum and subcallosal-periventricular lesions in multiple sclerosis: detection with MR. *Radiology*, 160, 363–7.

Simon JH (1993). Neuroimaging of multiple sclerosis. *Neuroimaging Clinics of North America*, 3, 229–46.

Simon JH, Jacobs L, Cookfair D, *et al.* (1995). The natural history of MS based on an annual MR snapshot: results from the MSCRG study of intramuscular recombinant interferon beta-1a. *Neurology*, 45(suppl 4), A418.

Sipe JC, Romine JS, Koziol JA, *et al.* (1994). Cladribine treatment of chronic progressive multiple sclerosis. *Lancet*, 344, 9–13.

Smith I, Beasley MG & Ades AE (1990). Intelligence and quality of dietary treatment in phenylketonuria. *Archives of Diseases of Childhood*, 65, 472–8.

Smith KJ, Blakemore WF, McDonald WI (1981). The restoration of conduction by central remyelination. *Brain*, 104, 383–404.

Smith KJ, Bostock H, Hall SM (1982). Saltatory conduction precedes remyelination in axons demyelinated with lysophosphatidyl choline. *Journal of the Neurological Sciences*, 54, 13–31.

Smith ME, Stone LA, Albert PS, *et al.* (1993). Clinical worsening in multiple sclerosis is associated with increased frequency and area of gadopentetate dimeglumine-enhancing magnetic resonance imaging lesions. *Annals of Neurology*, 33, 480–9.

Soderstrom M, Lindqvist M, Hillert J, *et al.* (1994). Optic neuritis: findings on MRI, CSF examination and HLA class II typing in 60 patients and results of a short term follow-up. *Journal of Neurology*, 241, 391–7.

Stadt D, Kappos L, Rohrach E, *et al.* (1990). Occurrence of MRI abnormalities in patients with isolated optic neuritis. *European Neurology*, 30, 305–9.

Stansbury FC (1950). Neuromyelitis optica (Devic's disease). *Archives of Ophthalmology*, 42, 292–335 and 465–501.

Steiger MJ, Tarnesby G, Gabe S, *et al.* (1993). Successful outcome of progressive multifocal leukoencephalopathy with cytarabine and interferon. *Annals of Neurology*, 33, 407–11.

Stevenson VL, Gawne-Cain ML, Barker GJ, Thompson AJ, & Miller DH, (1997). Imaging of the spinal cord and brain in multiple sclerosis: a comparison study between fast FLAIR and fast spin echo. *Journal of Neurology*, 244, 119–24.

Stewart WA, Hall LD, Berry K & Paty DW (1984). Correlation between NMR scan and brain slice data in multiple sclerosis. *Lancet*, 324, 412.

Stewart WA, Hall LD and Berry K (1986). Magnetic resonance imaging (MRI) in multiple sclerosis (MS): Pathological correlation studies in eight cases. *Neurology*, 36, 320.

Stewart WA, Alvord EC, Hruby S, *et al.* (1991). Magnetic resonance imaging of experimental allergic encephalomyelitis in primates. *Brain*, 114, 1069–96.

Stone LA, Frank JA, Albert PS, *et al.* (1995a). The effect of beta interferon on bloood–brain barrier disruptions demonstrated by contrast enhanced MRI in relapsing remitting multiple sclerosis. *Annals of Neurology*, 37, 611–19.

Stone LA, Smith ME, Albert PS, *et al.* (1995b). Blood–brain barrier disruption on contrast-enhanced MRI in patients with mild relapsing-remitting multiple sclerosis. Relationship to course, gender, and age. *Neurology*, 45, 1122–6.

Swirsky-Sacchetti T, Mitchell DR, Seward J, *et al.* (1992). Neuropsychological and structural brain lesions in multiple sclerosis: a regional analysis. *Neurology*, 42, 1291–5.

Sze G, de Armond SJ, Brant-Zawadzki M, *et al.* (1986). Foci of MRI signal (pseudolesions) anterior to the frontal horns: histologic correlations of a normal finding. *American Journal of Radiology*, 147, 331–7.

Sze G, Merriam M, Oshio K & Jolesz F (1992). Fast spin-echo imaging in the evaluation of intradural disease of the spine. *American Journal of Neuroradiology*, 13, 1383–92.

Tan EM, Cohen AS, Fries JF, *et al.* (1982). The 1982 revised criteria for the classification of systemic lupus erythematosus. *Arthritis and Rheumatism*, 25, 1271–2.

Tanner JE & Stejskal OE (1968). Restricted self diffusion of protons in colloidal systems by the pulsed-gradient, spin-echo method. *Journal of Chemistry and Physics*, 49, 1768–77.

Tas MW, Barkhof F, van Walderveen MAA, *et al.* (1995). The effect of gadolinium on the sensitivity and specificity of MR imaging in the initial diagnosis of multiple sclerosis. *American Journal of Neuroradiology*, 16, 259–64.

The IFNB Multiple Sclerosis Study Group (1993). Interferon beta- 1b is effective in relapsing-remitting multiple sclerosis. I. Clinical results of a multicenter, randomized, double-blind, placebo-controlled trial. *Neurology*, 43, 655–61.

The IFNB Multiple Sclerosis Study Group, University of British Columbia MS/MRI Analysis Group (1995). Interferon beta-1b in the treatment of multiple sclerosis: final outcome of the randomized, controlled trial. *Neurology*, 45, 1277–85.

The Multiple Sclerosis Study Group (1990). Efficacy and toxicity of cyclosporine in chronic progressive multiple sclerosis: a randomised, double-blind, placebo-controlled clinical trial. *Annals of Neurology*, 27, 591–605.

Thomas DJ, Penncock JM, Hajnal JV, *et al.* (1993). Magnetic resonance of the spinal cord in multiple sclerosis by fluid-attenuated inversion recovery. *Lancet*, 341, 593–4.

Thomas PK, Walker RWH, Rudge P, *et al.* (1987). Chronic demyelinating peripheral neuropathy associated with multifocal central nervous system demyelination. *Brain*, 110, 53–76.

Thompson AJ, Hutchison M, Brazil J, *et al.* (1986). A clinical and laboratory study of benign multiple sclerosis. *Quarterly Journal of Medicine*, 58, 69–80.

Thompson AJ, Smith I, Brenton D, *et al.* (1990a). Neurological deterioration in young adults with phenylketonuria. *Lancet*, 336, 602–5.

Thompson AJ, Kermode AG, MacManus DG, *et al.* (1990b). Patterns of disease activity in multiple sclerosis: clinical and magnetic resonance imaging study. *British Medical Journal*, 300, 631–4.

Thompson AJ, Kermode AG, Wicks D, *et al.* (1991). Major differences in the dynamics of primary and secondary progressive multiple sclerosis. *Annals of Neurology*, 29, 53–62.

Thompson AJ, Miller DH, Youl BD, *et al.* (1992). Serial gadolinium enhanced MRI in relapsing remitting multiple sclerosis of varying disease duration. *Neurology*, 42, 60–3.

Thompson AJ, Kermode AG, Moseley IF, *et al.* (1993a). Seizures due to multiple sclerosis. *Journal of Neurology, Neurosurgery and Psychiatry*, 56, 1317–20.

Thompson AJ, Tillotson S, Smith I, *et al.* (1993b). Brain MRI changes in phenylketonuria. Association with dietary status. *Brain*, 116, 811–21.

Thorpe JW, Kidd D, Kendall BE, *et al.* (1993). Spinal cord MRI using multi-array coils and fast spin echo. I: technical aspects and findings in healthy controls. *Neurology*, 43, 2625–31.

Thorpe JW, Halpin S, MacManus DG, *et al.* (1994a). A comparison between fast spin echo and conventional spin echo in the detection of multiple sclerosis lesions. *Neuroradiology*, 36, 388–92.

Thorpe JW, Barker GJ, MacManus DG, *et al.* (1994b). Detection of multiple sclerosis by magnetic resonance imaging. *Lancet*, 344, 1235.

Thorpe JW, MacManus DG, Kendall BE, *et al.* (1994c). Short tau inversion recovery fast spin-echo (fast STIR) imaging of the spinal cord in multiple sclerosis. *Magnetic Resonance Imaging*, 12, 983–9.

Thorpe JW, Kendall BE, MacManus DG, *et al.* (1994d). Dynamic gadolinium-enhanced MRI in the detection of spinal arteriovenous malformations. *Neuroradiology*, 36, 522–9.

Thorpe JW, Moseley IF, Hawkes CH, *et al.* (1994e). Brain and spinal cord magnetic resonance imaging in motor neurone disease. *Journal of Neurology, Neurosurgery and Psychiatry*, 57, 1298.

Thorpe JW, Mumford CJ, Compston DAS, *et al.* (1994f). The British Isles survey of multiple sclerosis in twins: magnetic resonance imaging. *Journal of Neurology, Neurosurgery and Psychiatry*, 57, 491–6.

Thorpe JW, Barker GJ, Jones SJ, *et al.* (1995). Quantitative MRI in optic neuritis: correlation with clinical findings and electrophysiology. *Journal of Neurology, Neurosurgery and Psychiatry*, 59, 487–92.

Thorpe JW, Kidd D, Moseley IF, *et al.* (1996a). Serial gadolinium-enhanced MRI of the brain and spinal cord in early relapsing/remitting multiple sclerosis. *Neurology*, 46, 373–8.

Thorpe JW, Kidd D, Moseley IF, *et al.* (1996b). Spinal MRI in patients with suspected multiple sclerosis and negative brain MRI. *Brain*, 119, 709–714.

Tien RD, Hesselink JR & Szumowski J (1991). MR fat suppression combined with Gd-DTPA enhancement in optic neuritis and perineuritis. *Journal of Computer Assisted Tomography*, 15, 223–7.

Tienari PJ, Salonen O, Wikstrom J, *et al.* (1992). Familial multiple sclerosis: MRI findings in clinically affected and unaffected siblings. *Journal of Neurology, Neurosurgery and Psychiatry*, 55, 883–6.

Timms SR, Cure JK, Kurent JE (1993). Subacute combined degeneration of the spinal cord: MR findings. *American Journal of Neuroradiology*, 14, 1224–7.

Tofts PS, Barker GJ, Simmons AMK, *et al.* (1995). Correction of nonuniformity in images of the spine and optic nerve from fixed receive-only surface coils. *Journal of Computer Assisted Tomography*, 18, 997–1003.

Trend P, Youl B, Sanders MD, *et al.* (1990). Vertical gaze palsy due to a resolving midbrain lesion. *Journal of Neurology, Neurosurgery and Psychiatry*, 53, 708–9.

Truyen L, Barkhof F, Frequin STFM, *et al.* (1994). A case-control study of epilepsy in multiple sclerosis using magnetic resonance imaging: implications for treatment trials with 4–aminopyridine. In: *Proceedings of The European Committee for Treatment and Research in Multiple Sclerosis*, 10th Congress, p. 38. Athens, University Studio Press.

Truyen L, van Waesberghe JHTM, Barkhof F, *et al.* (1995a). No demonstration of cyclic lesion formation on gadolinium-enhanced MRI in one-year follow-up of relapsing-remitting patients. *Journal of Neurology*, 242(suppl 2), S119.

Truyen L, van Waesberghe JHTM, Barkhof F *et al.* (1995b). Three year follow-up of hypointense lesions on T1 weighted SE images in MS: correlation with disease progression in secondary progressive patients. *Proceedings of The Society of Magnetic Resonance*, 1, 279.

Turner R, Le Bihan D, Maier J, *et al.* (1990). Echo-planar imaging of intravoxel incoherent motions. *Radiology*, 177, 401.

Uhlenbrock D & Sehlen S (1989). The value of T1-weighted images in the differentiation between MS, white matter lesions, and subcortical arteriosclerotic encephalopathy(SAE). *Neuroradiology*, 31, 203–12.

Valk J & van der Knaap MS (1989). *Magnetic Resonance of Myelin, Myelination, and Myelin Disorders*. Heidelberg, Springer Verlag.

van der Knaap MS & Valk J (1991). The MR spectrum of peroxisomal disorders. *Neuroradiology*, 33, 30–7.

van Walderveen MAA, Tas MR, Barkhof F, *et al.* (1994). Magnetic resonance evaluation of disease activity during pregnancy in multiple sclerosis. *Neurology*, 44, 327–9.

van Walderveen MAA, Barkhof F, Hommes OR, *et al.* (1995). Correlating MR imaging and clinical disease activity in multiple sclerosis: relevance of hypointense lesions on

short TR/short TE ('T1-weighted') spin-echo images. *Neurology*, 45, 1684–90.

Vermess M, Bernstein RM, Bydder GM, *et al.* (1983). Nuclear magnetic resonance (NMR) imaging of the brain in systemic lupus erythematosus. *Journal of Computer Assisted Tomography*, 7, 461–7.

Virapongse C, Mancuso A & Quisling R (1986). Human brain infarcts: Gd-DTPA-enhanced MR imaging. *Radiology*, 161, 785–94.

Visscher BR, Liv K-S, Clarke VA, *et al.* (1984). Onset of symptoms as predictors of mortality and disability in multiple sclerosis. *Acta Neurologica Scandinavica*, 70, 321–8.

Wang P-Y, Shen W-C, Jan J-S (1992). MR imaging in radiation myelopathy. *American Journal of Neuroradiology*, 13, 1049–55.

Waxman SG (1988). Biophysical mechanisms of impulse conduction in demyelinated axons. In: SG Waxman (ed.), *Advances in Neurology. Functional Recovery in Neurological Disease*, vol. 47, New York, Raven Press, pp. 185–221.

Weinshenker BG, Bass B, Rice GPA, *et al.* (1989a). The natural history of multiple sclerosis: a geographically based study. I. Clinical course and disability. *Brain*, 112, 133–46.

Weinshenker BG, Bass B, Rice GPA, *et al.* (1989b). The natural history of multiple sclerosis: a geographically based study. 2. Predictive value of the early clinical course. *Brain*, 112, 1419–28.

Whitaker JN, McFarland HF, Rudge P & Reingold SC (1995). Outcomes assessment in multiple sclerosis clinical trials: a critical analysis. *Multiple Sclerosis*, 1, 37–47.

Wicks DAG, Tofts P, Miller DH, *et al.* (1992). Volume measurement of multiple sclerosis lesions with magnetisation images: a preliminary study. *Neuroradiology*, 34, 475–9.

Wicks DAG, Barker GJ & Tofts PS (1993). Correction of intensity non-uniformity in MR images of any orientation. *Magnetic Resonance Imaging*, 11, 183–96.

Wiebe S, Karlik SJ, Lee DH, *et al.* (1990). Serial cranial and spinal cord quantitative MRI in multiple sclerosis: Clinical correlations. *Neurology*, 40(Suppl 1), 377.

Wiebe S, Lee DH, Karlik SJ, *et al.* (1992). Serial cranial and spinal cord magnetic resonance imaging in multiple sclerosis. *Annals of Neurology*, 32, 643–50.

Wiles CM, Omar L, Swan AV, *et al.* (1994). Total lymphoid irradiation in multiple sclerosis. *Journal of Neurology, Neurosurgery and Psychiatry*, 57, 154–63.

Willoughby EW & Paty DW (1988). Scales for rating impairment in multiple sclerosis: A critique. *Neurology*, 38, 1793–8.

Willoughby EW, Grochowski E, Li DKB, *et al.* (1989). Serial magnetic resonance scanning in multiple sclerosis: a second prospective study in relapsing patients. *Annals of Neurology*, 25, 43–9.

Wilms G, Marchal G, Kersschot E, *et al.* (1991). Axial vs sagittal T2-weighted brain MR images in the evaluation of multiple sclerosis. *Journal of Computer Assisted Tomography*, 15, 359–64.

Winer JB, Pires M, Kermose A, *et al.* (1991). Resolving MRI abnormalities with progression of subacute sclerosing panencephalitis. *Neuroradiology*, 33, 178–80.

Winfield JB, Shaw M, Silverman LM, *et al.* (1983). Intrathecal IgG synthesis and blood–brain barrier impairment in patients with systemic lupus erythematosus and central nervous system dysfunction. *American Journal of Medicine*, 74, 837–44.

Wolansky K, Bandini JA, Cook SD *et al.* (1994). Triple versus single dose gadolinium in multiple sclerosis patients. *Journal of Neuroimaging*, 4, 141–5.

Wolinsky JS, Narayana PA & Fenstermacher MJ (1990). Proton magnetic resonance spectroscopy in multiple sclerosis. *Neurology*, 40, 1764–9.

Wolff SD & Balaban RS (1989). Magnetization transfer contrast (MTC) and tissue water proton relaxation in vivo. *Magnetic Resonance in Medicine*, 10, 135–44.

Wong KT, Grossman RI, Boorstein JM, *et al.* (1995). Magnetization transfer imaging of periventricular hyperintense white matter in the elderly. *American Journal of Neuroradiology*, 16, 253–8.

Wroe SJ, Pires M, Harding B, *et al.* (1991). Whipple's disease confined to the CNS presenting with multiple intracerebral mass lesions. *Journal of Neurology, Neurosurgery and Psychiatry*, 54, 989–92.

Wullner U, Klockgether T, Petersen D, *et al.* (1993). Magnetic resonance imaging in hereditary and idiopathic ataxia. *Neurology*, 43, 318–25.

Youl BD, Kermode AG, Thompson AJ, *et al.* (1991a). Destructive lesions in demyelinating disease. *Journal of Neurology, Neurosurgery and Psychiatry*, 54, 288–92.

Youl BD, Turano G, Miller DH, *et al.* (1991b). The pathophysiology of optic neuritis: an association of gadolinium leakage with clinical and electrophysiological deficits. *Brain*, 114, 2437–50.

Youl BD (1992). *Magnetic Resonance Imaging Studies of Optic Neuritis*. MD thesis, University of Melbourne.

Young IR, Hall AS, Pallis CA, *et al.* (1981). Nuclear magnetic resonance imaging of the brain in multiple sclerosis. *Lancet*, 318, 1063–6.

Zimmerman RD, Fleming CA, Lee BCP, *et al.* (1986). Periventricular hyperintensity as seen by magnetic resonance: prevalence and significance. *American Journal of Radiology*, 146, 443–50.

Zuk T, Atkins S and Booth K (1994). Approaches to registration using 3D surfaces. In: Loew MH (ed,) *Medical Imaging 1994: Image Processing. Proceedings of the International Society for Optical Engineering*, 2167, 176–87.

Index

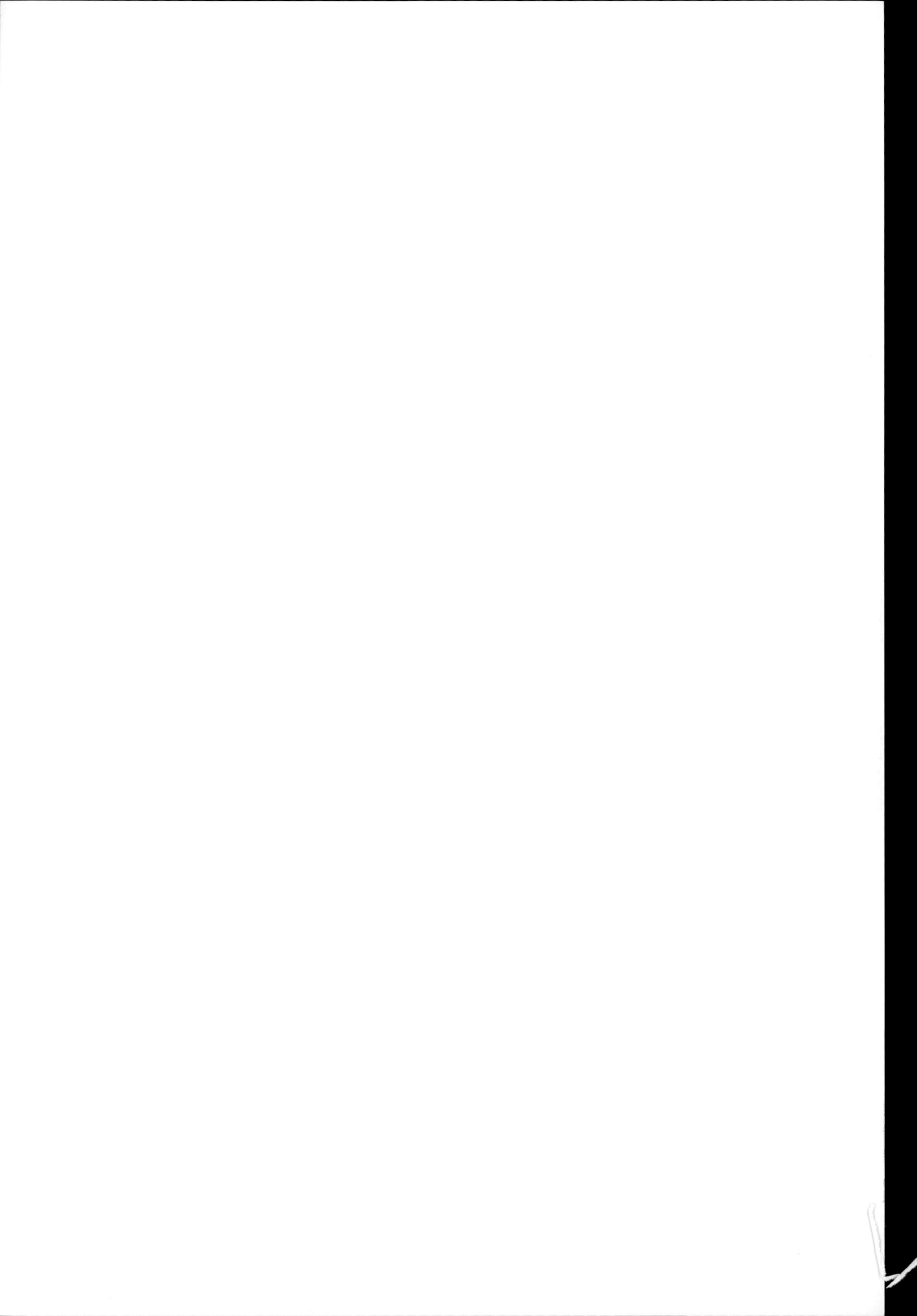